"As a woman who experienced trauma in childbirth when medicine was blind to its impact, I welcome this book. As a mother whose daughter's survival was precarious during pregnancy, I welcome this book. As an art therapist who has treated many women becoming parents, I thank Nora Swan-Foster for editing it."

**Judith A. Rubin**, PhD, ATR-BC, HLM, president, Expressive Media; Author, *Introduction to Art Therapy; The Art of Art Therapy*

"Picture a web, woven together by the intricacies of childbirth. That is what you will find in this anthology... a unique collection of knowledge, insight, and the reality of childbirth in present-day America. Without question, Swan-Foster has managed the extraordinary – bringing together critical information and perspectives for every art therapist, therapist, feminist, and/or practitioner who wants to better understand both the beauty and struggle of the perinatal period."

**Selena Shelley**, MA, LMHC – Psychotherapist, When Survivors Give Birth Trainer, and adjunct faculty in the Department of Midwifery at Bastyr University

"*Art therapy and childbearing issues* elegantly restores the childbirth process from one of a medically oriented procedure to its rightful place as a vital cosmic and archetypal experience – a profound threshold for the child and parents. The authors thoughtfully contribute their diverse perspectives, which bring forth a wealth of knowledge for the reader. Swan-Foster's text masterfully infuses the richness of participation in a primordial experience with contemporaneous relevance, a text sure to appeal to art therapists, students, and other mental health clinicians interested in the intersection of imagery and the emergent process of art and life."

**Michelle L. Dean**, MA, ATR-BC, LPC, CGP, Art Therapy Program director at Cedar Crest College, co-founder & director of The Center for Psyche & the Arts, LLC, and author of *Using Art Media in Psychotherapy*

"Swan-Foster is an organizing voice in the wilderness of women's political and psychic needs. These authors not only know the experience of art and its transformative value, but also bring this knowledge to women's growth and development at the crux of the childbearing and mothering experience. *Art Therapy and Childbearing Issues* is a must read for anyone working in the field, and an inspiring read to the lay person as well."

**Gayle Peterson**, LCSW, PhD, is author of *Birthing Normally, An Easier Childbirth* and *Making Healthy Families*. Gayle directs the training certification program "Peterson Childbirth Method" and has a private practice in Berkeley, CA

"*Art Therapy and Childbearing Issues* is a comprehensive collection of writings by outstanding scholars in the field. This timely book is superbly edited by Swan-Foster, a Jungian Analyst, Art Therapist and specialist working with the archetypal/initiatory experiences of women and how identity is solidified by the full circle of *matrescence*, a term borrowed from anthropology. Swan-Foster's expertise as an Art Therapist comes across in her selection of contributors with their breadth and depth of topics that show the value of using the expressive arts in work with all aspects of childbearing. This book is an invaluable contribution to the field that will leave the reader wanting more."

**Sondra Geller**, MA, LPC, ATR-BC, Jungian Analyst and Board Certified Art Therapist in private practice in Washington, DC

"*Art Therapy and Childbearing Issues* focuses on the very beginning: pregnancy, birth, postpartum, loss, palliative care, and mothering. As a trauma therapist working with very young abused children, I found the focus on early intervention immensely practical and hopeful as a preventative tool for a myriad of complex issues that expectant mothers face."

**Gussie Klorer**, PhD, ATR-BC, LCSW, LCPC, HLM, professor emeritus, Southern Illinois University Edwardsville. Author: *Expressive Therapies with Traumatized Children and Expressive Therapy with Troubled Children*

"Art Heals! Within the art of midwifery care, the Midwife listens deeply to guide and empower the client /family through their life transitions. Midwife means with women. What you are holding in your hands is a cutting edge treasure written by Art Therapist Midwives. It simply and powerfully elucidates how art therapy is the quintessential trauma informed, survivor led healing modality. This book reveals holistic and inclusive tools that will enable you to nourish and sustain your clients as they give birth to themselves on their journey to thriving."

**Teresa Robertson**, CNM-BC, MS, RN, SANE, adjunct clinical professor, Human Trafficking, Denver College of Nursing

"This text will surely be used in my own classroom as an example of how to use destigmatizing and agentic approaches that help mothers to explore, cope with, and shape their destinies for generations to come."

**Aurélie Athan**, PhD, Teachers College, Columbia University, Department of Counseling & Clinical Psychology, Reproductive & Maternal Wellbeing Certificate, New York, NY

# Art Therapy and Childbearing Issues

This text introduces readers to the diverse and unique ways art therapy is used with women who are undergoing various stages of the childbearing process, including conception, pregnancy, miscarriage, childbirth, and postpartum.

*Art Therapy and Childbearing Issues* discusses a range of topics including the role of transference/countertransference, supervision, attachment and maternal tasks, and neuropsychology. The book also addresses several motifs that are outside cultural norms of pregnancy and childbearing, such as racial and sociopolitical issues, grief and loss, palliative care, midwifery, menstruation, sex-trafficking, disadvantaged populations, and incarceration. Each chapter offers research, modalities, case studies, and suggestions on how to work in this field in a new way, accompanied by visual representations of different art therapy methods and practices.

The approachable style will appeal to a range of readers who will come away with a new awareness of art therapy and a greater knowledge of how to work with women as they enter and exit this universal, psychobiological experience.

**Nora Swan-Foster**, MA, ATR-BC, LPC, NCPsyA is a nationally registered and board certified art therapist who has used art therapy with childbearing issues for over 30 years. While adjunct faculty at Naropa University, she conducted prenatal art therapy research in a hospital setting. Also trained as a Jungian analyst, Nora is a member of the Inter-Regional Society of Jungian Analysts (IRSJA). Along with several publications, she is the author of *Jungian Art Therapy* and Co-Editor-in-Chief for the *Journal of Analytical Psychology*.

# Art Therapy and Childbearing Issues

Birth, Death, and Rebirth

Edited by Nora Swan-Foster

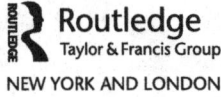
Routledge
Taylor & Francis Group

NEW YORK AND LONDON

First published 2021
by Routledge
52 Vanderbilt Avenue, New York, NY 10017

and by Routledge
2 Park Square, Milton Park, Abingdon, Oxon, OX14 4RN

*Routledge is an imprint of the Taylor & Francis Group, an informa business*

© 2021 Taylor & Francis

*Library of Congress Cataloging-in-Publication Data*
A catalog record for this title has been requested

ISBN: 978-0-367-43651-3 (hbk)
ISBN: 978-0-367-43650-6 (pbk)
ISBN: 978-1-000-17674-2 (ebk)

Typeset in Goudy
by Swales & Willis, Exeter, Devon, UK

To the sacred relationship between the Earth, the Moon, and the Sun

# Contents

# Acknowledgments

To the reader: As any creation that finds a form and takes a breath, the following collection of chapters was a labor of love, a *passion project*. We are grateful for your interest and hope you will take notice and find your own small way to participate in the necessary changes

To each contributing author: Your expertise is unquestionable as you investigated the shadow of our culture where living as a woman immersed in childbearing issues within the United States continues to hold hidden gifts, but not without the starkness of inequities and psychosocial challenges. I was endlessly inspired by your enthusiasm, and your willingness to write from your mind and heart, and to deliver chapters that speak with honest clarity and unending courage and compassion.

And to each person who remains confidentially disguised but whose story and images are included in this anthology: You made courage visible. This book would not exist without your generosity that deepens what we know to be true.

To Amanda Devine: As the Routledge editor, when you mentioned this topic, our conversation led to the necessary spark! You saw the need and I'm intensely grateful for your professionalism, steady dedication to the project and your support and belief in my vision for these authors' voices to be heard. Thank you too to Grace McDonnell, Sonnie Wills, and Ting Baker who were diligent and attentive to details and to everyone behind the scenes at Routledge who helped midwife this baby into the world.

To Jennifer Phelps: My deepest gratitude for your continuously generous and thoughtful professional polishing while maintaining the integrity of the individual voices—we all benefited from your gifts.

To my mother: Your own childbearing stories paved the way for thisbook to come into being. I'm forever influenced by your unwavering dedication to your creative process and your willingness to share the challenging stories.

And finally, to all those courageous women who came before us who were burdened by untold feelings and memories: Your childbearing stories have become part of the collective tipping point that influenced these authors. You are honored and remembered in the following pages.

# Contributors

## Editor and Contributing Author

**Nora Swan-Foster,** MA, ATR-BC, LPC, NCPsyA is a nationally registered and board certified art therapist who has used art therapy with childbearing issues for over 30 years. While adjunct faculty at Naropa University, she conducted prenatal art therapy research in a hospital setting. Also trained as a Jungian analyst, Nora is a member of the Inter-Regional Society of Jungian Analysts (IRSJA). Along with several publications, she is the author of *Jungian Art Therapy* and Co-Editor-in-Chief for the *Journal of Analytical Psychology.*

## Contributing Authors

**Mary Andrus,** DAT, LCAT, LPC, ATCS, is director of the Art Therapy Program in the Graduate School of Education and Counseling at Lewis and Clark. She spearheaded the historic art therapy legislation in Oregon and is committed to expanding the lens of the practice of art therapy, examining societal context, and creating equity in the relational wellbeing of clients.

**Casey Barlow,** MS, ATR-P, CTT, works as an art therapist with the FSU/FL DOC Art Therapy in Prisons Program. She specializes in the use of art therapy with incarcerated populations, with a particular focus on identity reconstruction, trauma transformation, and mindfulness. She earned her bachelor's degree from the University of Virginia and her master's degree from the Florida State University.

**Paula De Oliveira Santos,** MA, LPCC, has a master's degree from Naropa University in Transpersonal Art Therapy and a private practice in Boulder/Longmont, Colorado. Her passion is to enrich and empower individual's lives through creative modalities. Paula knows that our role as a therapist doesn't just end in the therapy room, but rather as therapists we must become advocates for a world that will support all of our clients.

**Valerie Epstein-Johnson,** MA, ATR-BC, LPC, is a registered and board-certified Art Therapist and Licensed Professional Counselor in private practice in the Denver, Colorado, area. She uses Art Therapy, Sandplay Therapy, and Acceptance and Commitment Therapy in her practice. Valerie specializes in working with grief, identity, values, and issues of motherhood—including pregnancy, infertility, pregnancy loss, and mothers without mothers.

**Fiona Swan Foster,** BA, MSc, has a master's with honors in Social Anthropology from the University of Edinburgh, Scotland, with research specializations in blood, food, and transformation. For over nine years she has conducted cultural research and created educational content in the United States and Europe. Fiona is a radio journalist for one of the only community-run stations in the US with a show focused on topics that impact community.

**Dave Gussak,** PhD, ATR-BC, is a professor for the Florida State University's (FSU) Graduate Art Therapy Program and project coordinator for the FSU/FL Dept of Correction's Art Therapy in Prisons program. He has presented and published extensively internationally and nationally on forensic art therapy and art therapy in forensic settings. These include, among others, *Art on Trial: Art Therapy for Capital Murder Cases* and *Art and Art Therapy with the Imprisoned: Re-Creating Identity*, and he co-edited *The Wiley Handbook of Art Therapy*. He serves on editorial boards including *Art Therapy: The Journal of the American Art Therapy Association*.

**Katherine A. Holbrook,** MA, ATR, LPC, is an art therapist and mental health counselor, recognized for her work in pediatric palliative care. She received her master's degree in Art Therapy and Counseling from Ursuline College, where she earned the academic excellence award. She has presented to National Medical Organizations. Katherine is in private practice in Charlotte, North Carolina.

**Jane Margaret Hunt,** MSW, is a Jungian analyst with a private practice in Ithaca, NY. A graduate of the Jung Institute of New England, she is also a member of IRSJA and the Jung Institute Zürich, where she is a training analyst. She founded an "-isms" peer supervision group focused on racism, homophobia, and misogyny in Ithaca in 2016.

**Juliet L. King,** MA, ATR-BC, LPC, LMHC, is an associate professor of Art Therapy at The George Washington University and adjunct professor of Neurology at the Indiana University School of Medicine. Professor King is currently pursuing a PhD in Translational Health Sciences with a focus on cognitive neuroscience. In 2016 she wrote and edited a textbook: *Art Therapy, Trauma and Neuroscience: Theoretical and Practical Perspectives*.

**Mary K. Kometiani,** MA, ATR-BC, LPCC, Art Therapy Heals, LLC, has over a decade of experience providing art therapy for survivors of sex trafficking, inpatient and outpatient pediatric medical patients and their families, and families of hospice patients and the bereaved. She is the editor of *Art Therapy Treatment for Sex Trafficked Survivors: Facilitating Empowerment, Recovery, and Hope* in addition to authoring several journal articles and book chapters.

**Rebecca Miller,** MA, ATR-BC, LCAT, CCLS, is a nationally registered and board-certified art therapist, artist, and art therapy educator. She is an assistant professor in the master of Arts in Art Therapy program at Saint Mary-of-the-Woods College in Terre Haute, IN, and is currently pursuing her PhD in Counselor Education and Supervision at the University of Missouri-St. Louis.

**Merryl E. Rothaus,** LPC, LMHC, ATR-BC, CHT, has a thriving private practice as a somatic art psychotherapist and clinical supervisor. Merryl was visiting core faculty in the Graduate Art Therapy department at Antioch University, Seattle, and is adjunct faculty in the Graduate Art Therapy department at Naropa University. She co-authored *Unity in Diversity; Communal Pluralism in the Art Studio and the Classroom* and authored the chapter *Hakomi Body-Centered Therapy and Art Therapy.*

**Shannon Schmitz,** MS-AT, is an art therapist who has worked within different forensics settings. She completed her undergraduate degree at Emporia State University and her master's degree in Art Therapy from Emporia State University. She is intensively trained in Dialectic Behavioral Therapy by Behavioral Tech and currently works in private practice utilizing art therapy in conjunction with DBT.

**Linda Siegel** is a licensed and board-certified creative arts therapist, a certified child and adolescent psychotherapist, parent–infant psychotherapist, psychoanalytic couple psychotherapist, a minister of spiritual counseling, and holds a doctorate degree in psychosocial studies. She is a full-time tenured professor at Pratt Institute, and has taught and presented her work nationally and in Argentina, Chile, the Dominican Republic, and the UK. She has maintained a private practice for over 30 years and is an exhibiting artist and published author.

**Alison Silver,** MPS, ATR-BC, CFTP, is a creative arts therapist in RWJBarnabas at Monmouth Medical Center's Perinatal Mood and Anxiety Disorder Outpatient Program in New Jersey and maintains a private practice. She is a graduate from Pratt Institute and has worked with diverse populations including: veterans, survivors of domestic violence, human/sex trafficking, and sexual abuse, brain injuries, and families undergoing medical hospitalizations.

**Ellen Speert** ATR-BC, REAT, directs the California Center for Creative Renewal, a therapeutic retreat center specializing in creativity, women's issues, loss, and spirituality since 1981. She is past president of SDATA and active with AATA and IEATA, presenting art therapy in Europe, Asia, and the Americas. She makes art, gardens, writes, and conducts workshops throughout the world, winning numerous awards as a public speaker.

**Denise R. Wolf** ATCS, ATR-BC, LPC, is the assistant director of graduate and undergraduate art therapy at Cedar Crest College, in Pennsylvania. She is an active member of the art therapy community including service to the Accreditation Council for Art Therapy Education and the AATA Scholarship Committee. Denise is a DBT trained art therapist who has worked with adolescents for over 20 years.

# Foreword

## Matrescence

In Nora Swan Foster's own introduction, she notes psychoanalyst D.W. Winnicott's perspective that the infant cannot become an infant without a mother. It is this suggestion that sets the stage for the rest of what is to come—the radical notion that without her own support a woman too cannot *become* a mother. This inversion of focus from what a mother does for her child, to what can be done for a mother is pivotal. Whether a practitioner, a policymaker, or a poet, readers will be called upon to shift their attention to the mother's inner experience, privileging her subjectivity, and her point of view above all other considerations. This may take considerable effort as the empathic thrust has not always been sent in this direction, and what may feel unnatural at first, must eventually become second nature if we are to transform society for the better.

Perhaps a more apt comparison for the critical life transition to motherhood would be *"matrescence* like adolescence." Using this catchy phrase, I revived the term matrescence first coined by medical anthropologist Dana Raphael (1975) so that our contemporary culture might also connect these important dots. Women who journey through preconception, pregnancy and birth, surrogacy or adoption, to the postnatal period and beyond, indeed experience an acceleration in personal growth true of any developmental push. By likening it to puberty, matrescence normalizes the natural disorientation and reorientation that occurs in nearly every domain: bio-psycho-relational-social-political-existential-spiritual. Unfortunately, research on mothers themselves has developed far too slowly unlike investigations into their children's outcomes, prompting a need for a new wave of theory, practice, and funding.

As is suggested in this art therapy anthology, becoming a mother is a true initiation into a new sense of being, an expanded identity, a lifelong search for meaning, and ultimate self-development. This 360° change requires the roundtable of disciplines that intersect its study to come together and offer creative approaches to wrap-around a mother and bolster her resilience. Yet, trainees lack resources to learn cutting-edge techniques applicable to diverse populations and circumstances.

A first in the field of art therapy to address childbearing issues, each chapter illuminates a path toward a woman's self-knowing—the autonomous, and spontaneous spirit that can lead her back to confidence and competence. Most of all, the core teaching of this art therapy book is the sacred work of facilitating space for a mother to activate her own inner guidance system with its unique set of orienting symbols. For an emerging mother, this is truly an opening, a beginning.

**Aurélie Athan, PhD**
Teachers College, Columbia University
Department of Counseling & Clinical Psychology
Reproductive & Maternal Wellbeing Certificate
New York, NY

## Reference

Raphael, D. (1975). Matrescence, becoming a mother, a "new/old" rite de passage. In: *Being female: Reproduction, power, and change* (pp. 65–71). The Hague, The Netherlands: Mouton.

# 1 Introduction

## Background Considerations for Childbearing Issues and Art Therapy

*Nora Swan-Foster*

The pediatrician and psychoanalyst D.W. Winnicott (1960) expressed that the infant cannot become an infant without a mother. This notion poignantly highlights the pivotal role of a woman's maternal identity and how art therapists can have an incredibly significant impact for women during this major life stage. The images that women create in art therapy, and their connection with other women, allows them to see parts of themselves not yet seen by the world. Caring for themselves during pregnancy and postpartum by making their internal world visible to themselves and others is an integral part of their maternal preparation and growth. Drawing from the creative and spiritual renewal found through art therapy, they can better see and provide care for their infants. This process is slightly different for mothers who endure losses —grief is more consciously interwoven into what it means to become a mother, to be restricted to only holding their babies, sometimes dead, sometimes in the care of others, in their minds and hearts. Childbearing issues form the center of a woman becoming a mother and yet her journey never unfolds perfectly. Instead, it is a collaborative endurance, and a creative and spiritual growth process called *matrescence*, an anthropological term that describes a holistic and compassionate acknowledgement of maternal growth and identity (Athan, 2017; Raphael, 1975). *Art Therapy and Childbearing Issues* examines a few of these important variations and ingredients.

When I lived in a Boston brownstone in the mid-1980s, our apartment was above a single mother who worked as a nurse midwife and saw patients at home in addition to working hospital shifts. I regularly met pregnant women in the foyer. And over tea, she told me her midwifery stories—the accounts of long sleepless nights, what helped, what did not, and the continuity of medical and psychosocial care between her, the midwife, and her medical team. While the fetus was always considered, I was impressed by the continuity of care for the physical and emotional adjustment of the mother and infant that begins early in pregnancy and extends six to eight weeks into postpartum. Women who lost their babies were also given this continuity of care.

During this time, I received an informal training in medical terms, procedures, celebrations, disappointments, and grief associated with childbearing issues. I saw how an experienced midwife handled uncertainty with time, responded to unexpected events with confidence, and handled her life with both grace and authority. I learned what she considered to be normal or an emergency, and how certain events unfolded from a mismanaged pregnancy or birth. She regularly negotiated with doctors and nurses in the hallways of the hospital and supported her patients to express their feelings and make educated choices. Her home was a community where oral stories could be told with dignity, absent of shame or rebuke. Modeled by the midwifery community, I saw that when antenatal care is collaborative, it benefits both maternal and infant mental health.

As I trained and worked in maternal/infant/child mental health, I began using art therapy with pregnant women and learning about the benefits. Unlike today, art therapy was only used with those with handicaps and mental illness, but I was curious about the supposed "normal" yet hidden nature of pregnancy and childbearing issues. No matter what the outcome of the conception and gestation, I observed how the midwifery web supports and nourishes the pregnant woman's journey and I saw how some doctors were also able to support their patients with compassionate listening ears.

My own pregnancies were life-changing events. Certainly, I encountered moments of joy, peace, and satisfaction, but there was loss, and incorporating a new identity into my life led me deeper into prenatal emotions and thoughts that arose from the collision with change and uncertainty. We packed and moved, and searched for affordable apartments and new birth communities that matched what I had left behind. I found new friends, new mothers, but spent many hours alone, pregnant, with an infant, and later with an infant and a curious toddler. I worked in adolescent treatment and child residential because of financial stress and a desire to stay connected to my professional identity. What saved me in the darkest hours was my routine with art, writing, and dreams that led me towards the illumination of symbolic connections and personal meaning; the images held and formed my uncontained uncertainty, worries, and fears. I quickly learned that the answers to my questions were not as much physical as emotional. There were turning points: I risked speaking my truth to a woman with medical authority, I switched birth providers in the eleventh hour and discovered support in an unexpected place with two compassionate male doctors. I rejected certain protocols, and my second birth was more difficult than my first birth, which contradicts traditional wisdom that it gets easier. Pregnancy, childbirth, and postpartum do not necessarily get easier. They are labors of love, sacrifice, and devotion that are concerned with curiosity and process. Uncertainty and imperfection become the moments for reflection and maturation.

What truly impacts a woman is her relationship with her partner and/ or her antenatal support team. This is the web of knowledgeable support woven around the pregnant woman with supple but solid threads made of love, confidence, and encouragement. It should be this way for every single woman no matter who she is, the color of her skin, or where she lives. So essential were the family, friends, nurses, and midwives who stood beside me for long hours like they do with so many women, it is appropriate to celebrate that the World Health Organization declared 2020 to be the year to acknowledge nurses and midwifes. Perhaps the US will continue to learn from other countries on how a compassionate and caring antenatal model, with the inclusion of the creative arts therapies, can be seamlessly and economically integrated into our childbearing system that serves all people who are creating families. This is an ideal. A dream. But we should aim for no less when it comes to women, infants, and their families.

In the meantime, the collection of chapters in *Art Therapy and Child-bearing Issues* illustrate how women are the canaries in the coal mine—if they are in trouble, then we are all in trouble. In 1978 the United States Senate passed the Pregnancy Discrimination Act (PDA) in the attempt to eliminate pregnancy-based discrimination. Although I was well aware that inequalities prevailed and women's reproductive rights are endlessly debated in the United States, childbearing issues remain mostly a hidden topic not only within art therapy, but within the American culture. I was not naïve to the fact that the mother is either idealized and glorified or taken for granted, stereotyped, blamed, and rejected. I was aware of systemic discrimination, and yet, when I began compiling this book, I had not yet fallen so deeply into the weeds of the disturbing facts on social justice and toxic stress issues (Lakhani, 2019), or the dramatic statistics on surgeries and medical interventions (or lack thereof), maternal mortality rates (Lakhani, 2019), and the criminalization of pregnancy, childbirth, and postpartum in the US, which is determined by predominately white male legislators.

This anthology gathers clinically experienced art therapists and other professionals who care about and/or work with women and childbearing issues and cross various divides to do their work. With the support of literature, statistics, clinical examples, personal narratives, and visual art, these authors bring the woman's perspective and maternal voices out from the shadows and they contribute their services to our communities. Through their unique lenses and experiences, the contributing art therapists provide insight into appropriate and ethical application and theory as well as future potential areas of research, clinical attention, and professional collaboration.

Certainly, there are other art therapists who are doing this work across America, gathering the stories and making visible the joys and hardships associated with childbearing issues and those areas that currently haunt a woman's mental health and physical freedom in the United States. This book is but a heartfelt opening, a beginning—the first of its kind in this country—to focus solely on art therapy and childbearing issues. The timing is powerfully synchronistic for many reasons. Not only has the #MeToo movement ushered in a new wave of collective awareness that rises above shame and fear, but there are increasing news reports and books in this country that reveal the complicated discrimination and severity of neglect of women, and in particular, childbearing women in this country. Finally, just as this book was submitted to the publishers, the United States was impacted by the COVID-19 global pandemic with "stay at home" orders that required social distancing, masks, and a sudden interruption of celebrating the many maternal threshold crossings of the childbearing stage. The invisible but virulent virus has brought the honest truth of medical, racial, and social inequities to light and revealed in greater detail aspects of the unsupported, underfunded, confusing, and divided medical system that begs for restructuring. Additionally, childbearing women have suddenly experienced heightened anxiety, fear, and grief resulting from an abrupt lack of clear medical knowledge, and increased isolation and restrictions during prenatal, childbirth, and postpartum periods. Also, it will be remembered that mothers, or family members, have been unable to actively support their daughters as new mothers and are restricted from holding their grand-babies because of social distancing. As one mother said to me, "my baby will be grown before anyone gets to know him." Becoming a mother requires that both mother and baby are witnessed, but the quarantine has torn asunder some of these precious shared moments of intimacy and trust that cannot be replaced through internet contact. Further, with maternal and infant deaths, families have been prohibited from comfort from touch and shared grieving rituals. While we were unable to include these stories, I recognize that this pandemic will leave behind complicated reports of joy and creativity alongside emotional and physical wreckage. Undoubtedly, future research will show that the stories of maternal/infant relational trauma and grief associated with fear, anxiety, distance and separation, lack of touch, masked maternal and paternal faces, severe interruptions and losses will all cause un-worded wounds that will one day tell an important story through art therapy.

Indeed, this book illustrates how art therapy contributes to the prevailing conversation of women and childbearing issues in a significant and creative way. As a treatment it is neither alternative nor radical; nor is art therapy a marginalized profession lacking evidence of humanizing results that build communities (AATA, 1999). Art therapy is rooted in thousands of years of humanity that has used art to honor humanity's transitions, now joined with psychological and social theories. Those trained in the field have a solid base of theoretical knowledge, clinical experience, artistic training, knowledge of materials and professional collaboration within communities. Furthermore, art therapy is integrated and highly visible in some parts of the medical and psychosocial communities in this country, led by professionals who have devoted their life to a field that is over 70 years old. The American Art Therapy Association (AATA) recently celebrated 50 years as a professional association and that is because it has the unique and commanding ability to reveal the mythic lives that people, and in this case women, are living. Encouraging the use of the imagination, the creative process and drawing on the psychological and emotional aspects of process and product, as well as interventions and spontaneous imagery, art therapy brings fresh awareness and consciousness to the human journey. The creative process facilitates a connection between her body and her emotions and this has a subtle but clear impact on a woman's self-esteem, her ability to articulate her thoughts and moods, and her capacity to learn that vulnerability is a strength that leads to relationships with others as she works to expand her future identity to include the identity of forever being a mother no matter the context or the outcome.

Despite the dramatic physical changes that show in the external world, childbearing women still live in the shadows. *Art Therapy and Childbearing Issues* encourages the subversive act of making art. In this small act, a woman has an effect, an influence, not just in her personal world, but on others in her community when she so bravely makes choices to express her inner emotions and thoughts, and address issues that matter to her and to others. But where she lives in the US matters, so let us consider just a few of the powerful divisions and their impact on motherhood.

## The United States Are Divided States for Motherhood

With its 50 states and handful of territories, the United States is one unified country that defines itself as a democracy with a constitution that protects individual rights. It's a country originally guided by the inspiring image of the towering beauty, the Statue of Liberty, that calls out: "Give me your tired, your poor, Your huddled masses yearning to breathe free" (Lazarus, 1883/2019). While a democracy depends upon individuals fighting for their rights, in America not everyone is equally cared for nor granted the dignity they deserve as human beings. The poetic invitation casts a shadow: this country is complicated, widely divided, and intensely diverse. In her discussion of motherhood, Rothman (2000) considered three main threads that define America's current climate: patriarchy, technology, capitalism. Twenty years later, fundamentalism makes a fourth thread. The intricate power structure is often fed by complex, hideous, sociopolitical, racial, religious and geographical perspectives that are deeply and systemically ingrained and enforced by the ruling hegemony. In the US, *Forbes Magazine* reported 600 billionaires (Kroll & Dolan, 2019)—the highest number worldwide—who directly or indirectly benefit from these four main threads, while the middle class and the poor struggle in exhaustion to make ends meet. The income discrepancy is unquestionably the worst it has ever been.

Women make up over 50% of the population and a high number are living as single mother heads of households. Any woman who is perceived as stepping outside of society's conception of the ideal caregiver and mother is specifically marginalized, scrutinized, stigmatized, and more recently criminalized in America.

Moreover, despite the declared unity, the country has complicated environmental and cultural regions, individual state legislation, and deep roots in greed and racial discrimination of indigenous populations and immigrants; prosperity was built from a slave history and traumatic wounds that continue from before the Civil War. Psychosocial services and public health are so overwhelmed and underfunded that they may disregard the intersectionality of ethnic diversity, socioeconomic status, and the gender and age disparities that are unique in one state or region of the country but not in another. Additionally, if the federal government maintains one view, this may not always concur with local legislation on such critical issues as health insurance and medical benefits. For instance, the trend is to decrease Medicaid benefits, but one state may offer increased Medicaid benefits while the neighboring state will refuse these federal benefits because of political allegiances. These decisions affect women and children in a multitude of complex and overlapping ways.

## Women's Healthcare in America

The lack of low-cost and comprehensive healthcare and a woman's role as a major provider for her family, despite earning less than men, remains one of the greatest stressors and areas of vulnerability (Gunja et al., 2018). Most women in the United States do not seek medical support for fear of cost until they are forced to go to the emergency room. While the Affordable Care Act has provided women with a safeguard, medications and medical services are not always fully covered and the uncertainty of hidden costs for necessary or emergency procedures can leave women at tremendous financial risk. On average women aim to have two children, which means they spend three or more years attempting to conceive, pregnant or in postpartum. Three decades of their life women try to avoid pregnancy (Guttmacher, 2019).

According to the radio broadcast "Calling the Shots" (Zwillich, 2020) there is a predicted shortage of nurses, particularly in rural areas, that has already led to stressful work environments. The broadcast admitted that America could learn about successful healthcare, particularly for childbearing women from other developed nations where collaborative teams, which include community midwives, are built to support maternal/infant health. Consequently, as a cost-efficient model, American hospitals and obstetric practices are beginning to integrate midwifery as it is already a highly respected profession that so many other countries have long depended upon with exceptional benefits.

Unfortunately, the United States continues to lag behind other developed countries regarding childbearing and women's access to affordable and reliable healthcare, including high rates of C-sections, poor access to prenatal care, and high rates of obesity, diabetes, and heart disease (Gunja et al., 2018). The disquieting fact is that the US has the highest maternal mortality rates when compared to other wealthy nations (Gunja et al., 2018) and while other countries' numbers decreased by 44%, America's rose by 34% in 2015 (Dangi-Garimella, 2018). American women's emotional stress is also the highest compared to other nations, and, although demographic facts like race (particularly black women) contribute to this statistic, the stress is further compounded by poor access to safe and respectful antenatal care.

Women continue to find themselves caught in statistics that are discouraging and reflect the ongoing incessant power of the patriarchy, leaving them in dire situations to find their own way. Perinatal women in the US skip care because of unknown costs, stigma, and uncertainty surrounding preexisting conditions and the criminalization of pregnancy. This would be unheard of in other developed nations. So what is available for US women and families thus far?

## Family Medical Leave Act (FMLA)

In order to rectify a universal gap for employed women with children, a nine-year fight to support families led to the passage of the 1993 Family Medical Leave Act (FMLA) in the United States. This act included provisions for pregnant women, including guaranteed job protection and 12 weeks off from work per year for specified health and family caregiving reasons. However, by including pregnancy as part of a medical *disability*, the inference is that the antenatal period is not a natural human process, but one of exception, dysfunction, and sickness, or—what insurance companies took advantage of until 2010 and the Affordable Care Act—that maternity is a preexisting condition and an additional insurance rider needs to be purchased for coverage. Sadly, the issue of preexisting condition is once again now up for debate.

While the FMLA was a significant first step for the United States, it is important to note that the 12 weeks are unpaid and not comprehensive for all working women; those who are eligible must use accrued paid leave (sick time or vacation) as income for their time off. Once the 12 weeks are up, women are guaranteed their jobs for full pay and previous benefits. However, because not all women qualify for such job protection, one in four women return to work just ten days after childbirth (Hiles, 2018), meaning that FMLA remains an elite benefit in America where millions of women and their children are stranded if they do not qualify for Medicaid benefits. In one of the wealthiest nations in the world, this policy is inadequate and only further divides us as a nation when we could be joining together to support all families. In recognition of this deficiency, several states have expanded upon the FMLA with state-specific legislation that offers increased benefits. More recently, companies see the need and are providing their own maternal and family leave benefits, but again, this does not solve the larger problem for which other countries around the world have already considered and implemented moral and ethical solutions.

## Developed Nations Support Mother/Infant Health

It's well known that Canada, Sweden, and Japan currently have the best maternity leave laws, all of which provide a year's paid leave. When I was traveling in Europe, over a meal, a group of women and I conversed about maternal leave laws around the world. The American women were silent as they listened to a woman from the UK talk about 52 weeks of maternity leave with 39 weeks of full pay. She started her leave 11 weeks before she delivered and in the end, she explained that she had a year leave with a percentage of her salary. A German woman said her leave included the option for her husband to take a portion of it. She took six weeks off work before her due date and then had a whole year that was paid at 65% of her salary. She explained that women are *required by law* to take eight weeks off after birth. The time extends if a woman experiences a premature birth, a multiple birth, or a Cesarean birth. An Australian woman noted she had required time off and pointed out the maternity leave requirements in Scandinavian countries. In Norway, women can take 35 weeks at full pay or 45 weeks at 80% pay and fathers are part of the equation. Sweden has the most generous maternity for a couple with a required 16 months that are available to use in any amount until the child is eight years old. When an American woman explained that the only way she could take maternity leave was to save her money ahead of time and then quit her job to be home with her child, the European women were shocked. Another American woman said she had 12 weeks with her company, but it was not paid leave and she needed to accumulate her vacation and sick leave. While paid leave does not mean a full salary, women in other developed nations receive at least 65% of their salary for up to a year that does not come out of vacation or personal time, and are guaranteed to have their jobs upon their return. If they leave their jobs, they owe their employer for the time. American women who choose to stay home because child-care stretches beyond their paycheck sacrifice both their finances and their career mobility despite pregnancy discrimination laws. Therefore, it's no surprise that some women face painful choices and their pregnancy becomes unwanted simply because the economic burden can dump them further into poverty.

## Unwanted Pregnancies

Statistics show that approximately 50% of American pregnancies are unwanted (Finer & Zolna, 2016) and yet, criminalizing abortion in the United States does not correlate with lower abortion rates. Rather, since abortion was legalized in 1973, US abortion rates reached a historic low in 2017 because of an increase in publicly funded and freely available healthcare for childbearing women. Further, a five-year study across 21 states concluded that 95% of American women believe they made the right decision to abort and the long-term predominant feeling was relief (Aratani, 2020). This research discredits the anti-abortion groups and the socially conservative political message that abortion is a challenging decision so women need mandatory counseling and waiting periods. Statistics show that in 2014, white women accounted for 39% of abortion procedures, black women for 28%, Hispanic women for 25%, and that race and location have a strong influence on the availability of abortion services sought by heterosexual or straight women (Jerman, Jones & Onda, 2016).

It is clear that striking inequalities arise when we look at the levels of access to services that are offered state by state, as well as the differing levels of intersectional discrimination, such as the criminalization of pregnant women. Furthermore, while women who suffer from incest, rape, partner abuse, early childhood sexual abuse, severe trauma and dissociation, postpartum psychosis, or other chronic mental illness greatly benefit from and often require increased mental healthcare—as not all pregnancies are wanted or successful—these issues rarely receive appropriate attention (Geiser, 1990; Simkin & Klaus, 2004).

## Healthcare in America

Although a wide range of research, clearly and without question, demonstrates marked benefits of comprehensive affordable medical and mental healthcare for antenatal women and their infants, the majority of women still receive limited and demographically inconsistent care. Lack of antenatal care results in an increase of perinatal mood and anxiety disorders (PMADs), medical interventions, maternal death, preterm labors, low birth weights, and postpartum risks (Chasse, 2016; Davis-Floyd, 1992/2003). Further, early fetal loss or miscarriage, defined as before 20 weeks of pregnancy, is often medically dismissed as a genetically compromised fetus that would not survive outside the womb; this factual explanation offers little emotional comfort to the bereft woman. Losses following the 20 weeks are defined as stillbirths and often the woman is required to go through childbirth and return home with empty arms. No matter the timing, all perinatal loss leads to grief and a psychobiological process driven not just by hormones but also time and emotions. Despite the messages to "move on" or "try again," perinatal loss results in what Kersting and Wagner (2012) name as "complicated grief." How she is treated at the time of the loss and socioeconomic, gender, and race issues influence the diverse styles of grieving. Women of color, lower socioeconomic status, or women who experience perinatal depression, perinatal losses, drug addiction, sex trafficking, or incarceration will endure greater neglect and assaults by the system that can humiliate and dehumanize women as was the case of Ms. Sanchez who gave birth alone in her jail cell and was documented on video (Padilla, 2019). This brings us to a difficult and unbidden question within prenatal art therapy.

## Who Has Rights: Woman or Fetus?

*Roe v. Wade* was a landmark decision passed in 1973 that protected the pregnant woman's physical health and safety and the liberty to choose an abortion without government restriction. This was the beginning of reproductive rights, contraception and the freedom for women to make reproductive choices and live a fuller life. In reaction to a woman gaining a constitutional right to choose (which also gave equal rights to women to *not* choose an abortion), "personhood" laws or "fetal protection" laws have been introduced in each of the 50 states with tactical language that classifies fertilized eggs, zygotes, embryos, and fetuses as "persons" that must be granted full legal protection under the US Constitution, including the right to life from the moment of conception. The aim of these laws is to steadily undermine a woman's rights, because the "personhood" laws criminalize abortion across the board and prohibits some forms of contraception, in vitro fertilization (IVF) and healthcare for pregnant people. This is important because in a few states where these laws have passed, the "personhood" laws show a "dangerous trend of criminalizing pregnancy, by mandating that women who terminate a pregnancy may be even imprisoned because of the supposed injury done to a separate 'person'—namely, the fetus" (Rewire, 2018). The report explains that the so-called fetal homicide laws have been used in several states to arrest and prosecute individuals who are viewed as "harming the fetus" through miscarried pregnancies or being blamed for the delivery of a stillborn. These laws also lead to actions that disregard a woman's legal privacy rights such as giving her a pregnancy test without her knowing.

Effectively, federal mandates and Constitutional Amendments are continuously challenged state by state in reaction to *Roe v. Wade*. Supporting maternal and infant health is morally legitimate and beneficial, but using criminalization to promote public health and well-being is ineffective, discriminatory, and has dire consequences for our society. According to Amnesty International (2017),

In 38 states, fetal assault laws define the embryo or fetus as being the potential victim of a crime. In 23 states, these laws apply from the moment of fertilization. In most states, these laws may be applied to pregnant women.

(p. 5)

These laws have driven pregnant women further into hiding, neglect, and danger and leave them without medical care, where they sometimes give birth to their babies alone. Further, these laws are no longer just impacting poor black women, as was the case in the 1980s and 1990s with the epidemic of crack cocaine babies, but with the current opioid crisis in America, the notion of "white privilege" doesn't protect women who struggle with opioid addiction revealing the powerful "intersection of other categories of disadvantage" (Bridges, 2020, p. 851). Amnesty International Ltd (2017) notes that when drug dependency is not treated as a health condition but a crime, the woman fails to receive adequate medical treatment and is then further punished for her health condition. The state of Texas not only has the highest maternal mortality rate of all developed nations (Goodwin, 2020), but the state is amassing punitive discriminatory reproductive laws that are deliberately meant to undermine the Constitutional Amendment of *Roe v. Wade*. In some cases, the impact is so hideous that a woman in a coma or who is brain dead is used to keep the fetus alive even if her body is not functioning and her husband and family have requested that she be medically pronounced dead because her body is decaying (Goodwin, 2020).

If we pay attention, we will learn that the criminalization of pregnancy is a slow and steady process that places childbearing aged women across America at risk (Goodwin, 2020). A woman who hemorrhages with a miscarriage assumes that her hospital treatment will be based on medicine, not on religious doctrine, but one in six hospital beds in America are owned by Catholic hospitals (ACLU, 2016) and medicine is directed by Catholic doctrine. There are such procedures as "contraception, sterilization, infertility treatments and abortion, even when a woman's life or health is jeopardized by a pregnancy" (ACLU, 2016), meaning a miscarriage may be medically mismanaged based on religious doctrines that preserve a heartbeat at all cost, even at the risk of the mother's life. Further, withholding emergency medical care has occurred when women are perceived as poor and unable to pay; in other words, if you're a woman of color your chances of not receiving treatment greatly increase.

Why does this matter for art therapists and other mental health workers interested in childbearing issues? For several reasons. First, because the care of childbearing women, including the policing and criminalization of pregnant and postpartum women, is happening in every neighborhood and seeping into medical policy, sometimes controlling doctors and nurses in the privacy of the medical room. Further, it is clear that intersectional discrimination is inextricably linked with other factors that affect women, so it is vital for therapists to be informed about trauma as well as educated on the facts of systemic discrimination. Not recognizing social injustices is potentially ethical and moral neglect by the art therapist because such degradation of maternal and infant care in America continues to impact *all women* who sit in our offices, agencies, groups or other art therapy sites. Becoming conscious of the complicated and subtle injustices enacted upon pregnant and postpartum women is an ethical responsibility that will certainly deepen the therapeutic relationship (Potash, 2019). Finally, women have often been labeled as hysterical, overly emotional or dramatic when expressing their feelings, particularly when it comes to anger or grief. Because art therapy channels bodily sensations and emotions into expressive forms and images, this modality can be experienced as a powerful intervention that advocates for women to claim their subjective experiences, stand solid in their authority about their thoughts and feelings and find support to make choices for their bodies and their infants. For some women, the personal becomes political because the political is certainly personal. Knowing that what is discovered through art therapy can change a woman's life, this brief sociopolitical and economic overview becomes integral to our work as mental health providers particularly when we encounter complicated psychosocial issues during the childbearing phase in our patients' lives.

## Why Art Therapy and Childbearing Issues?

Images and the creative process have been the center of human expression for thousands of years. In 1913, Jung began his work on *The Red Book* (2009); when it was finally published, his work brought the image and the creative process front and center, further enhancing the field of art therapy as a viable therapeutic modality to address emotions and imagination. He encouraged others to do the same because he understood that the image led him into the depths from which he discovered the model of analytical psychology that art therapists know today (Swan-Foster, 2018). Artists, teachers, and art therapists have always known that art is healing, which is why the field of art therapy has grown and found its way into American culture as a respected profession.

*Art Therapy and Childbearing Issues* aims to inspire art therapists, creative arts therapists, and others who work in mental health and medical fields in the United States to continue to envision collaborative clinical services that are specifically focused on maternal/infant health, including conception, pregnancy, postpartum, perinatal loss, and various medical conditions and social justice issues. The focus on the emotional and psychological development of the woman through art therapy validates the major transformation of her identity and her maternal development. All too often overlooked, a childbearing woman is locked in by stereotypes, projections, and social expectations that set her up for failure and a disconnection from herself. Art therapy is a viable and creative approach where a woman can pause in her daily life to break the silence, interrupt the double binds and find and speak her truths; through the art therapy process, she can discover tangible images that document her incredible journey. She brings a new consciousness to who she is, who she wants to become, and how she might creatively integrate this new identity into her life. While her fetus and infant attract attention from the external world, a woman may not have the living evidence of her hard-won work, know her pregnant self or resonate with her maternal identity without engaging in art therapy. Each woman endures challenges and survives difficult events that are remembered by her body, heart, and mind. Art therapy is just beginning to show the benefits for the childbearing phase of a woman's life; the landscape is vast and mostly uncharted, but the following chapters illustrate some powerful examples of work being carried out in the United States.

## Map of the Chapters

*Art Therapy and Childbearing Issues* offers various perspectives on topics related to women and their childbearing experiences through the lens of clinically experienced and socially dedicated art therapists. The manuscript is divided into four sections: Pregnancy, Postpartum, Grief and Loss, and Special Topics of Childbearing Women. Childbirth is not overlooked but referred to in several chapters.

### Part I: Art Therapy: Pregnancy

In Chapter 2, "The Juxtaposition of Rupture and Repair," Wolf and King introduce art therapy as a powerful and supportive intervention for trauma and post-traumatic growth. In particular, the authors consider how the rhythm of trauma facilitates the development of a maternal identity through a construction and deconstruction process supported by the creative process. Swan-Foster further explores how the initiation model supports the maternal development of the pregnant woman. She uses clinical vignettes to illustrate motifs that spontaneously arise through dreams and art that express the feminine initiation process in Chapter 3, "Prenatal Art Therapy and Feminine Initiation." Next, Miller shines a light on the pregnant therapist in her chapter "Supervising the Pregnant Art Therapist." She uses three models of arts-based supervision (ABS) that encourage the pregnant art therapist to better understand her pregnancy and its impact on her clients illustrated by supervisee material. In "Using Art to Prepare for Birth as a Doula-Grandmother," Hunt's storytelling and painting process unwraps her role as a doula-grandmother immersed in her daughter's childbirths. Guided by a midwifery model rather than a traditional medical model, Hunt emphasizes the transformational process that is available for those who support women during childbirth.

## Part II: Art Therapy: Postpartum

In "Going on Being: Losing and Finding a New Identity in the Early Phases of Treatment with Postpartum Mothers" Siegel poetically explores the psychological process that a woman undergoes during this life stage and how these states reflect the early development of symbolization that is necessary for motherhood. She elaborates on how kinesthetic art therapy can be sensitively incorporated to hold and encourage a gradual unfolding of a woman's maternal identity during postpartum. "Perinatal Mood and Anxiety Disorder" is considered in Chapter 7 by Silver who illustrates how a creative arts therapy approach complements a medically oriented environment to support women and families who struggle with complex trauma and perinatal mood disorders. She shares with us her diligent work with a couple that is grappling with postpartum issues, complex birth trauma, and how that couple prepares for a second childbirth through a specific trauma protocol. Further information on postpartum can be found in Appendices.

## Part III: Art Therapy: Grief and Loss

Rituals are rarely emphasized in America when it comes to perinatal loss, but Rothaus poignantly weaves together ritual and somatic art therapy in Chapter 8 "Cultivating Aliveness after Pregnancy Loss." She intimately shares her own story of babyloss and, through a clinical example, illustrates how somatic art therapy can reveal aliveness after loss. In Chapter 9, "Honoring the Process," Kometiani and Holbrook introduce us to how art therapy can be clinically implemented within a hospital milieu while emphasizing the therapeutic alliance that sensitively supports mothers of pediatric palliative care patients shortly after childbirth. Authors' response art is considered alongside a clinical illustration of how the creative process allowed a mother and her family to express their grief. A significant loss that is rarely considered is creatively addressed in "Motherhood Rounds It Out" by Epstein-Johnson. She demonstrates how art therapy benefits women grappling with their grief associated with the loss of a mother figure while at the same time trying to process the complexities of their own childbearing issues. In Chapter 11 "The Use of Japanese Ritual and Art Therapy in Healing from Pregnancy Loss" Speert adapted a powerful ritual to form contemplative art therapy groups in the US for people dealing with perinatal loss and offers reflection on how to better honor perinatal grief and loss.

## Part IV: Art Therapy: Special Topics of Childbearing Women

Blood is an integral and significant topic for childbearing women. The sight of it can bring grief or immense relief. It can also signify unbearable worry, pain, danger, and even foreshadow criminalization. In Chapter 12 "Where It All Begins" Foster, a cultural anthropologist, introduces us to some of her research on blood and transformation. She introduces us to cultural views on menstruation and examines three modern populations that experience menstruation stigmatization and speculates on where art therapists might intercede to improve reproductive literacy within our society. In Chapter 13, "Penalizing More Than One," Barlow, Schmitz and Gussak introduce us to the penal system and the massive degradations and challenges for women who are pregnant or have recently given birth. The authors show that within this environment art therapy has clinical effectiveness when addressing issues of maternal identity and motherhood, particularly the complicated and consequential losses that incarcerated mothers live with on a daily basis. De Oliveira Santos addresses Latina mothers and immigration in her chapter "Working with the *Huecos*." Drawing on her countertransference, she questions the savior complex of art therapists, highlights social justice issues, and prioritizes the metaphor as an acceptable image that may pave the way to a respectful therapeutic relationship. In Chapter 15, "Infertility to Motherhood," Andrus grapples with several reproductive topics: infertility, loss, pregnancy, and motherhood through an art therapy group for underserved pregnant women and a film project focused on pregnancy loss. Confronting social constructs requires meaningful communities for women to hear their own voices and for their inside experience to be seen and heard by others. Lastly, when motherhood and sex trafficking converge, art therapy is a powerful intervention as Kometiani poignantly explains in "Addressing Motherhood Issues of Sex Trafficking." The author offers her expertise when working with the complexity of exploited and marginalized women who face difficult childbearing dilemmas by emphasizing the importance of a trauma-informed approach.

Collecting these noteworthy chapters into one book showcases not just the variety of articulate voices within art therapy, but also where art therapy seamlessly fits with ease and brilliance into process and product, both of which offer renewal for antenatal individuals and communities within the United States. These chapters also remind us that the education of boys and men is essential if we want to see holistic and deep change for a diverse and inclusive society. Certainly, art therapy has the potential to expose and repair the ruptures and divides between populations often known to us as statistics, but as we become more familiar with individuals and knowledgeable of the colorful, textured intricacy of their everyday challenges, women of all shapes and colors have the opportunity to listen, speak, and support each other. In this process, they reflect on their lives and participate in planting seeds of compassion so as to harvest a kinder and more respectful future.

## Conclusion

Childbearing issues are archetypal and the issues of feminine transformation permeate the mythology and literature of virtually every human society and provide rich symbolic imagery that expands upon the personal experience. The dramatic changes that occur to a woman's body begin with the growth of breasts and the flow of menstrual blood at puberty and then move to the swelling of the abdomen during pregnancy, the labor and act of giving birth, followed by the cessation of blood in menopause; each dramatic event is visible to those around her and puts her at risk of being objectified. Loss of a pregnancy or infant can intersect at various points and interrupt her journey, marking unforgettable junctures that leave her bereft. Fairy tales and myths depict these stages in a woman's life, offering metaphors, images, and symbols that illuminate the loss, ambivalence and challenges rising within the psyche that are potentially attended to through an art therapy process. May the following chapters inspire the guidance and protection from the moon and the diverse stories of our feminine ancestors who planted, tilled, and carried the harvested load before us.

## References

American Art Therapy Association (AATA). (1999). *Art Therapy Research Initiative [Brochure]*. Mundelein, IL: The American Art Therapy Association. [Google Scholar].

American Civil Liberties Union (ACLU) (2016, May 5). Women who have been denied medically necessary health care at Catholic hospitals speak out. Retrieved from: www.aclu.org/press-releases/new-report-reveals-1-6-us-hospital-beds-are-catholic-facilities-prohibit-essential

Amnesty International Ltd. (2017). *Criminalizing pregnancy: Policing pregnant women who use drugs in the USA*. London: Amnesty International. https://www.amnesty.org/download/Documents/AMR5162032017ENGLISH.pdf.

Aratani, L. (2020). Most women do not regret having an abortion, study finds. *Guardian*, Sunday 12. Retrieved from: www.theguardian.com/world/2020/jan/12/abortion-women-do-not-regret-study

Athan, A. (2017, Oct 3). Matrescence: Self development in motherhood. [Presentation given to Every Mother Counts]. Retrieved from: www.matrescence.com/blog/2018/4/10/matrescence-self-development-in-motherhood

Bridges, K. (2020). Race, pregnancy, and the opioid epidemic: White privilege and the criminalization of opioid use during pregnancy. *Harvard Law Review 133*(3), pp. 770–851. https://harvardlawreview.org/wp-content/uploads/2020/01/770-851_Online.pdf

Chasse, J.D. (2016). Prenatal depression risk reduction & education program. *Journal of Prenatal and Perinatal Psychology and Heath 30*(4), Summer, pp. 279–296.

Dangi-Garimella, S. (2018, June 15). 5 updates on maternal health in the United States. *Newsroom*. Retrieved from: www.ajmc.com/newsroom/5-updates-on-maternal-health-in-the-united-states

Davis-Floyd, R. (1992/2003). *Birth is an American rite of passage*. Berkeley, CA: University of California Press.

Finer, L.B. & Zolna, M.R. (2016). Declines in unintended pregnancy in the United States, 2008–2011. *New England Journal of Medicine 374*(9), pp. 843–852. doi:10.1056/NEJMsa1506575.

Geiser, R.M. (1990). When a mother kills her child. *Art Therapy 7*(2), pp. 86–93. doi:10.1080/07421656.1990.10758898.

Goodwin, M. (2020). *Policing the womb: Invisible women and the criminalization of motherhood*. Cambridge, UK: Cambridge University Press.

Gunja, M.Z., Tikkanen, R., Seervai, S., & Collins, S.R. (2018, Dec 19). What is the status of women's health and health care in the U.S. compared to ten other countries? *The Commonwealth Fund*. Retrieved from: www.commonwealthfund.org/publications/issue-briefs/2018/dec/womens-health-us-compared-ten-other-countries

Guttmacher Institute. (2019, January). *Unintended pregnancy in the United States*. Retrieved from: www.guttmacher.org/fact-sheet/unintended-pregnancy-united-states

Hiles, C. (2018). How U.S. maternity leave policy stats up to the U.K. and Germany. *The Penny Hoarder*, August 23, 2018. Retrieved from: www.thepennyhoarder.com/save-money/maternity-leave/#:~:targetText=Germany%20and%20the%20U.K.%20are,87%20weeks%20of%20paid%20leave.

Jerman, J., Jones, R.K., & Onda, T. (2016). *Characteristics of U.S. Abortion Patients in 2014 and Changes Since 2008*. New York: Guttmacher Institute. Retrieved from www.guttmacher.org/report/characteristics-us-abortion-patients-2014.

Kersting, A. & Wagner, B. (2012). Complicated grief after perinatal loss. *Dialogues Clinical Neuroscience* June 14(2), pp. 187–194.

Kroll, L. & Dolan, K. (2019, March 5). Billionaires: The richest people in the world. *Forbes*, March 5. www.forbes.com/billionaires/#58db674f251c

Lakhani, N. (2019). America has an infant mortality crisis: Meet the black doulas trying to change that. *The Guardian* November 25, 2019. Retrieved from www.theguardian.com/us-news/2019/nov/25/african-american-doula-collective-mothers-toxic-stress-racism-cleveland-infant-mortality-childbirth

Lazarus, E. (1883/2019). The new colossus. Retrieved from www.libertystatepark.com/emma.htm

Padilla, M. (2019). Woman gave birth in jail cell alone, lawsuit says. September 1, *New York Times*.

Potash, J. (2019). Relational social justice ethics for art therapists. *Art Therapy: Journal of the American Art Therapy Association 35*(4), pp. 202–210.

Raphael, D. (1975). Matrescence, Becoming a mother, A "new/old" rite de passage. In D. Raphael *Being female: Reproduction, power, and change* (pp. 65–71). The Hague: Mouton Publishers.

Rewire. (2018, Nov 7). Legislative Tracker: Personhood. *Rewire.News*. Retrieved from: https://rewire.news/legislative-tracker/law-topic/personhood/

Rothman, B.K. (2000). *Recreating motherhood*. New Brunswick, NJ: Rutgers University Press.

Swan-Foster, N. (2018). *Jungian art therapy: Dreams, images and analytical psychology*. New York, NY: Routledge.

Simkin, P. & Klaus, P. (2004). *When survivors give birth*. Seattle, WA: Classic Day Publishing.

Winnicott, D. W.(1960). The theory of the parent-infant relationship. *The International Journal of Psychoanalysis 41*, 585–595. https://icpla.edu/wp-content/uploads/2012/10/Winnicott-D.-The-Theory-of-the-Parent-Infant-Relationship-IJPA-Vol.-41-pps.-585-595.pdf.

Zwillich, T. (Host) (2020, Jan 14). Calling the shots in the year of the nurse and midwife [Radio Broadcast]. In M. Harven (producer). 1A. Washington, DC: Radio WAMU. Retrieved from: https://the1a.org/audio/#/shows/2020-01-14/calling-the-shots-in-the-year-of-the-nurse-and-midwife/119745/@00:00

# Part I
# Art Therapy
Pregnancy

# 2 The Juxtaposition of Rupture and Repair

## Exploring Trauma and Resilience with Women on the Paths of Childbearing, Birth, and Motherhood

*Denise R. Wolf and Juliet L. King*

In the nature of human creation and existence there is a series of rupture and repair. The process of childbearing and motherhood is subject to many small "t"s and large "T"s as well, although these are often not consciously processed. This chapter explores how the normative experience of trauma can be considered through a non-pathological lens and offers art therapy as a resourceful method to foster resilience and post-traumatic growth (PTG).

## Art Making as a Birth

The physical act of making art has often been referred to as an act of giving birth, offering a metaphor for rupture and repair. The concept of natalism, or the dynamic experience of birth and the resultant relationship between child and caregiver, is well documented through history and culture (Groff, 1985; Irving, 1989; Verny & Kelly, 1988). Dr. Irving, a sculptor and therapist, has been described as a world leader in developing the theory of natalism, which identifies parallel processes between creative expression and birth experiences (Irving, 2019). From Botticelli and da Vinci to Cassatt and Sherman, artists have portrayed the complicated role of motherhood that serves to hold an ongoing narrative about its often conflicted role. This primary trauma is "registered in the psyche, and for the artist, later projected into art, ritual and myth" (Irving, 1989, p. 84). Viewing visual art productions that express natilistic themes may offer opportunity to attend to, explore and resolve one's own personal pre or perinatal history (Pelowski, Markey, Lauring, & Leder, 2016). Visual art carries archetypal themes and templates to help consciously articulate subjective experiences.

Artworks and aesthetics allow us to connect our minds and experience through the witnessing of another's story. Archetypal imagery has emerged throughout centuries to provide us with a template to understand ourselves and embrace a universality of womanhood. Childbirth is a powerful, dramatic ritual where "paintings of the mother giving birth, with the exposed child still connected to her via the umbilical cord are found throughout the Cro-Magnon caves" (Sjoo & Mor, 1987, p. 47). At times bold and engaging, or disturbing or unsettling, the symbolism and stories told through the art allow for a dialogue and potential reframe of our own experience. The process of childbearing and birth can be a triggering experience for women and may be accompanied by a range of emotional and cognitive responses that are not always assimilated. Do the physical effects of trauma supersede the subjective experience? Does the body know the difference?

## Rupture and Repair

Women live their lives through ongoing construction, deconstruction, and reconstruction in their monthly cycles alone. Hormonal shifts impact cognitive and emotional functioning from early teenage years through menopause and older adulthood. These bio-physio-psychological changes create a series of perceptual changes that are further pronounced through the pregnancy and birthing process. Here we might see that a woman's traumatic experiences are those of embodiment, where creativity becomes a resourceful healer, and traumatic hindrance is seen as growth. PTG is associated with a positive psychological change emergent from traumatic experiences (Tedeschi & Calhoun, 2004) and the experience of trauma is seen as a natural phenomenon. Traumatic memories are fragmented and displaced into areas of our psyche that we have less conscious access to, and while this may create a disruption of overall homeostasis, responses may also become reparative. Dekel, Mandl, and Solomon (2011) noted the importance of considering PTG in an otherwise pathogenic clinical perspective of trauma and share the value of this progressive outlook in the healing process. In particular, the loss of control associated with the traumatic experience may lend itself to a revitalized perspective of ones' evolutionary capacities.

Threat and response to threat is where growth happens. We respond to the threat and we grow, and if not, we stagnate. A vivid memory can be recalled of how the growth model of "homeostasis and threat" was once introduced in middle school science class. First the teacher drew a staircase on the board, pointed to the horizontal stair tread, and named it "homeostasis." "This," he said, pointing to the intersecting vertical line, "is a threat. The organism can respond to the threat, adapt or assimilate, and grow." "GROW!" he exclaimed! With this, he dramatically traced the vertical rise upward to the next tread. "Or," he said, "the organism stagnates." With this, he circled the lower tread. In other words, there is no change without a destruction of what was (Spielrein, 1994). This can be thought of as a model for growth, and more specifically PTG: the homeostasis, threat, response, and resilience that accompany this process. Growth. Repeat. Rupture and repair. We are designed to respond to threat, and this is how we grow and learn lest we stagnate and regress. This is our destiny as humans and our story of origin. As a colleague of Freud and Jung in the early 1900s, Spielrein (1994) offered this as a biological fact, where "during reproduction, a union of female and male cells occurs. The unity of each cell thus is destroyed and from this product of this destruction, new life originates" (p. 156). Like art, science offers an opportunity to explore dimensions of being that branch beyond conscious thought.

How effective we are in managing our emotional experiences is due to many factors that include genetic predisposition, past experiences, and a creative outlook (LeDoux, 1996). The brain's capacity to revise one's narrative can be described through the scientific fact of neuroplasticity, which essentially means the brain's ability to rewire itself. While experiences shape the anatomical structure of the brain, through mindful engagement and relational exchange there is great capacity to reframe perspectives (Siegel, 2007). Neuroplasticity contributes to PTG and offers evidence-based data to support a person's liveliness and ability to re-write their own story. The brain's ability to shift and change through relationships is evident throughout the lifespan and energized from the very beginning. Mahler (1972) identified the rapprochement phase as a normative stage of child development where a separation from caregiver takes place, managing the anxiety of abandonment, to develop a singular sense of identity. This may be seen as rupture and repair—a seeking of identity without the other, a new formation of self that manifests repeatedly throughout our relationships. We are hard-wired for homeostasis following any challenge to the system and our psyches follow the wisdom of our bodies through interactions with others. Contemporary theory suggests that this cyclical rupture and repair is one of regulation as well as attachment, which offers deeper connections in understanding the healing process throughout the therapeutic relational exchange (Schore & Schore, 2008).

## Birth as Trauma

Trauma is commonly understood as an experience of intense fear and/or perceived threat to self or loved one, where typical coping skills are insufficient (Boorman, Devilly, Gamble, Creedy, & Fenwick, 2014; Chapman, 2014; Herman, 1997; King, 2016; Talwar, 2007). Does childbirth fit the facts? A recent study revealed that as many as 43% of mothers reported their birth experience as traumatic (Alcorn, O'Donovan, Patrick, Creedy, & Devilly, 2010).

> During any trauma, one's illusion of personal control, autonomy and individuality is stripped away. Whether this is through natural disaster, sexual assault, physical accident, war, or indeed childbirth, the effect on the self is consistent, a person's identity is shaken as the self is reduced or objectified through the vulnerability of trauma.
>
> (Byrne, Egan, MacNeela, & Sarma, 2017, p. 10)

While the literature is ripe with information regarding the effects of motherhood stress and mental health on unborn children (Cozolino, 2014) there is less to be found that speaks to a woman's perception of self in the mothering process as it pertains to stress and trauma. Viewing the experience of pregnancy, childbirth, and motherhood as parallel to a traumatic experience offers art therapists a supportive, feminist, and restorative lens and approach to wellness. By understanding the needs of the woman through a trauma lens we can offer opportunities for growth and repair through the symbolic nature and relational exchange involved in art therapy processes.

Art making in the context of the therapeutic relationship can aid in the processing of distressing events and the attendance to complexities of the relational exchange are crucial (Hass-Cohen, Findlay, Carr, & Vanderlan, 2014). Art therapists have witnessed countless experiences of the benefits of the creative process to foster resilience, self-awareness, and the amelioration of stress and anxiety. A neuroscientific approach has shown that art therapy (1) Facilitates the organization and integration of traumatic memories; (2) Reactivates positive emotions and serves as a vehicle for exposure and externalization of difficult content; (3) Reduces heightened arousal responses; (4) Enhances emotional self-efficacy and maintains a space for the exploration of self-perception and psychic integration; and (5) Enhances the development of identity (King, 2015, p. 84). Participating in art therapy offers an ability to explore oneself through an active and engaged relationship.

According to Rubin (1984), "Childbearing requires an exchange of a known self in a known world for an unknown self in an unknown world" (p. 52). As trauma therapists, we might think of this as, "Who am I now that this event has happened (to me) and how do I understand this new world that holds the event?" These two components of identity reconstruction have been the centralized focus of a specific approach to trauma treatment, which has successfully informed each unique approach with a client. Demecs, Fenwick, and Gamble (2011) identified a cultural shift towards viewing childbirth as a medical event, with decreasing attention paid to the emotional aspects of pregnancy and childbirth. This appears as a dangerous shift; although birth is a medical event it is also constitutes a rupture to identity and integrated sense of self, which warrants attention and support towards repair and growth.

## Maternal Identity

In their paper "Debating Natalism," Harari and Kroul (2019) encouraged their readers to reflect on the cultural and social importance of motherhood and natalism. Contemporary culture seems to be moving towards the repression of a woman's choice to express and explore her interpersonal responses to childbearing and parenthood as an integral part of life. However, history suggests this need is both pervasive and ancient. Through history, and around the world, "the symbolic expression of birth and prenatal consciousness can be found in art, mythology, and creative expression" (Irving, 1989, p. 83). This juxtaposition presents itself in the therapeutic space, for example, when mothers are conflicted with feelings of inauthenticity, guilt, fatigue, shame for being tired, and grieving the loss of their maternal identity and body.

For her graduate thesis, art therapist Jewelie Sluzas (2012) investigated *The Development of Maternal Identity and Awareness of the Primiparae in Transition Through Pregnancy into Motherhood*. This qualitative research examined the artwork of three first-time mothers who gave birth at a local birthing center. Each participant in the study created imagery in response to the following three prompts: self before pregnancy, self during pregnancy, and self after giving birth. Participants made verbal associations to their artwork through a series of open-ended questions, which Sluzas identified for common themes. In a recent interview, Sluzas expanded upon her motivation to begin the research, "I don't think women are fully seen through this process. The life changing experiences in and around childbirth have been minimized. How could this huge event in our lives not change who we are?" (J. Sluzas, personal communication, September 28, 2019). In her thesis (2012), Sluzas noted that Swan-Foster was the only art therapist writing about this overlooked topic, mentioning her 1989 article as well as a co-authored article (Swan-Foster, 1989; Swan-Foster, Foster, & Dorsey, 2003). Sluzas further supported the experience of contemporary culture denying collaborative experiences for pregnant and postpartum women to share their personal narratives (J. Sluzas, personal communication, September 28, 2019). This need for narration has existed in both prenatal experiences and trauma theory. Irving (1989) supported the idea that through history and culture we see many images and metaphors that depict the process of birth, which are largely unconscious. Boorman et al. (2014) conducted a study that explored ways childbirth fits the criteria for a traumatic event. They, too, identified the need for women to speak about their birth experiences. Herman (1997) recognized the power of the narrative towards meaning making in trauma therapy. She identified the importance of expressing not just the event, but the response of "survivors," as well as the response of those people close to her. Perhaps this speaks to the need to reintegrate, or repair, one's identity pre and post-partum? This directly relates to the named pre and postnatal experiences of women asking the same questions, "Who am I now? What is this world that holds both me and this baby? What now are my personal, professional and social identities?"

## Making the Nonverbal Verbal

Identity was also one of the salient themes identified by Sluzas (2012). She suggested that the loss or change in identity happens earlier than birth. Other themes identified in Sluzas' research (2012) included change, self in the world, and use of symbol and metaphor. Through her study, her participants identified previously unnamed feelings related to the birthing experiences, including shifting expectations from self and others. She posited that the art therapy process allowed the expectations to be brought to the surface, named, and reflected upon towards gaining insight, reintegrating identity, and connecting with others. "Like a fishing line cast into a deep pool, what needs to be seen will emerge" (J. Sluzas, personal communication, September 28, 2019).

Utilizing art therapy processes makes the nonverbal verbal. If we understand birth as a traumatic event, we understand that experiences surrounding birth are stored in the brain in an area that is not only resistant to verbal identification and expression, but more respondent to artistic expression. The art becomes a symbolic container of the person's experience and assists in the reconsolidation of memories and fragmented emotional responses (Tripp, 2007). This traumatic experience of birth may be further denied expression due to cultural and social expectations that birth does not "fit the facts" as a traumatic experience. This limits space for expression, exploration, and repair. The traumatic memory is stored as imagery; art therapy can allow for processing and resolution (Chapman, 2014; King, 2016; Talwar, 2007).

Demecs et al. (2011) explored the experience of women attending a creative arts program during pregnancy. They identified a growing body of literature that supports the need for and value of women connecting to "cultural knowledge" about birth. Their study further revealed four themes expressed in the artwork of the participants: seeking support, connecting to others, finding a place to share, and finding balance. These needs seem to align with trauma treatment researcher Dr. Judith Herman's (1997) four stages of trauma recovery and offer a conceptual parallel for the use of creative arts therapies to treat (see Table 2.1):

*Table 2.1* Themes in Artwork Aligned with Stages of Trauma Recovery

| Themes emergent in artwork (Demecs et al., 2011) | Stages of trauma recovery (Herman, 1997) |
| --- | --- |
| Seeking support | Safety and stabilization |
| Finding a place to share | Remembrance and mourning |
| Connecting with others | Reconnection and integration |
| Finding balance | Reconnection and integration |

## A Feminist Approach

A feminist approach to art therapy for maternal wellness can offer a space for reflection and repair, a place for nonverbal communication with both self and others. This can foster the development of a narrative as well as create opportunities for connection and validation as Marstine (2002) explained: "Current trauma theory posits that trauma exists not through the encounter, but through surviving the encounter and being unable to understand it" (p. 633). Sluzas (2012) saw art therapy as a way to both reflect and reinterpret the world and experience of pregnancy and childbirth. Art is a primary means to connect with, and relate to preconscious and unconscious experiences (Appleton, 2001; Chapman, 2014; Irving, 1989). Nonverbal forms of expression like drawing or painting offer opportunities to transform or repair the traumatic memory so that it can be integrated into the life story (Herman, 1997). In discussing healing ruptures through recognition, Charles (2017) emphasized, "It is our willingness to look at what is happening and try to make meaning" (p. 186).

Birth is a normative experience of rupture and repair. What if we viewed pregnancy and birth through a lens of cultural humility and feminism that honors a woman's desire to have control of herself throughout pregnancy and birth while holding the knowledge that these experiences may be out of her control and traumatic? Art therapy is well suited to hold a space that "negotiates a safe passage between the twin dangers of constriction and intrusion" (Herman, 1997, p. 176). Or, as Charles (2017) stated,

> Facilitate movement into an external world in which there is the possibility of being received, accepted and valued without losing one's sense of self when the outer regard is lacking ... the past loosens its hold on us when we can find ourselves within in and talk with one another about it.
>
> (p. 193)

Sluzas (2012) asked why, when art therapy theory is largely reliant on understanding identity formation through artistic expression, it is not more present as an approach towards maternal wellness and understanding birth experiences. Can we remove the judgment from the term "trauma" and understand it as a maternal disruption to identity that warrants care? Can we view this as a normative experience of rupture and repair and an opportunity for post-traumatic growth?

Likening pregnancy and childbirth to trauma has great potential for misunderstanding and criticism. Trauma is a frequently used term, often misused and overly simplified. Women may feel criticized for experiencing birth as a trauma, viewing it as "one more thing women are doing wrong." Trauma is a natural part of life; the very genesis of life is a rupture. It is a part of how we live and grow. We have an emergent understanding of what constitutes a traumatic experience and how the brain and body are impacted. We know how to approach this clinically as Sluzas (2012) noted: "Through art therapy processes, women can uncover and explore conflicts, and work toward building a cohesive sense of self as her identity shifts. For mothers, art making provides a nonlinear format of expression and much needed personal space" (p. 169). Recognizing birth as a normative traumatic experience would further opportunities to normalize this experience for mothers and culture at large, providing opportunities for psychoeducation. Psychoeducation about trauma can help to shape interventions appropriate to the stage of the stress response, depathologize normative and transient responses, and decrease stigma (Vasterling, Daly, & Friedman, 2011). This creates a culture that supports the mother in moving forward, while honoring the loss of her previous identity and providing support to manage ongoing change.

## References

Alcorn, K. L., O'Donovan, A., Patrick, J. C., Creedy, D., & Devilly, G. J. (2010). A prospective longitudinal study of the prevalence of post-traumatic stress disorder resulting from childbirth events. *Psychological Medicine*, 40(11), 1849–1859.

Appleton, V. (2001). Avenues of hope: Art therapy and the resolution of trauma. *Art Therapy*, 18(1), 6–13.

Boorman, R. J., Devilly, G. J., Gamble, J., Creedy, D. K., & Fenwick, J. (2014). Childbirth and criteria for traumatic events. *Midwifery*, 30(2), 255–261.

Byrne, V., Egan, J., MacNeela, P., & Sarma, K. (2017). What about me? The loss of self through the experience of traumatic childbirth. *Midwifery*, 51, 1–11.

Chapman, L. (2014). *Neurobiologically informed trauma therapy with children and adolescents: Understanding mechanisms of change*. New York, NY: W.W. Norton & Company.

Charles, M. (2017). The promise of love revisited: Healing ruptures through recognition. *Psychoanalytic Psychology*, 34(2), 186.

Cozolino, L. (2014). The impact of early stress. In L. Cozolino (Ed.), *The neuroscience of human relationships: Attachment and the developing social brain* (pp. 258–277). New York, NY: W.W. Norton & Company.

Dekel, S., Mandl, C., & Solomon, Z. (2011). Shared and unique predictors of post-traumatic growth and distress. *Journal of Clinical Psychology*, 67(3), 241–252.

Demecs, I. P., Fenwick, J., & Gamble, J. (2011). Women's experiences of attending a creative arts program during their pregnancy. *Women and Birth*, 24(3), 112–121.

Groff, S. (1985). *Beyond the brain: Birth, death, and transcendence in psychotherapy*. Albany, New York: Suny Press.

Harari, D., & Kroul, G. (2019). Debating natalism: Israeli one-woman shows on experiencing childlessness. *New Theatre Quarterly*, 35(2), 121–134.

Hass-Cohen, N., Findlay, J. C., Carr, R., & Vanderlan, J. (2014). "Check, change what you need to change and/or keep what you want": An art therapy neurobiological-based trauma protocol. *Art Therapy, 31*(2), 69–78. doi:10.1080/07421656.2014.903825

Herman, J. (1997). *Trauma and recovery: The aftermath of violence from domestic abuse to political terror.* New York, NY: Basic Books.

Irving, M. (1989). Natalism as pre and perinatal metaphor. *Journal of Prenatal & Perinatal Psychology & Health, 4*(2), 83.

Irving, M. (2019). Retrieved from www.irvingstudios.com/artist.htm

King, J. L. (2015). Art therapy: A brain based profession. In M. Rosal & D. Gussak (Eds.), *The handbook of art therapy* (77–89). Hoboken, NJ: John Wiley & Sons.

King, J. L. (2016). *Art therapy, trauma, and neuroscience: Theoretical and practical perspectives.* New York NY: Routledge, Taylor & Francis Group.

LeDoux, J. (1996). A few degrees of separation. In J. LeDoux (Ed.), *The emotional brain: The mysterious underpinnings of emotional life* (pp. 139–178). New York, NY: Simon & Schuster.

Mahler, M. S. (1972). Rapprochement subphase of the separation-individuation process. *The Psychoanalytic Quarterly, 41*(4), 487–506.

Marstine, J. (2002). Challenging the gendered categories of art and art therapy: The paintings of Jane Orleman. *Feminist Studies, 28*(3), 631–654.

Pelowski, M., Markey, P. S., Lauring, J. O., & Leder, H. (2016). Visualizing the impact of art: An update and comparison of current psychological models of art experience. *Frontiers in Human Neuroscience, 10*, 160.

Rubin, R. (1984). *Maternal identity and the maternal experience.* New York, NY: Springer.

Schore, J. R., & Schore, A. N. (2008). Modern attachment theory: The central role of affect regulation in development and treatment. *Clinical Social Work Journal, 36*(9), 9–20. doi:10.1007/s10615-007-0111-7

Siegel, D. (2007). Brain Basics. In D. Siegel (Ed.), *The mindful brain: Reflection and attunement in the cultivation of well-being* (pp. 29–50). New York, NY: W.W. Norton & Company.

Sjoo, M., & Mor, B. (1987). *The great cosmic mother. Rediscovering the religion of the earth.* New York, NY: HarperCollins.

Sluzas, J. G. (2012). *The development of maternal identity and awareness of the primiparae in the transition through pregnancy into motherhood as expressed in artwork and interview: A phenomenological study* (Unpublished master's thesis). Drexel University, Philadelphia, PA.

Spielrein, S. (1994). Destruction as the cause of coming into being. *Journal of Analytical Psychology, 39*(2), 155–186.

Swan-Foster, N. (1989). Images of a pregnant woman: Art therapy as a tool for transformation. *The Arts in Psychotherapy, 16*, 283–292.

Swan-Foster, N., Foster, S., & Dorsey, A. (2003). The use of human figure drawing with pregnant women. *Journal of Reproductive and Infant Psychology, 21*(4), 293–307.

Talwar, S. (2007). Accessing traumatic memory through art making: An art therapy trauma protocol (ATTP). *The Arts in Psychotherapy, 34*(1), 22–35.

Tedeschi, R., & Calhoun, L. (2004). Posttraumatic growth: Conceptual foundations and empirical evidence. *Psychological Inquiry, 15*(1), 1–18. doi:10.1207/s15327965pli1501_01

Tripp, T. (2007). A short term approach to processing trauma: Art therapy and bilateral stimulation. *Art Therapy, 24*(4), 176–183.

Vasterling, J. J., Daly, E. S., & Friedman, M. J. (2011). Posttraumatic stress reactions over time: The battlefield, homecoming, and long-term course. In J. I. Ruzek, P. P. Schnurr, J. J. Vasterling, & M. J. Friedman (Eds.), *Caring for veterans with deployment-related stress disorders* (pp. 35–55). American Psychological Association. doi:10.1037/12323-002

Verny, T., & Kelly, J. (1988). *The secret life of the unborn child.* New York, NY: Dell Publishing.

# 3   Prenatal Art Therapy and Feminine Initiation[1]

## When Pregnant Imagination Gives Birth to Maternal Identity

*Nora Swan-Foster*

### Pregnancy

Pregnancy is an archetypal event. When it is viewed as an initiation it offers women an alternative and yet medically compatible lens for understanding in greater depth the power of how this archetype reshapes their lives. Jung (1960/1972) noted that initiations bring "the realization of a part of the personality which has not yet come into existence but is still in the process of becoming" (p. 293). Neumann (1955/1974, p. 31) noted that pregnancy as the second blood mystery transforms the woman's personality prior to the next archetypal constellation of childbirth. Indeed, a pregnant woman is both being and becoming through specific initiatory tasks. The fetus symbolizes the potential for a new consciousness, a new maternal attitude that grows and expands towards birth. I have noted that "intense dreams and fears are common during pregnancy but the pregnant woman holds them as silently as she holds her growing baby" (Swan-Foster, 1989, p. 284) until art therapy facilitates the birth of her prenatal images that visibly allow her to find meaning and incorporate the important aspects of pregnancy into her personality. As her body changes with the growing fetus, "[p]sychically, the baby is implanted in the soil of her unconscious ... gaining substance from her fantasies, influenced by and influencing the climate of her psychic reality" (Raphael-Leff, 1993, p. 14). Prenatal art therapy reveals these depths and clarifies her journey as both personal and archetypal; the images support her emotional integration and preparation for childbirth and motherhood.

Alongside her medical care, a modern woman may view pregnancy as a time-limited opportunity for greater psychological and spiritual growth. What unfolds emotionally is often invisible to the outside world particularly as "standard obstetric procedures" have become the modern "rituals" that are "managed" through new technology (Davis-Floyd, 1992/2003, 2001, 2019a, 2019b). While not all pregnant women are conscious of their potential to both *reflect* and *effect* individual paradigm shifts (Davis-Floyd, 1992/2003), a woman may intuitively gravitate towards a collaborative approach where her inner voice is honored and valued. The term "conscious pregnancy" or an "initiation-oriented pregnancy"[2] (Swan-Foster, 2012) has been proposed to acknowledge this approach. Finally, the pregnant woman is an archetypal image for universal processes such as conception, incubation, gestation, and death/rebirth that amplify an inherent structure within the reproductive journey that parallels the creative process in art therapy.

Over the years, I have viewed prenatal art therapy as an early intervention modality (Swan-Foster, 1989, 2001, 2010, 2012; Swan-Foster, Foster, & Dorsey, 2003) that invites a woman to reflect upon her pregnant self. Art therapists and prenatal art therapy are easily integrated into educational and preventative programs, hospitals, agencies, and private practices, offering a viable and respected clinical approach, particularly to address nonverbal prenatal emotions. Prenatal mental health and well-being is integral to a woman's maternal identity and development with a plethora of research validating the value and long-term benefits of emotional support for antenatal women. The following literature review considers how anthropology, psychology, and art therapy are collaborative paradigms that value the transformation, dignity, and emotional well-being of the pregnant woman. Clinical examples will illustrate how the initiatory stages of pregnancy are reflected through women's art work.

Finally, our culture has evolved into a time where gender identity is seen as fluid, illustrated by trans-men giving birth to babies and courageously creating families (Hempel, 2016; Silva, 2016). In this new decade, the requests for acceptance, support, and peaceful recognition actually deserve cultural celebration. Rooted in the hegemony of heterosexuality, psychosocial challenges exist for nonconforming prenatal subgroups whose experiences could be explored through art therapy. Because conception requires the opposites (X and Y chromosomes) to join together and implant within a uterus to form a fetus, the psychobiological experience and gender term "woman" will continue to be used. The biological fact does reject the gray and fluid spaces that are integral to a diverse culture that accepts people with fluid gender identities with equally complex childbearing issues.

## Literature: Anthropology, Psychology, and Prenatal Art Therapy

### Anthropology

Anthropology has considered pregnancy as a feminine initiation and have related fear and anxiety to creativity, cosmos, blood, and death. More precisely, a feminine initiation honors the woman's sacrifices and transformation. She turns towards her dramatic physical transformation

that ignites the immersive journey where personal and cultural complexes and archetypal patterns are confronted. Female rites are less
documented, perhaps because early research was undertaken by men or
the cultural complexes associated with feminine blood were complicated
and women maintained a private space with their rituals.

Initiations are a three-part structure that begin with "hearing the
call." This is followed by specific ordeals or tasks that risk death,
followed by the initiand's return to the community with a gift and
a new name. The stages remain germane today: **pre-liminal** (separation
from one's environment), **liminal** (a non-ordinary state of consciousness related to thresholds), and **post-liminal** (an incorporation into
a new world) (van Gennep, 1960). Within this structure, van Gennep
(1960) noted childbearing as a *rite of passage*; however, unlike the male
initiand who strips down, leaves home and crosses territorial boundaries, the female initiand turns inwards to focus on the territory of
her body, psyche, and spirit. Within all rites of passage is a state of
*liminality* that Turner (1967/1979) described as "likened to death,
being in the womb" (p. 95) or no longer of the old and not yet made
new. In fact, some tribal communities isolated a pregnant woman
because she was thought to be dangerous, contaminated, and likely
to infect those around her (Westermarck, 1906/2010). Behaviors
rooted in the superstition and fear of the power of blood gave the
woman hidden powers over her husband and men in the tribe and led
to her isolation. Specifically, the Hova tribe in Madagascar considered
the pregnant woman dead from conception until she gave birth, at
which point she was considered resurrected (van Gennep, 1960, p. 43),
illustrating a death/rebirth motif found in modern pregnancy and the
creative process.

Lincoln (1981) researched the rites of five different cultures and noted
four preliminary actions of the female initiation used in various combi-
nations: body mutation, identification with a mythic heroine, cosmic
journey, and play of opposites (p. 94). By identifying with a heroine, the
initiand's temporal situation shifts to *atemporality* where she becomes,
through creative acts, someone who is "beyond death, beyond aging,
beyond time" (p. 96). The following vignettes illustrate how a creative
unfolding of not just time, but also space where the mythic and cosmic
journey can liberate the pregnant woman from her locale to travel the
heavens and the seas using her creative imagination. The woman's cosmic
importance is also expressed through her daily life, her body and her
relationships with other women, perhaps at times offering a "religious
compensation for a sociopolitical deprivation" (p. 105). The play of
opposites are perhaps the most difficult to characterize, but "the resolution of opposites always involves a move from separation to unity,
tension to harmony, and limitations to totality ... the nature of her
very being is radically transformed" (p. 98) and that "each time a woman

is initiated, the world is saved from chaos, for the *fundamental power of creativity is renewed in her being* [emphasis added]" (p. 107).

Importantly, feminine initiations do not bring women increased social status or hierarchal power, but instead, her compensation is a "cosmic status" (Lincoln, 1981, p. 105) because she has "transcended the bounds of her mundane existence ... jolted out of her immediate locale and introduced to the universe" (p. 97). She is adorned to emphasize her special status and the cosmic prenatal journey "changes [her] fundamental being ... A woman does not become more powerful ... but *more creative* [emphasis added], more alive, more ontologically real" (p. 104).

In modern culture, Davis-Floyd (1992/2003) considered antenatal rites with respect to American standards and determined that "technocratic" medical protocols and hospital births do the opposite of what Lincoln noted, creating "separation and segmentation (better known as 'specialization') so pervasive in our society today ... there is complete denial of the fundamentally female power of creativity" (pp. 285–286). Further, with managed care, malpractice threats, and high medical and insurance costs, "[w]omen in American society have been deprived, not only of social 'equality' but also of their cosmic significance as birth-givers, transformed even in the transformation of giving birth into mere machines to be manipulated and repaired" (pp. 285–286). Further, the lack of relationship mixed with inequality may stimulate an emotional regression in which she relinquishes her adult self within the paternal medical environment that determine the rituals.

Amplifying this perspective are the dramatic statistics that reveal socioeconomic and racial/ethnic disparities in America with a growing number of health concerns and pregnancy-related mortality rates for women of color, particularly black women (Lakhani, 2019; Petersen et al., 2019). These women consistently face institutionalized racism with severe psychosocial inequalities, inhumane discrimination, and disparities within medical antenatal care, and high levels of unaddressed toxic stress and health issues that impact birth outcomes (Ely & Driscoll, 2019; Guardino & Schetter, 2014; Lakhani, 2019). Reports are that if a woman is not white or does not speak English, she will be harshly treated during medical visits and childbirth. Traumatic moments during pregnancy and childbirth are absorbed as body memory and interrupt the process of a woman becoming an emotionally well-attuned mother, interrupting the period of *matrescence* (Athan, 2017; Athan & Miller, 2005; Raphael, 1975), or maternal development, especially if "women ... end up with many regrets after their birth experiences. Some regrets are so obvious that women can name and understand them, but regrets get buried in the cells of women's bodies and unconscious minds" (Çoker, Karabekir, & Varlik, 2019, p. 121) as nonverbal and potential long-term health issues. Creative and spiritual work through art therapy can often repair these regrets and ruptures.

From her research, Davis-Floyd (1992/2003) defined the dominant source of reproductive knowledge in America as *mechanistic* and *techno-cratic*. Knowledge once held by an elder and sought by the initiand is managed or withheld by a physician who maintains an expertise that the pregnant woman depends upon; focused on test results, she is distracted from her own internal locus of knowing and collaboration. "In spite of the uniqueness of each birth and each woman who gives birth, standardized obstetrical procedures give ... the reassuring appearance of sameness and conformity to the socially dominant reality model" (p. 66), which suggests less diverse, flexible or creative options. Because antenatal care has become more "managed," Davis-Floyd (2019a) proposed four cognitive stages to evaluate how we *know* and *think* about the antenatal process, which includes listening to the pregnant woman (p. 2). In a hierarchal developed society such as the United States, "most pregnancy pre- and proscriptions emerge from the medical domain ... the primary source of culturally-recognized 'authoritative knowledge'" (Davis-Floyd & Georges, 1996, pp. 1014–1016), which provides essential care and comfort for some women in some situations, but as a single form of treatment, it lacks flexibility and collaboration, marginalizing the woman's unique psychosocial story.

While anthropology observed various authoritative sources of knowledge, the point is not to return to unsafe superstitions and ancient shamanic practices, but to evaluate how the dominant culture controls and potentially traumatizes the individual when she is in a liminal state and easily misunderstood or disregarded and how practices such as midwifery and doula support create an environment of collaboration (Davis-Floyd, 2019a, 2019b; Merchant, 2012; Raphael, 1975).

Davis-Floyd's observations of the American model of pregnancy and childbirth amplify how the modern pregnant initiand is easily objectified and marginalized. Rather than pathologizing or marginalizing her liminal state, because she is no longer who she was and not yet who she will become, when the medical team resists authoritative measures for respectful collaboration instead, the woman locates an inner strength to engage with the transformation of her identity.

It is not easy to trust the deconstruction and reconstruction of an un-worded liminal state that is initially known through complexes associated with normal ambivalence, disorientation, fear, and vulnerability surrounding her own separation or death, the separation and death of her fetus, or the separation and death of her partner. But perhaps we can trust her prenatal fears as the seeds for potential psychological transformation and maternal maturation and allow her to affect how we *think* and what we *know* about her as she connects to a new relational life of creativity, imagination, unity and wholeness driven by her changing body. A feminine initiation model during pregnancy invites us to hold a larger perspective that greatly benefits maternal/infant outcomes (Davis-Floyd, 2019a, p. 2).

*Psychology*

The foremother of psychoanalysis, Karen Horney, separated from Freud because his theory excluded half of the population.

> [A]s a woman, [I] ask in amazement, and what about motherhood? And the blissful consciousness of bearing a new life within oneself? And the ineffable happiness of the increasing expectation of the appearance of this new being? And the joy when it finally makes its appearance and one holds it for the first time in one's arms? And the deep pleasurable feeling of satisfaction in suckling it and the happiness of the whole period when the infant needs her care?
>
> (1926, p. 329)

Although somewhat idealized, her sensitive recognition of motherhood as a vital characteristic of some female experiences brought recognition and dignity to a woman's reproductive process. Helene Deutsch (1944) also dispelled the notion that psychological work with pregnant women was dangerous, a diversion from her male colleagues. Benedek (1959) viewed pregnancy as a somatic "psychological crisis" while Bibring, Dwyer, Huntington, and Valenstein (1968) noted three important stages of maturation: receiving, retaining, and releasing. While most pregnancies are not problematic, a differentiation between normal and special aspects of pregnancy were explored by Nadelson (1978) who outlined pregnancy and postpartum and specific signals for obstetricians. As preventative Peterson (1984, 1991) researched and implemented a pioneering holistic approach towards prenatal emotions and childbirth. Colman and Colman (1991) emphasized the developmental stages of pregnancy as significant emotional markers that deserved attention. The psychoanalyst Raphael-Leff (1991, 1993) viewed the womb as a symbolic "container" for emotional material and emphasized the pregnant woman's temporary *permeability*, or a loosening of internal barriers, as a time-limited emotional growth opportunity.[3] Noteworthy is that this permeability for early sexual abuse survivors often requires trauma-focused approaches (Simpkin & Klaus, 2004/2018).

Certain rites of passages are no longer used in modern times, but dreams and their various motifs show how the pregnant initiand is doing and offer a differentiated way to understand her psyche (Abt, Bosch, & MacKrell, 2000). Woman's childbearing issues were ritualized, honored, and made sacred by spontaneous archetypal images and dreams in Jungian analysis, revealing the innate feminine initiation patterns (Beane Rutter, 1993/2009, 2011). Côté-Arsenault, Brody, and Dombeck (2009) emphasized the rite of passage as a significant structural model for pregnancy and childbirth when following perinatal loss, while the obstetrics doctor Kortendieck-Rashee (2011) applied an initiation model using the myth of Persephone and the dreams from immigrant pregnant women in Germany. Pregnancy as a distinct period of initiation was conceptualized in greater depth through myth, dreams, and art therapy (Swan-Foster, 2010, 2012).

## Prenatal Art Therapy

Prenatal art therapy is a powerful clinical approach that compliments the pregnant woman's emotional availability and makes visible her rite of passage through creative work. In my early research (1989, 1991), I used four specific drawings with a small group of pregnant women to replicate a creative birthing process (draw yourself pregnant, draw a fear, transform the fear, and closing mandala).[4] The drawings addressed and stabilized underlying prenatal emotions such as fear, loss, and anxiety. Several future topics were identified for prenatal art therapy, including specific populations and research areas. Responding to how tension and fear impact childbirth outcomes (Dick-Read, 1953), the fear of childbirth and transforming that fear, demonstrated that art therapy successfully exposes underlying emotions and reinforces maternal confidence (Swan-Foster, 1991). In a quantitative study of fear of childbirth (FOC), 30 women were divided into two random groups: one offering psychoeducation and the other art therapy (Sezen & Ünsalver, 2019). The results showed art therapy decreased depression, anxiety, and FOC in the third trimester. Prenatal fear of childbirth[5] was investigated with greater focus and depth by midwives who used art with patients with positive results (Wahlbeck, Kvist, & Landgren, 2018). Wardi-Zonna (2017) advocated for art therapy, as an alternative for prenatal depression and anxiety to claim their own voice and decrease symptoms. Using the Bird Nest Drawing to investigate attachment issues of pregnant women, Overbeck (2002) sampled a small group of high-risk women and found important incongruences between drawing indicators and verbal reports. This finding may highlight comorbidity of postpartum mood and anxiety disorders (PMADs) with unresolved initiation tasks inhibited by psychosocial economic challenges. Research investigating high-risk pregnancies in a level five Denver hospital[6] used the FEATS[7] art therapy scale to score the Human Figure Drawing or "draw yourself pregnant" from the original drawing series (PATII) (Swan-Foster, 2001). Results suggested that high risk inpatient (HRI) drawings scored less for depression, pointing to benefits from medical predictability, technology, and obstetrics' authoritative knowledge for high-risk populations (Swan-Foster et al., 2003). A prenatal human figure drawing was viewed as a concise clinical assessment tool where maternal "emotions can be brought into graphic form concurrent with medical care" (p. 305). An art therapy self-study was used to prepare for being a single mother by choice (Henderson, 2000). Using dreams, art, and meditation, Henderson's research structure during pregnancy was found to have a positive influence on postpartum. Hocking (2007) asked a small group of first-time mothers to reflect back on their pregnancies and create self-symbols as they recounted their prenatal narrative. Through a Jungian lens, the symbols illustrated a clear, unfolding path of transformation through form and color, which visually documented maternal development. Sluzas (2012) further investigated maternal development in three first time pregnancies using specific art therapy drawings and found particular themes associated with loss of identity.

Prenatal art therapy is also a nonthreatening approach used for prenatal groups and has many benefits. In 1996, I introduced prenatal art therapy into a Colorado obstetrics practice in collaboration with childbirth classes. Collage materials were used to facilitate group discussion of prenatal anxiety and fears associated with pregnancy and childbirth and the birth educator/nurse was available for medical questions. This process allowed couples to reflect and actively investigate and transform their emotional concerns through art therapy and couples benefitted from sharing emotions and building cohesion within the group model.

In other instances, Anand and Baker (1997) used group art therapy with addicted, pregnant, and parenting women in an innovative 12-step art therapy treatment program in Mississippi where antenatal women struggling with addiction were profoundly underrepresented and underserved. Complicated issues that arose from traumatic histories were: powerlessness, sexual abuse, violence, anger, depression, and economic and vocational issues. Stiles and Mermer-Welly (1998) applied art therapy interventions in disadvantaged environments with pregnant adolescents who believed their pregnancy would resolve adolescent challenges, fill an inner emptiness or lead to re-bonding with their mothers. Wadeson (2000) included clinical examples of hospitalized pregnant women and noted challenges and parameters of prenatal art therapy with severe mental health. Hogan (2003) emphasized the feminist perspective surrounding images of pregnancy and motherhood and conducted qualitative art therapy research with prenatal and post-natal women who shared feelings regarding maternal development and postnatal adjustment. While difficult feelings arose, including violent impulses towards the fetus or baby, and fear of being judged, Hogan (2003) saw art therapy as an opportunity to discover a new sense of self. Hogan (2006, 2013) discussed motherhood and antenatal issues, noting how the misogynistic discourse within psychology oppresses and violates a women's self-expression and her body. Demecs, Fenwick, and Gamble (2011) defined specific themes from creative art therapy groups for pregnant women: prenatal well-being, connection with their fetus, maternal confidence and connection with other pregnant women. Herman-Lemelin (2016) created a six-week art therapy group for pregnant women at a local maternity center; art making and creativity supported a cohesive and ongoing community for women to consider several issues including the ambiguity of motherhood.

Pregnancy is described as an initiation with three stages: Gateway (preparing for conception), Attending (prenatal maternal tasks), and Passage (preparing for birth) (Swan-Foster, 2010, 2012, 2018). I will consider these stages of pregnancy as a feminine initiation through clinical art therapy examples.

## Gateway

*Gateway* suggests a door-like structure, a hole or opening (Ayto, 1990, p. 250) that illustrates the initial stage of expectancy and preconception. The image of a gate also defines a future space that a woman imagines into through her *pregnant imagination* (Swan-Foster, 2012). She considers personal emotional vicissitudes of pregnancy such as having something living within her, dependent upon her, and the adjustments or sacrifices she'll make regarding her future pregnancy. Psychologically, she may desire a personal transformation, imagine a pregnancy will cure her emotional emptiness, or the idea of something living inside her may constellate anxiety, dissociation or even repugnancy.

**Rey.** Depending upon the woman, the initiation sometimes *calls* from within through a dream, an inner voice or an image. Before conceiving her second child, Rey had the following dream:

> I was walking down a very dark and large hill and I looked up and saw the moon. It was absolutely massive in the sky. I could only see the top half and a stranger kept trying to tell me to see it, but I already did. It was so huge and detailed it scared me and I wanted to keep walking down the hill. I did and then I could see the whole thing but there were images of children all around it.

When she painted the dream, the relationship between the earth and the moon was made visible, facilitating a growing connection between the ego and the unconscious (Figure 3.1) that echoes the evolving attachment process. In the dream, Rey walked towards a threshold where her lunar (feminine) consciousness allowed her to see an image of unity, or "the whole thing." With this lowering of ego consciousness, she could momentarily experience the mystery of the Great Mother archetype. Moreover, it is common that aspects of the woman's psyche/soma are expressed through archetypal dreams or images before she is aware of them and these numinous experiences ignite a woman's respect for her intuition and promote a confidence in her pregnant imagination.

At the time of this dream, Rey had a son, but was concerned about conceiving and raising a daughter because she was adopted; she worried that her difficult relationship with her adoptive mother might impact her

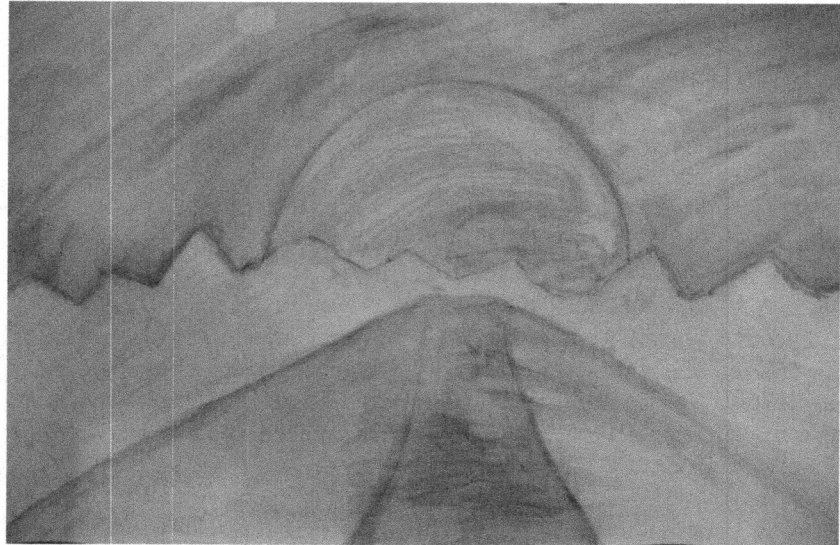

*Figure 3.1* Moon watercolor.

maternal sensibility. Rey imagined that a daughter would bring emotional repair and, while she had some trepidation, she desired the opportunity to work on a healthy mother/daughter relationship.

Symbolically, the moon expresses her connection with a *matriarchal consciousness* (Neumann, 1955/1974), a tremendous force within nature that is expressed through the relationship with the earth and the daily tides, and through the monthly cycles of menstruation that depend upon the uterus as a container. The mythic and cosmic connection to nature provided a spontaneous symbol that both documented and influenced her initiation journey. When Rey learned she was pregnant, the dream was reconsidered; not long after, Rey had a dream of walking in a foursome and seeing moons multiplying, suggesting the "splitting up of the archetype" so that parts of it can be psychologically incorporated and made conscious (Neumann, 1955/1974). The lunar archetypal rhythm of reproduction with the progressive movement of psychic energy was becoming physically coalesced through conception, implantation, and gestation. With the symbolic guidance of the moon and the possibility of mothering a daughter, Rey experienced a deconstruction of her identity and a renewed purpose as she awaited the arrival of her baby, at which point she learned she had indeed conceived a daughter.

**Anne and Maria.** For some women, Gateway is a place of mourning and longing; she has the painful initiatory knowledge of danger, death and suffering as she patiently waits in the unknown; her unbearable

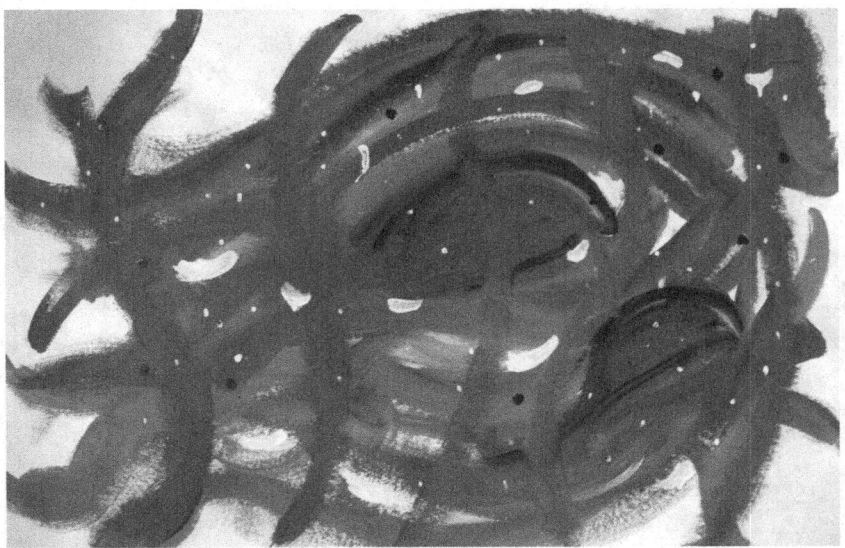

*Figure 3.2* Anne's "Dolphins" painting.

psychological and physical emptiness benefits from art therapy rituals. After her visit with a fertility specialist, Anne felt hopeful and asked to paint. Using her favorite colors of blues and greens on a large piece of paper, she focused on a water scene where she discovered dolphins that symbolize the source of life and the center of many creation myths.

She declared: "This is my favorite painting so far ... I'm fully committed to blue and green." Several weeks later, she learned she was pregnant without the medical intervention she had sought. She reflected back on the dolphins with admiration, demonstrating that the symbol had expressed her new attitude towards her maternal self (Hocking, 2007).

After Maria met up with a garden snake that touched both feet she decided the snake blessed her for a pregnancy that had not yet become conscious. Maria had playfully made a fertility talisman (Schaverien, 1992) (Figure 3.3) she carried in the Gateway phase; it was slightly reminiscent of the large, flat wooden Akua'ba fertility doll from Ghana that a woman might carry for conception and protection of her pregnancy.

Each of these women were touched by personal symbols from the unconscious, but not until after they were pregnant did they reflect upon and claim the images as personal symbols that conveyed their new maternal consciousness. In other words, the pregnant woman can be unconsciously drawn into the initiatory process, which spontaneously and autonomously presents itself in the form of an image or symbol that

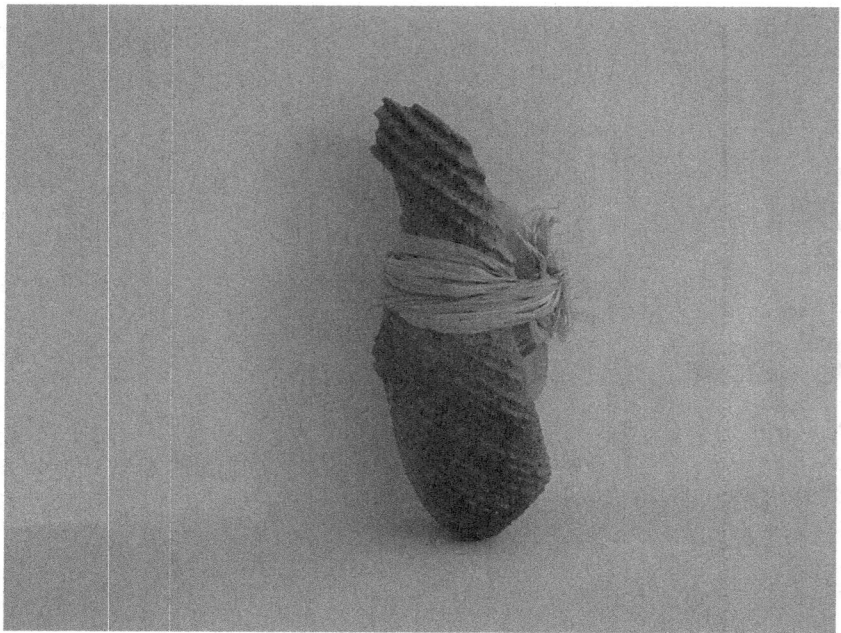

*Figure 3.3* Maria's wood talisman.

expresses the unification of opposites and the depths of her prenatal landscape (Jung, [1916]/1958/1972).

## Attending

The Attending phase commences with a woman confirming her pregnancy and encompasses the nine months preceding the onset of early labor. "Attend" is to *stretch*, listen, or direct the mind toward something. Related to *tenere*, it means to hold and contain and to care for with a religious quality (Ayto, 1990, p. 42), accurately describing the psycho-biological aspects of pregnancy. *Stretching towards* evokes the pregnant body that stretches to make room for the growing fetus, but also there is an emotional and archetypal stretching towards the future. To find meaning and a new consciousness, she is pulled inwards to contemplate the transformation of her inner landscape, her identity, and to cultivate a relationship with the Self[8] through the mythic and cosmogonic meaning of her pregnancy (Lincoln, 1981). Within the Attending phase, I used myths to illustrate four archetypal bi-polar patterns within the mythic journey of pregnant woman: wandering/home, contained/container, abandoned/related and conquered/conqueror (Swan-Foster, 2010, 2012). Additionally, the myth of *Eros and Psyche* was drawn upon to highlight prenatal tasks that awaken the woman's instinctive nature and facilitate the growth of her maternal identity.

Three key psychological components of the shadow[9] describe the focus during Attending: she confronts and accepts the physical changes in her body and the fetus as a separate being, she is immersed in the opposites, searching for integration, and she engages with simultaneity through personal symbols that carry psychic energy, creative expression, and influence her mythic journey and cosmic status.[10] These broad but specific initiatory tasks allow for the uniqueness of the pregnant woman to explore such issues as her maternal role, her partnership, her relationship with her mother, her changing body, past childbearing issues, her creative/spiritual work, and her role as a woman in her community.

While exceptionally difficult, psychological growth requires an acceptance and integration of shadow material. In attempts to avoid the shadow through emotional "cushioning" because of loss or regret (Côté-Aresenault & Donato, 2011), the pregnant initiand may be overwhelmed with feelings and then reject traditional rituals and gifts that honor her importance. Integrating shadow content is not only essential, but as her ego consciousness softens and she has more permeability, new information can revitalize the pregnant initiand, build her emotional resiliency, and give roots to her maternal identity.

### The Pregnant Body

Shadow may become known first through the physical intrusion of the fetus that forces the initiand to face the uncertainty and unknown. "To accept this intrusion and incorporate it successfully is the first adjustive task of the pregnant woman" (Bibring et al., 1968, p. 15). Maturation emerges from a growing maternal preoccupation with bodily sensations, unavoidable emotional changes and impingements that are reinforced with quickening, hearing the heartbeat and ultrasounds to a completely transformed psyche/soma that slows down, softens, and expands for childbirth.

**Arianne** was a 35-year-old married woman who experienced periods of anxiety and obsessive compulsive disorder (OCD). Her first pregnancy ended in an early abortion. Art therapy as a form of meditation, connecting mind and body through multimodal expression (Siegel, 2019), anchoring her in the moment by calming her thoughts. She said:

> I have been honoring this time that is so uncomfortable, constantly nauseous, feelings of uncertainty … facing my anxieties and fears, holding hopes, and reflecting on my faith—and sometimes lack thereof—in my body's ability to grow, heal and create something this magical.

In her second trimester she reflected: "I was almost grateful for the physical feelings I had initially because they reminded me that I was pregnant. I focused my mind away from the previous loss and my fear of seeing blood again." Hearing the resiliency of the heartbeat calmed her worries, and decreased intrusive thoughts of blood. "I thought he was stardust ... before he was forming he was a little star inside me—I had an image to meditate on, hold the unknown vastness of the universe." When her pregnant imagination was used productively through art making her anxiety decreased, marking the mythic and cosmic elements of her initiation journey.

Using the color red that was initially associated with blood, Arianne painted a comforting image of her heart and the baby's heart held by two hands to signify support of their vibrant "red life force" (Figure 3.4). In the bottom right corner (Aloe plant with multiple roots) is a personal

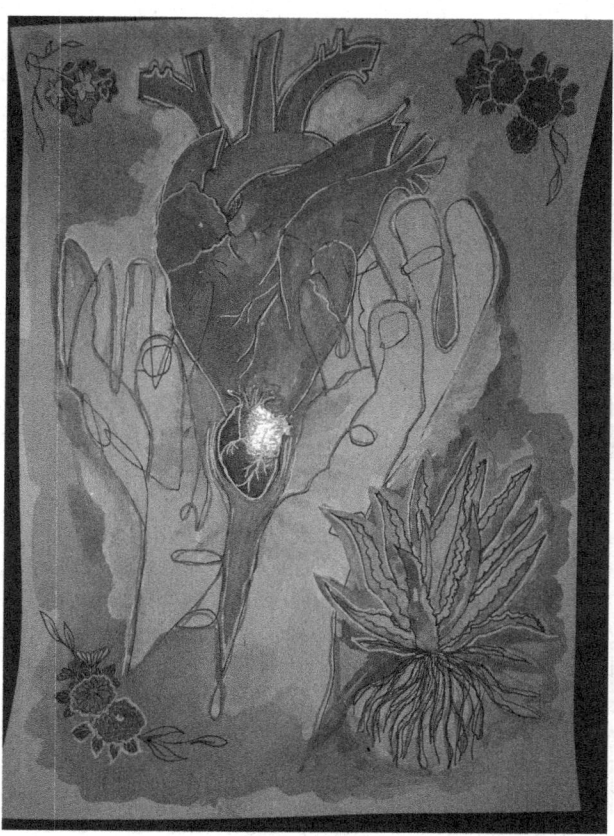

*Figure 3.4* "Two Hearts Beating Together" watercolor and ink.

symbol of protection and "universal protection, connecting with something bigger," such as her ancestors. After an ultrasound, Arianne saw "somebody real ... who yawns and stretches—we're a little team." Illustrating their separateness but connectedness, Arianne saw beyond her physical ordeals to wonder about the baby's personality and her ability to mother it. Less preoccupied with her body, Arianne focused on her emotional relationships. "Oddly, I feel fear about the future, about death, my mortality and missing out—I have no control—that scares me. I think the more love I have the more vulnerable and fearful I am." Arianne used art and meditation to interrupt her repetitive thoughts and created an image of herself calmed by nature symbols that expressed personal meaning and connected her to the journey (Figure 3.5). This painting was "everything in her imagination; holding the light and dark with the different realms of life. It was a visual blessing with the white

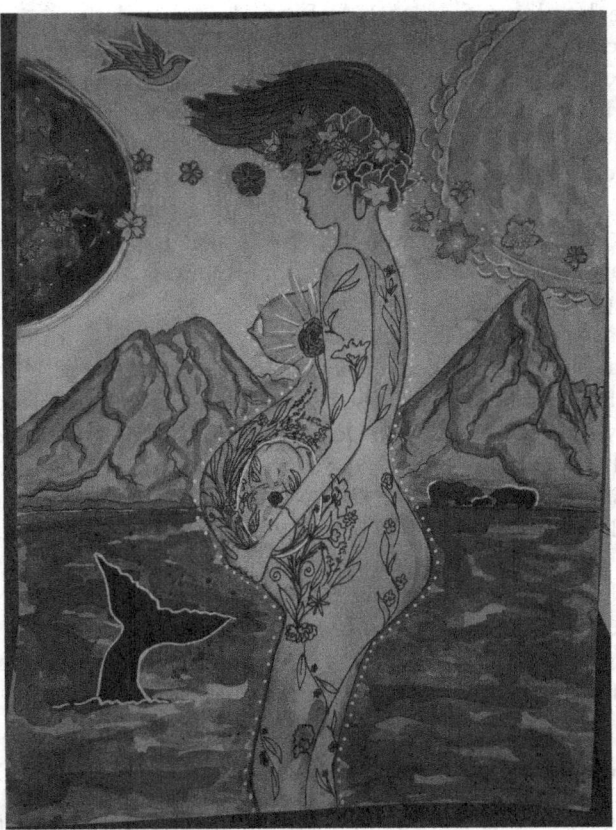

*Figure 3.5* "Pregnant Self" watercolor and ink.

dots of energy for protection ... she is very spiritual and full of life," said Arianne. We might imagine the figure is facing the past, or perhaps turning away from the temporal world to embrace the inner opposites and to "weather whatever may come as life is unpredictable, with an open heart." The flowers flow in both directions offering unification and a sense of continuity and totality. The various creatures are isomorphic representations of her own instinctual wisdom, but also denote the co-existence of time and space and the sustaining presence of nature's elements.

**Penny** was 35 years old and she did not want to be *fixed*, but sought to know her pregnant self. In art therapy she named what she had sacrificed and she mourned her losses; her anxiety settled because the deadened parts of her psyche and body were attended to without judgment or fixing. For Penny, permeability was an opportunity. "I'm in a state of mild panic ... I'm physically nauseous, but ... also emotionally nauseous with panic." Her physical symptoms became emotional metaphors: she tore paper to create a mandala that described her emotional "spinning" and feeling untethered in life. The colored papers and glue paradoxically anchored her so that she could face her loss of control, lack of choice, and the uncertainty of motherhood. Penny learned that "The difference we make between the psyche and the body is artificial ... psyche is as much a living body as body is living psyche: it is just the same" (Jung, 1998, p. 114). It's clinically noteworthy that these women had the ego strength to use their anxiety and prenatal permeability as doorways into their pregnant imagination (metaphors and symbols) for reflection and effecting their worlds. This is not always the case and although archetypal images may naturally emerge in women's artwork, treatment and art therapy interventions should remain clinically appropriate and never imposed.

**Lynn** was a 40-year-old single mother by choice in her third trimester. She was a teacher and had always wanted a child. She drew herself pregnant (Figure 3.6) and discussed how pregnancy had transformed her, particularly how she handled shadow projections (the figure faces right) of shame and vulnerability regarding not having a partner. "Don't feel sorry for me," she said. "I'm proud of my pregnancy." Lynn considered how her critical thoughts about her body image had evaporated for appreciation, love, and protection. Although she initially struggled to draw herself, by the end she conveyed satisfaction, illustrating that she was learning to value herself and her pregnancy. Lynn's ability to prioritize her decisions during pregnancy was the beginning of claiming her maternal identity and preparing for childbirth and postpartum.

## Play of Opposites

As the pregnant initiand grows into her second and third trimester, she is more physically visible, yet she may also feel emotionally invisible, alone and cognitively dead. The play of opposites expresses the emotional

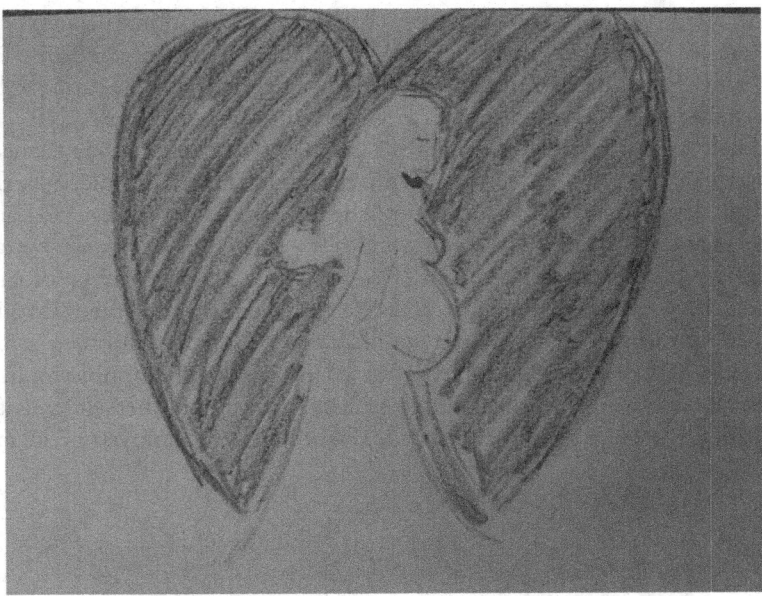

*Figure 3.6* "Pregnant" water crayons.

complexity that prenatal art therapy deliberately addresses with the aim to experience the spontaneous images of transformation (Swan-Foster, 2018). Mixed media, wet and dry, watercolors, and the process of tearing rather than cutting paradoxically encourages the pregnant woman to accept an imperfect process or to process childbirth trauma and physical alterations (Swan-Foster, 2018, p. 170). Tearing paper or cutting with scissors may replicate medical interventions or surgeries, including perineum tears or "snips." Thread and needle offer ways to metaphorically repair medical interventions. Through the creative process, she engages in an undoing and redoing that repairs whatever mutations or traumas her body endured and finds wholeness within her changed body through telling her story and perhaps finding a personal symbol. High risk hospitalized pregnant women who endure increased medical interventions appreciate beading, stitching, or tearing. Tangible objects for people at home help them feel connected and useful. Examples of the opposites are seen in Figures 3.1, 3.2, and 3.3 through colors or contrasting symbols. Specifically, in Figure 3.3 the notion of death/rebirth are held in the reframing of the color red and the motif of two hearts.

Prenatal worry and fear are natural maternal tasks as she integrates aspects of her new identity and responsibilities. She may fear separation or death—the separation and death of her fetus or the separation and death of her partner—leaving her isolated and alone. These motifs contain unique symbolic meaning found through image, metaphor, and visual symbol, and pave the way for greater emotional clarity and confidence. When an initiand can acknowledge that the opposites (i.e. light and dark, life and death) sit side-by-side, the images support her maternal identity; she can mourn her past without self-rebuke.

Sometimes a pregnant woman feels intimidated, irrelevant or silenced, but retreats to *privately* connect with her mythic and cosmic maternal identity. The bind is if she speaks up, she'll be teased or disregarded and/ or feel abandoned, but if she is silent and relies solely on herself, she betrays herself by not asking for support. Double binds create psychobiological tension between the opposites and are revealed and released through spontaneous images that pinpoint conflicts that deserve attention.

**Alexa.** A play of opposites arose for Alexa caught in a double bind. In her third trimester of her second pregnancy, Alexa drew herself pregnant and added written and magazine words (Figure 3.7). She enjoyed pregnancy

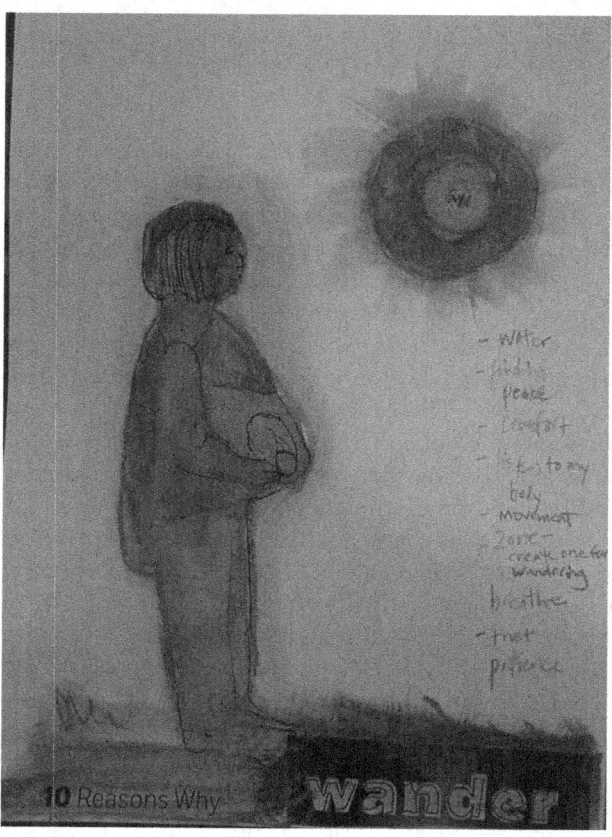

*Figure 3.7* "Wandering" mixed media.

because she had an excuse to wander emotionally, but she also felt physically trapped and vulnerable; the picture focused on her desire for freedom, a compensation for decreased mobility. The tension between her adult self and her baby self was conflicting shadow material that led Alexa to express her desire to wander during childbirth without hospital rules, but the emotional layers were present in her affect. When we unpacked her emotions, she expressed discomfort about speaking to her doctors because she might be labeled as "demanding." As she made a mandala with mostly black and blue inks, we unpacked the narrative of violence in her family, and the fear of physical pain when she remained still. Significant was that Alexa had the space to emotionally differentiate the energy of violence from the archetypal energy of childbirth. When she shared the drawing with her doula and midwife, they encouraged her to communicate with her physician, which led to collaboration, emotional resiliency, and maternal confidence.

Alexa's drawing is an "embodied drawing" rather than a "diagrammatic" drawing (Schaverien, 1992) because of her investment in the creative and emotional process. It illustrates several opposites: mixture of cool and warm colors, magazine words and handwritten list (collective/personal) and a sun in the top corner suggesting the presence of archetypal energies that contain the opposites (yellow/blue, warm/cool, mother/father).

### Simultaneity

Simultaneity describes a reflective and contemplative place of both being and becoming. The word refers to things being similar or happening at the same time (Ayto, 1990, p. 478). As with Alexa's drawing, transparencies (simultaneity) in pregnant women's drawings "may signify an integrated psychosomatic understanding of psychological permeability illustrated through an isomorphic representation" (Swan-Foster et al., 2003, p. 302). The image of the Russian nesting dolls illustrates how the pregnant initiand moves fluidly between various inner emotional states and comes to recognize these states as having purpose and meaning. Her expanded sense of imagination and a creative trust in both the liminality of being and becoming (and death/rebirth) during the Attending phase furthers the unfolding mythic and cosmic journey. The transparencies in Figures 3.4 and 3.6 illustrate the layered emotional experiences with the baby, her naked body, her clothing and surrounding space. A strict medical model treats pregnancies as linear, (beginning, middle, and end), and structured by three trimesters; however, with an initiation lens, a pregnant woman's ego softens to include multiple states of consciousness, enlivening her pregnant imagination and facilitates her maternal confidence.

Furthermore, symbols express multiple meanings—a moon, dolphin or aloe plant signify specific energic variations of an emotional experience that, within a still place of opposites and simultaneity, further unifies an experience through visual documentation. When the woman tolerates the tension between a waiting stillness and stretching towards to make room for *other*, prenatal art therapy honors her sacrifices and discovers a cohesive structure or definition to her mythic journey.

## Passage

The word "passage" suggests a hallway or passageway that takes us through a transitional tight space. Passage also describes the final phase of pregnancy when the pregnant initiand feels a shift in psychic energy as her body now prepares for the events of labor and the end of pregnancy. In this post-liminal stage, she is not having active contractions so she can engage with last-minute issues and reflect back on her pregnancy as she prepares for childbirth. Sometimes a woman requests an art therapy session specifically focused on childbirth; she uses materials to confront remaining fears, release feelings, and embrace a creative physical process. This is often the last chance for belly casts (Swan-Foster, 2018). The German term *Zwischen*, translated as "between," is an expression of early labor, a time of waiting and wondering (Studelska, 2012). The pregnant woman is encouraged to immerse herself in the process of relaxing and opening:

> Write it down, sing ... go commune with nature ... I tell [them] ... to let go of their worry; this is an early sign of labor ... sequester ... if they need space ... go out if they need distraction ... give them permission to follow the instinctual gravitational pulls that are at work within them, just as real and necessary as labor.
>
> (Studelska, 2012)

Essentially, in the last weeks of pregnancy, a woman may emotionally prepare for childbirth and post-partum before the Passage phase comes to an end and active childbirth begins.

## Final Reminders for the Art Therapist

Pregnancy constellates a compelling archetypal countertransference in the therapeutic relationship. The art therapist is brought into a prenatal "liminal field" of transformation where the core themes of initiation can influence and dominate the antenatal dyadic relationship. "All those who participate in her initiation accompany her into the mythic atemporality" (Lincoln, 1981, p. 96). When working with antenatal women using the initiation model, art therapists can consider specific issues found in the Appendices.

## Conclusion

Viewing pregnancy as a feminine initiation provides a theoretical foundation that acknowledges the creative archetypal nature of what is viewed as a major feminine transition and gives further credence to collaborative modalities that serve the well-being and mental health of a pregnant individual. By including a nonverbal modality, art therapy can unveil normal or critical antenatal issues while bringing creativity, dignity and value to the pregnant woman's unique path. Further, when stress, anxiety, and depression are screened for through individual or group art therapy, the creative and birth-giving capacity is reclaimed. The art therapy model offers viable and integrative approaches easily implemented within a holistic medical setting, agency, birthing center or private practice, helping to overcome the stigma of mental health issues, particularly if prenatal art therapy is integrated into regular screening programs and research projects for specific and vast prenatal issues and topics, including social justice and discrimination issues. Finally, when we are curious and listen to a woman's emotional concerns, encourage her ability to make decisions and build collaboration amongst medical systems, she grows conscious about her maternal responsibility that has particular value within community. Essentially, the pregnant woman living within the liminal space has the ability to transform the consciousness of those supporting her along the way. When we give the pregnant individual the love, encouragement, respect and dignity she deserves for her creative and birth-giving capacity, she internalizes the moments not as regret, shame, or powerless vulnerability but as acceptance, empowerment, strength found in her vulnerability, and success. This acknowledgment translates into a more conscious and confident mother who holds the future in her arms.

## Notes

1 Portions of this chapter were first published in the *Journal of Prenatal and Perinatal Psychology and Health* 26(4), Summer 2012
2 A "conscious pregnancy" or "initiation-oriented pregnancy" recognizes the archetypal nature of pregnancy; the woman engages with her pregnancy as an emotional, psychological and spiritual opportunity for significant personal growth and individuation as a mother.
3 Raphael-Leff defined three mothering styles: regulator, facilitator, and reciprocator (1991, 1995).
4 This series was identified as the *Prenatal Art Therapy Intervention and Inventory* (PATII). Further information is found in the Appendices.
5 *Tokophobia* is an extreme version of childbirth fear
6 A tertiary level five hospital has specialists and receives referrals from surrounding states.
7 Research was modeled on and adapted in part from the Formal Elements Art Therapy Scale (FEATS) © 1990, 1998, Linda Gantt, written permission of Gargoyle Press, 314 Scott Avenue, Morgantown, WV 26,508, USA.

8 Analytical psychology specifically uses the term "Self" to describe that aspect of the psyche that connects to the cosmos, spirit, God or wholeness.
9 Shadow was C.G Jung's term for unconscious material that is disavowed, unseen, or unknown.
10 See description in *Jungian Art Therapy* as to how Jung's notion of the transcendent function applies to art therapy.

## References

Abt, R., Bosch, I., & MacKrell, V. (2000). *Dream child: Creation and new life in dreams of pregnant women*. Einsiedeln, Switzerland: Daimon Verlag.

Anand, S. A., & Baker, F. (1997). Art therapy with addicted, pregnant, and parenting women. *AATA 28th Annual Conference*, conference proceedings, November 12–16. Milwaukee, WI.

Athan, A. (2017, Oct 3). Matrescence: Self development in motherhood. [Presentation given to Every Mother Counts]. Retrieved from: www.matrescence.com/blog/2018/4/10/matrescence-self-development-in-motherhood

Athan, A., & Miller, L. (2005). Spiritual awakening through the motherhood journey. *Journal of the Motherhood Initiative for Research and Community Involvement*, 7(1), 17–31.

Ayto, J. (1990). *Dictionary of word origins*. New York: Arcade Publishing.

Beane Rutter, V. (1993/2009). *Changing woman: Feminine psychology re-conceived through myth and experience*. New Orleans, LA: Spring Journal Books.

Beane Rutter, V. (2011). Saffron offering and blood sacrifice: Transformation mysteries in Jungian analysis. In V. Beane Rutter & T. Singer (Eds.), *Ancient Greece, Modern psyche archetypes in the making* (pp. 39–83). New Orleans, LA: Spring Journal Books.

Benedek, T. (1959). Sexual functions in women and their disturbances. In S. Arieti (Ed.), *American handbook of psychiatry* (Vol 1. pp. 727–748) New York: Basic Books.

Bibring, G., Dwyer, T., Huntington, D., & Valenstein, A. (1968). A study of the psychological processes in pregnancy and the earliest mother-child relationship. In *The psychoanalytic study of the child*, (Vol. XVI pp. 9–23) New York, NY: International Universities Press, Inc.

Çoker, H., Karabekir, N., & Varlik, S. (2019). Birth with no regret in Turkey. *Journal of Prenatal and Perinatal Psychology and Heath*, 34(2), Winter, 114–128.

Colman, L., & Colman, A. (1991). *Pregnancy: The psychological experience*. NY: Noonday Press.

Côté-Arsenault, D., Brody, D., & Dombeck, M. (2009). Pregnancy as a rite of passage: Liminality, rituals and communitas. *Journal of Prenatal and Perinatal Psychology and Health*, 24(2), 69–87.

Côté-Arsenault, D., & Donato, K. (2011). Emotional cushioning in pregnancy after perinatal loss. *Jounral of Reproductive and Infant Psychology*, 29(1), 82–92.

Davis-Floyd, R. (1992/2003). *Birth is an American rite of passage*. Berkeley, CA: University of California Press.

Davis-Floyd, R. & Georges, E. (1996). On pregnancy. In *Encyclopedia of Cultural Anthropology*, New Haven CT: Human Relations Area Files, pp. 1014–1016. Retrieved from: http://www.davis-floyd.com/wp-content/uploads/2016/11/Entry-on-Pregnancy.pdf.

Davis-Floyd, R. (2001). The technocratic, humanistic, and holistic models of birth. *International Journal of Gynecology & Obstetrics, 75*(Supplement No. 1), S5–223.

Davis-Floyd, R. (2019a). Open and closed knowledge systems, the four stages of cognition, and the cultural management of birth: Part 1. *Journal of Prenatal and Perinatal Psychology and Heath, 34*(1), Fall, 1–19.

Davis-Floyd, R. (2019b). Open and closed knowledge systems, the four stages of cognition, and the cultural management of birth: Part 2. *Journal of Prenatal and Perinatal Psychology and Heath, 34*(2), Winter, 1–19.

Demecs, I. P., Fenwick, J., & Gamble, J. (2011). Women's experiences of attending a creative arts program during their pregnancy. *Women Birth*, Sep, 24(3), 112–121. doi: 10.1016/j.wombi.2010.08.004. Epub 2010 Sep 24.

Deutsch, H. (1944). *The psychology of women.* New York, NY: Grune and Stratton.

Dick-Read, G. (1953). *Childbirth without fear.* New York, NY: Harper.

Ely, D., & Driscoll, A. (2019). Infant mortality in the United States, 2017: Data from the period linked birth/infant death file. *National Vital Statistics Report, 10*(68), 1–19.

Guardino, C., & Schetter, C. D. (2014). Understanding pregnancy anxiety: Concepts, correlates, and consequences. *Zero to Three.* March, 12–21.

Hempel, J. (2016). My brother's pregnancy and the making of a new American family. *Time Magazine.* September. https://time.com/4475634/trans-man-pregnancy-evan/

Henderson, A. B. (2000). *Single woman's dream images during first pregnancy: A psychological preparation for motherhood.* (Unpublished Master's Thesis). Naropa University, Boulder, CO.

Herman-Lemelin, J. (2016). *Landscapes of motherhood: Art therapy support group for women's transformative journey into parenthood.* (Unpublished Master's Thesis). Kutenai Art Therapy Institute, Kutenai, Canada.

Hocking, K. (2007). Artistic narratives of self-concept during pregnancy. *The Arts in Psychotherapy, 34*(2), 163–178.

Hogan, S. (2003). A discussion of the use of art therapy with women who are pregnant or who have recently given birth. In S. Hogan (Ed.), *Gender issues in art therapy* (pp. 148–172). London: Jessica Kingsley.

Hogan, S. (2006). The tyranny of the maternal body: Maternity and madness. *Women's History Magazine.* Women's History Association, 54, 21–30.

Hogan, S. (2013). Your body is a battle ground: Art therapy with women. *The Arts in Psychotherapy, 40*(4), 415–419.

Horney, K. (1926). The flight from womanhood: The masculinity-complex in women, as viewed by men and by women. *International Journal of Psychoanalysis,* (7), 324–339.

Jung, C. G. (1960/1972). On the nature of dreams. In *Collected works. Vol. 8* (pp. 281–297). Princeton, NJ: Princeton University Press.

Jung, C. G. (1998). *Jung's seminar on Nietzsche's Zarathustra.* (J. Jarret, Ed.). Princeton, NJ: Princeton University Press.

Jung, C. G. ([1916]/1958/1972). The transcendent function. In *Collected Works Vol 8* (pp. 67–91). Princeton, NJ: Princeton University Press.

Kortendieck-Rashe, B. (2011). Coming home to Demeter: Reflections on pregnancy as a natural initiation in the dreams of immigrant women. In V. Beane Rutter & T. Singer (Eds.), *Ancient Greece, Modern psyche archetypes in the making* (pp. 85–98). New Orleans, LA: Spring Journal Books.

Lakhani, N. (2019). American has an infant mortality crisis: Meet the black doulas trying to change that. *Guardian.* November 25. Retrieved from www.theguar dian.com/us-news/2019/nov/25/african-american-doula-collective-mothers-toxic-stress-racism-cleveland-infant-mortality-childbirth

Lincoln, B. (1981). *Emerging from the chrysalis: Rituals of women's initiation.* New York, NY: Oxford University Press.

Merchant, J. (2012). *Shamans and analysts: New insights on the wounded healer.* New York, NY: Routledge.

Nadelson, C. (1978). "Normal" and "special" aspects of pregnancy: A psychological approach. In M. T. Notman & C. C. Nadelson (Eds.), *The woman patient: Medical and psychological interfaces Volume 1: Sexual and reproductive aspects of women's health care* (pp. 73–86). New York, NY: Springer Publishing.

Neumann, E. (1955/1974). The great mother: An analysis of the archetype. Princeton, NJ, Princeton University Press.

Neumann, E. (1955/1974). *The great mother: An analysis of the archetype.* Princeton, NJ: Princeton University Press.

Overbeck, L. (2002). *A pilot study of pregnant women's drawings.* (Unpublished master's thesis). Eastern Virginia Medical School, Norfolk, VA.

Petersen, E. E., Davis, N. L., Goodman, D., Cox, S., Mayes, N., Johnston, E., ... Barfield, W. (2019). Vital signs: Pregnancy-related deaths, United States, 2011–2015, and strategies for prevention, 13 states, 2013–2017. *Morbidity and Mortality Weekly Report, 68,* 423–429.

Peterson, G. (1984). *Birthing normally: A personal growth approach to childbirth.* Berkeley, CA: Mindbody Press.

Peterson, G. (1991). *An easier childbirth: A mother's workbook for health and emotional well-being during pregnancy and delivery.* Los Angeles, CA: Jeremy Tarcher, Inc.

Raphael, D. (1975). Matrescence, Becoming a mother, a "new/old" rite de passage. In D. Raphael (Ed.), *Being female: Reproduction, power, and change* (pp. 65–71). The Hague: Mouton Publishers.

Raphael-Leff, J. (1991). *Psychological processes of childbearing.* New York, NY: Chapan & Hall.

Raphael-Leff, J. (1993). *Pregnancy: The inside story.* Northvale, NJ: Jason Aronson, Inc.

Raphael-Leff, J. (1995). *Pregnancy: The inside story.* Northvale, NJ: Jason Aronson, Inc.

Schaverien, J. (1992). *The revealing image: Analytical art psychotherapy in theory and practice.* London, UK: Routledge.

Sezen, C., & Ünsalver, B. O. (2019). Group art therapy for the management of fear of childbirth. *The Arts in Psychotherapy, 64*(3), 9–19.

Siegel, L. (2019). Drawing breath: Breathing into the rhythm and form of art therapy. *American Imago, 76,* 251–267. https://time.com/4453134/when-trans-men-want-to-give-birth/

Silva, B. (2016). When trans men want to give birth. *Time Magazine.* September 1.

Simpkin, P., & Klaus, P. (2004/2018). *When survivors give birth: Understanding and healing the effects of early sexual abuse on childbearing women.*

Sluzas, J. G. (2012). *The development of maternal identity and awareness of the primiparae in the transition through pregnancy into motherhood as expressed in artwork and interview: A phenomenological study* (Unpublished master's thesis). Drexel University, Philadelphia, PA.

Stiles, G. J., & Mermer-Welly, M. (1998). Children having children: Art therapy in a community-based early adolescent pregnancy program. *Journal of the American Art Therapy Association, 15*(3), 156–176.

Studelska, J. (2012). The last days of pregnancy: A place of in-between. *Mothering.* April 2012, Retrieved from www.mothering.com/articles/the-last-days-of-pregnancy-a-place-of-in-between/

Swan-Foster, N. (1989). Images of pregnant women: Art therapy as a tool for transformation. *The Arts in Psychotherapy, 16*(4), 283–292.

Swan-Foster, N. (1991). Transforming fear. In Gayle Peterson (ed.). *An easier childbirth: A mother's workbook for health and emotional well-being during pregnancy and delivery* (pp. 159–163). Los Angeles, CA: Jeremy Tarcher, Inc.

Swan-Foster, N. (2001). Research Using a Prenatal Art Therapy Intervention and Inventory (PATII). *AATA 32nd Annual Conference, conference proceedings,* November, Albuquerque, NM.

Swan-Foster, N. (2010). *Pregnancy as a feminine initiation: Personal and archetypal.* (Unpublished Thesis).

Swan-Foster, N. (2012). Pregnancy as a feminine initiation. *Journal of Prenatal and Perinatal Psychology and Health, 26*(4), Summer, 207–235.

Swan-Foster, N. (2018). *Jungian art therapy: Dreams, images, and active imagination.* New York, NY: Routledge.

Swan-Foster, N., Foster, S., & Dorsey, A. (2003). The use of the human figure drawing with pregnant women. *Journal of Reproductive and Infant Psychology, 21*(4), 293–307.

Turner, V. (1967/1979). *The ritual process: Structure and anti-structure.* Hawthorne, NY: Aldine de Gruyter.

van Gennep, A. (1960). *The rites of passage: A classic study of cultural celebrations.* Chicago, IL: University of Chicago Press.

Wadeson, H. (2000). *Art therapy practice: Innovative approaches with diverse populations.* New York, NY: John Wiley Inc.

Wahlbeck, H., Kvist, L. J., & Landgren, K. (2018). Gaining hope and self-confidence: An interview study of women's experience of treatment by art therapy for severe fear of childbirth. *Women Birth, August, 32*(4), 299–306.

Wardi-Zonna, K. (2017). Pregnancy reclaimed: Art therapy as intervention for depression and anxiety. *Journal of the Motherhood Initiative, 8*(1–2), 251–270.

Westermarck, E. (1906/2010). *The origin and development of moral ideas* (Vol. I & II). Charleston, SC: Nabu Press.

# 4 Supervising the Pregnant Art Therapist

## Integrating Reflective Developmental and Arts-based Supervision Approaches

*Rebecca Miller*

An art therapist's pregnancy introduces a personally revealing and continually evolving dynamic into therapy spaces and relationships, with definite implications for client treatment and outcomes. Yet, as reviewed by Miller and Giffin (2019), literature examining the topic has been sparse (Hurdman, 1999; Skaife, 2012; ter Maat & Vandersyde, 1995). This is curious, given evidence that women continue to comprise the overwhelming majority of practicing art therapists in the United States (Elkins & Deaver, 2015), United Kingdom (Health and Care Professions Council, 2019), Canada (Lee, 2010), and likely elsewhere. Even less examined has been the role of clinical supervision in supporting pregnant supervisees, with scant attention paid to the topic in the broad psychotherapy literature (Baum, 2009; Goldberger et al., 2003; Imber, 1995) and nearly absent consideration in art therapy literature (Miller & Giffin, 2019).

Institutional practices in the United States shape a prevailing view of pregnancy as mainly a physical and medical experience (Swan-Foster, 2012). However, it is well understood that pregnant women also experience changes involving emotional, psychological, and social functioning. Professional and working women, including art therapists and other clinicians, must necessarily sort through the impact of pregnancy to professional duties, roles, and responsibilities. For art therapists who continue active practice throughout pregnancy, the personal and the professional may unavoidably intertwine, placing professional identity issues at the forefront. Thus, pregnant art therapists may benefit from a holistic approach to supervision that goes beyond clinical skill development and case conceptualization, to also include attention to personal growth, professional identity concerns, and self-care needs.

This chapter presents theory and strategies for supervising pregnant art therapists at a time when increased professional support may be paramount. Supervision theory emphasizing reflectivity as a core task of supervision (Frawley O'Dea & Sarnat, 2001; Frolund & Nielsen, 2009; Ladany, Friedlander, & Nelson, 2005; Neufeldt, Karno, & Nelson, 1996) will be integrated with arts-based supervision strategies (Deaver & Shiflett, 2011; Fish, 2017; Ishyima, 1988; Miller, 2012; Shiflett & Remley Jr., 2014) to further the pregnant supervisee's professional and personal development. This includes case conceptualization skills, managing transference and countertransference, exploring the supervisor–supervisee relationship and practicing self-care and well-being. Specific examples of arts-based supervision strategies that may be used to further supervisee reflectivity around the impact of pregnancy are discussed. Finally, consideration to potential practical and ethical issues are also explored.

## Art Therapist Pregnancy and Implications for Clinical Supervision

In their explorations of art therapist pregnancy, Hurdman (1999) and ter Maat and Vandersyde (1995) provided rich depictions of client transference reactions believed to have been elicited by the art therapist's pregnancy. This included discussion of a range of client responses that emerged through interpersonal dynamics or artwork, such as loss, denial, abandonment, and envy, and the ways these feelings and reactions were worked through in treatment. Yet, the therapist's own countertransference reactions were only minimally addressed. Skaife (2012) focused attention on the pregnant art therapist's countertransference, but did not delve into the impact of pregnancy on the personal and professional development of the art therapist or the role of supervision in supporting the pregnant art therapist.

Miller and Giffin's (2019) heuristic inquiry examined a unique circumstance of simultaneous pregnancy within a supervisory dyad, highlighting the use of a reflective developmental approach to clinical supervision that emphasized mutual education, inquiry, and support. In particular, they focused on three main areas experienced as having significant impact on clinical dynamics and that occurred largely in tandem with the three trimester stages of pregnancy: pregnancy disclosure; managing interpersonal boundaries and self-care; and facilitating closure in clinical and supervisory relationships. Through discussion of supervisory dynamics and client case illustrations, Miller and Giffin deemed continuous reflectivity to the impact of the art therapist's pregnancy on the clinical and supervisory work as essential, indicating that it ultimately "served to strengthen the supervisory alliance, build clinical skills, increase self-confidence and promote practices of self-care at a time when these were crucial" (p. 100). They concluded that clinical supervision may have a critical role to play in supporting pregnant art therapists, calling for further inquiry and research in this vastly under-explored area.

## Reflective Developmental Approaches to Supervision

Supervision is a distinct professional activity in which education, training, and support are utilized to develop competent, ethical, and effective practitioners (Bernard & Goodyear, 2019; Ladany et al., 2005). Supervisors may vary in style, theoretical orientation or the specific supervision model or activities utilized. Although reflective processes may be encouraged in supervision contexts generally, the use of continuous and focused reflective inquiry has been regarded as an essential skill in the development of clinical expertise across several different professional fields (Calvert, Crowe, & Grenyer, 2017; Cheng, LaDonna, Cristancho, & Ng, 2017; Ronnestad & Skovholt, 2013) and comprises a central component of several well-known developmental models of psychotherapy supervision (e.g., Holloway, 2016; Ladany et al., 2005; Loganbill, Hardy, & Delworth, 1982; Stoltenberg & McNeil; 2010).

Bernard and Goodyear (2019) characterized the use of reflective inquiry as "inherently developmental" (p. 37) in that it positions the reflective learning cycle as endemic to the supervisee's development of both basic clinical skills and more complex interpersonal, affective and expressive relational competence skills (Calvert et al., 2017; Fouad et al., 2009). As such, reflective approaches require attunement to inner cognitive and emotional experiences, including the ability to tolerate and process ambiguous phenomena in spontaneous and genuine ways (Jenkins, 2010). Grounded in the work of early theorists in education and other fields (Dewey, 1933; Kolb, 1984; Schon, 1983), at the heart of reflective practice is the belief that one does not learn by simply doing; rather, one must also deliberately and intentionally reflect on the meaning of one's experiences in order for professional growth and development to occur.

Schon's work (1983) has been especially influential in the development of psychotherapy supervision models that champion use of reflective processes. Schon differentiated between two types of reflective processes believed to enable professional growth: *reflection-on-action*, which consists of reflection after an experience in order to examine what went well or could have been done differently, and *reflection-in-action*, or reflectivity that occurs in the experiential moment. Neufeldt et al. (1996) acknowledged the utility of both types of reflectivity for supervisory work, indicating that supervisee reflectivity is usually stimulated in response to a specific trigger followed by a sequential process of active searching to understand and make meaning of an experience. This, in turn, yields a demonstrable consequence in terms of supervisee perceptual or behavioral change. Thus, supervisee reflectivity is an iterative process similar to Kolb's (1984) experiential learning cycle, which typically leads to further repetition of the cycle, and ideally, long-term growth over time. Moreover, they indicated that intervening conditions play an important role in either facilitating or restraining reflective practice, which include supervisee factors (e.g., personality and cognitive complexity), environmental conditions (e.g., practice setting), and supervisor factors. Among supervisor factors, both the quality of the supervisory alliance and the supervisor's modeling of reflective strategies may be especially important (Orchowski, Evangelista, & Probst, 2010).

## Supervision Strategies that Promote Supervisee Reflectivity

Clinical supervision literature contains discussion of a wide variety of supervisory interventions and strategies intended to promote supervisee reflectivity. As reviewed by Bernard and Goodyear (2019) and others, the most commonly suggested interventions include: video review through Interpersonal Process Recall (IPR; Kagan, 1980); intentional and systematic questioning (Holloway & Carroll, 1999; Moffett, 2009); journal writing (Neimeyer, Woodward, Pickover, & Smigelsky, 2016; Orchowski et al., 2010); the supervisor's modeling of "thinking aloud" and collaborative participation in reflexive dialogue (Borders & Brown, 2005; Calvert et al., 2017); and a wide variety of creative and arts-based strategies, such as metaphoric drawing, visual journaling, sandtray, and psychodrama (e.g., Amundson, 1988; Anekstein, Hoskins, Astramovich, Garner, & Terry, 2014; Deaver & McAuliffe, 2009; Fish, 2017; Graham, Scholl, Smith-Adcock, & Wittman, 2014; Guiffrida, Jordan, Saiz, & Barnes, 2007; Ishyima, 1988; Shiflett & Remley, 2014). Strategies may be used in-session, post-session, or out-of-session (Deaver & Shiflett, 2011; Fish, 2017; Malchiodi & Riley, 1996), and may involve administrative aspects of supervision, including intentional reflection on the supervision contract (Neufeldt, 1999; Orchowski et al., 2010).

Art-based supervision (ABS) approaches have been increasingly recognized for their utility in increasing supervisee reflectivity and learning towards the goal of effective clinical practice. Although ABS methods have been less prominent in counseling and psychotherapy generally, within the profession of art therapy, ABS approaches have a long and rich history (see Fish, 2017 for a comprehensive review). Deaver and Shiflett (2011) posited ABS as inherently reflective, delineating three main areas around which ABS should occur: (a) case conceptualization, (b) processing of transference and countertransference, and (c) developing the supervisor–supervisee relationship. Additionally, both Fish (2017) and Miller and Robb (2017) regarded personal and professional growth and identity development dimensions as squarely within the scope of important reflective emphases that might be addressed using ABS methods.

In addition to development of clinical skills, exploration of intersections between the personal and the professional may be particularly important for the pregnant art therapist supervisee, especially given political and social realities that often complicate the pregnancy journey for working women in the United States. This includes discrimination in work and academic spaces experienced by pregnant women and working mothers (Collins, 2019; National Partnership for Women & Families

[NPWF], 2016) and high rates of perinatal intervention, infant mortality and maternal mortality when compared to other industrialized countries, especially among low income and minority women (Gunja, Tikkanen, Seervai, & Collins, 2018).

## Three ABS Approaches with Pregnant Art Therapist Supervisees

Three ABS approaches may be particularly useful in supervision with pregnant art therapists: *visual case processing* (VCP; Ishyima, 1988; Shiflett & Remley, 2014), *reflective visual journaling* (RVJ; Deaver & McAuliffe, 2009) and the *El Duende One Canvas Process Painting* approach (EDOCPP; Miller, 2012). These approaches meet the criteria of effective reflective supervisory foci as outlined by Deaver and Shiflett (2011). In the following section, I pair visual case processing, reflective visual journaling and EDOCPP with the first, second and third trimesters of pregnancy, respectively, in order to highlight how unique characteristics of each ABS approach may meet salient professional and personal growth needs at a particular trimester stage. However, supervisors may gravitate towards using any one of these or other reflective approaches as a consistent practice given theoretical overlap or their own ways of working. The case examples offered are of supervisees who agreed to be identified by first name only. It should be noted that not all examples reflect individuals who were pregnant; in the first example, the case presented only provides illustration of this particular ABS method.

### Visual Case Processing

Originating from the field of counseling, visual case processing (VCP) is a metaphoric arts-based supervision approach that primarily focuses on the development of supervisee case conceptualization skills within group supervision (Amundson, 1988; Ishyima, 1988). Ishiyama's (1988) operationalization of metaphoric case drawing for both clinical practice and research outlined four main steps to this approach. First, the supervisee reflects on a case through written response to six sentence stems. Next, the supervisee generates metaphoric images or symbols in response to the completed sentences. Third, the supervisee creates a visual representation of the case in association with the metaphoric images and symbols, usually in the form of a drawing. Finally, the supervisee presents the case in group supervision.

Research findings indicate that supervisors and supervisees alike perceived VCP favorably regarding its structure and ability to increase supervisee cognitive complexity, including the ability to "think more abstractly and critically" (Shiflett & Remley Jr., 2014, p. 47).

Ishyima (1988) also believed that the increased structure of this approach over other case drawing methods would serve to decrease supervisee anxiety around using art in tandem with case conceptualization. Research concurs that high structure supervision approaches tend to be viewed more favorably than low structure approaches by supervisees in training and newer professionals (e.g., Hart & Nance, 2003; Usher & Borders, 1993).

Supervisors may find VCP beneficial in work with art therapy supervisees in the earliest days of their pregnancy, as it places direct and explicit focus on clients during a time when self-immersion and internal attunement is often heightened (Miller & Giffin, 2019). This may aid the pregnant supervisee in remaining anchored and connected to the clinical work. Additionally, the highly structured nature of this ABS method may be perceived as more psychologically safe by supervisees experiencing increased emotional vulnerability or anxiety. It should be noted that because it is common practice among women in the United States to keep pregnancy private until reaching the second trimester (Ross, 2015), supervisors may not be aware of supervisee pregnancy until after this stage has ended. This highlights the essential nature of privacy needs for many women at this stage, further underscoring use of approaches that keep supervision tasks directly focused on client needs and concerns. The following example illustrates the VCP method only; it does not provide an example of a pregnant art therapy supervisee. Nevertheless, the use of VCP shows how a supervisee might effectively utilize this approach to develop case conceptualization skills.

Lauren, an art therapy supervisee, was interning at a residential treatment facility that served adolescents with psychiatric diagnoses, often concurrent with severe trauma and abuse. She used the VCP method to better conceptualize her work with "Red," a 15-year-old African American girl with a long history of self-harm and suicidal ideation subsequent to chronic sexual abuse endured in childhood. Figure 4.1 shows Lauren's completion of six sentence stems for step one of the VCP method.

This step helps supervisees reflect in an intentional way about their perceptions of a client, both holistically and in relation to a specific session. They may choose to focus on a recent session or one in which something significant occurred within the relational dynamic. Next, Lauren used the completion of these sentence stems as a primer for the creation of metaphors, images or symbols to describe the case in step two (Figure 4.2).

In the third step, Lauren created a collage to symbolize dynamics of the case generated through steps one and two. Her image (Figure 4.3) depicted the central paradox that she experienced in working with Red, with one side symbolizing setbacks and the other an engaged and nurturing relational dynamic. A bird flying towards the client as she

| Sentence Stem | Lauren's Response |
|---|---|
| What I see as the client's main concern is: | that she is very self-destructive and willing to self-harm at any given moment according to staff. Red has been on and off Q10's & 1 to 1.'s. |
| The way the client interacted with me is: | very talkative in the first session and then very calm and emotional in the second session. She was also in one my groups, so we have begun to build a solid rapport. |
| What I was trying to do in this session was: | begin to understand Red's personal needs for art therapy while getting to know more about her and why she felt the need to self-destruct her hard work on her treatment. |
| What I felt or thought about myself as a therapist during this session was: | feeling like I did well by handing myself although I was very concerned with her image. |
| The way this session went is: | positive. Red was surprised by my memory and I believe that it made our therapeutic bond stronger and she opened up to me in the session. |
| What I think the client gained from this session was: | Red recognizing that she is a key part of her treatment progress and that the staff and resident's care and are concerned for her well-being. |

*Figure 4.1* Visual case processing, step one—Lauren's completed sentence stems.

| Metaphor, Image, or Symbol Generation Sentence Stem | Lauren's Response |
|---|---|
| The way I perceive the client with his or her concern may be characterized by a metaphor like... | watching someone you know personally go down the wrong path and being unsure how to help them. |
| The way the client responded to me and felt toward me during this session may be characterized by a metaphor or an image like... | in grade school when you first began to warm up to that one teacher that really showed interest in your well-being. |
| The way I conducted myself during this session may be characterized by a metaphor or image like... | that gut feeling of feeling sad although you put on a brave face. |
| The way this session went may be characterized by a metaphor or an image like... | an added piece to the puzzle to establish a foundation for our building therapeutic relationship. |

*Figure 4.2* Visual case processing, step two—Lauren's metaphors, images, and symbols.

contemplated going the "wrong way" seemed to serve as a bridge, connecting and integrating the two images.

In step four, Lauren presented the image to her supervision group. She described her feelings of powerlessness as she watched Red oscillate between progress and setback. Yet, she also relayed her sense that Red was slowly becoming more receptive to treatment, describing Red's

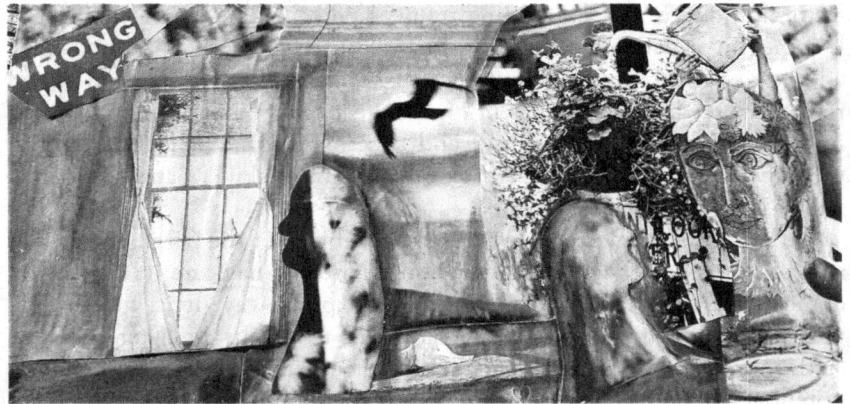

*Figure 4.3* Visual case processing, step three—Lauren's completed image.

noticeable astonishment and softening of demeanor when Lauren had remarked on patterns in Red's artwork, conveying that she was paying close attention to Red and her creative process. The visual case processing method enabled Lauren a better overall understanding of the case, including the important relational role that she played in Red's treatment.

Although the art therapy supervisee in this example was not pregnant, it is clear that the highly structured nature of VCP ensured that supervisee reflection centered the client's treatment goals and concerns. Such an approach may be ideal for supervisees in the first trimester of pregnancy who, at a time of intense change, need clear structure and grounding to maintain focus on clients' needs, while also developing case conceptualization skills. As per Shiflett and Remley (2014), supervisors may increase effectiveness of VCP with pregnant supervisees who show reluctance or anxiety by "emphasizing the creative process over the completed product, clarifying the technique directive, adapting the process according to individual needs, and monitoring and facilitating group response to the visual case presentation" (p. 44).

### Reflective Visual Journaling

Visual journaling refers to the practice of combining words and image, typically within a contained book format, and is commonly used in art therapy (Capacchione, 2002; Deaver & McAuliffe, 2009; Durkin, Perach, Ramseyer, & Sontag, 1989; Ganim & Fox, 1999; Malchiodi & Riley, 1996). Relative to supervision, Deaver and McAuliffe (2009) defined reflective visual journaling (RVJ) as a "constructivist educational strategy" that combines focused art making and responsive writing to increase trainees' development of critical reflection skills, self-awareness, and professional growth (p. 616). Their qualitative study revealed that both art therapy and counseling trainees perceived RVJ as beneficial in helping them gain new insights, increase case conceptualization skills, address and explore countertransference, and for purposes of stress reduction. Additionally, intentional reflection to imagery and words involves integration of cognitive and affective realms, believed to aid in the supervisee's development of complex clinical skills (Batten & Santanello, 2009; Tangen, 2017).

In the second trimester, the increased visibility of the pregnancy to self and others requires the art therapy supervisee to navigate its impact on clinical and supervisory dynamics in an explicit way. It is widely held that therapists should disclose pregnancies to clients no later than the sixth month of pregnancy to enable sufficient time to work through any potential impact on the clinical work (as reviewed by Miller & Giffin, 2019). This includes issues pertaining to transference and countertransference, as well as the therapist's own management of personal and professional boundaries in relation to self-care needs. As anxiety and emotionality tends to lessen for many pregnant women in proportion to increased contentment in the second trimester of pregnancy (Dyson & King, 2008), the pregnant art therapy supervisee may also be more ready to engage in exploration of transference and countertransference than in earlier stages.

RVJ allows the supervisee choice and autonomy concerning the creating and sharing of reflective expression. As a metaphor for containment, the book format dovetails well with the prevalent focus to interpersonal boundaries in the second trimester, and its portability makes it highly adaptable for use in-session, post-session or out-of-session. It may be useful in exploring transference and countertransference related to clinical dynamics and occurring in parallel between supervisor and supervisee. It can also be easily paired with reflective writing, such as intentional questioning or imaginal dialogue, as in the following example.

I served as an off-site supervisor for Sara, an art therapist who worked at an alternative middle school in a rural setting. Our supervision transpired the length of her pregnancy. I encouraged Sara to use RVJ, in part, to help her understand when her own emotional reactions stemmed from idiosyncratic countertransference (i.e., her own personal issues) vs. homogeneous countertransference that tends to be common in work with adolescents and is often an indication of the client's needs or concerns. Figure 4.4 is a page from Sara's visual journal in which she reflected on themes of personal protection for herself, her unborn child, and the loss of protection that many of her clients had experienced. Sara used imaginal dialogue, writing "I am the one who surrounds you, keeps you safe, the incubator, the nurturer. I give you sustenance so you can thrive. You needed protection too. Are you jealous that I give it to her?"

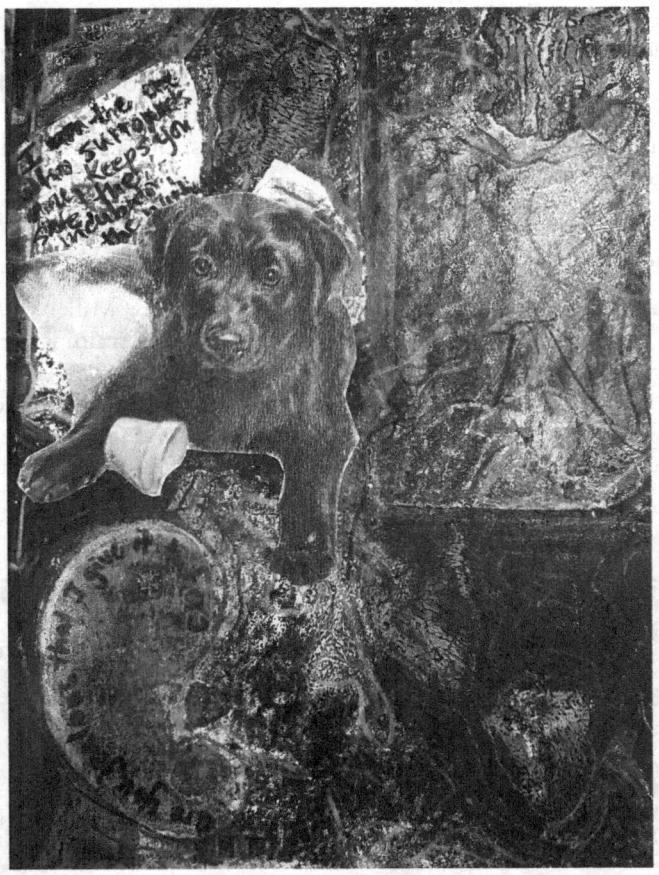

*Figure 4.4* Reflective visual journaling, Sara's journal.

RVJ enabled Sara to differentiate between intrapersonal and interpersonal dynamics so that countertransference feelings would not inadvertently and negatively impact the clinical work. Supervisors may also benefit from using RVJ to explore their own responses to the supervisory work, including emotional reactions, countertransference or other practical concerns. This may be especially necessary when supervising pregnant clinicians, especially when it is the first time doing so. By joining the supervisee in using ABS processes, the supervisor demonstrates belief in the value of the aesthetic dialogue, fosters reflectivity by modeling it, and encourages art making for purposes of self-care as a professional responsibility. Just as with clients, however, the supervisor should exercise judgment and caution when sharing their own response art with the supervisee; the supervisor's RVJ that does not have a clear relationship to the supervisee's needs, goals or professional development is better reserved for exploration elsewhere. Figure 4.5 depicts a response art image created in my visual journal in relation to my supervision of Sara. I shared with Sara that it reflected my desire to be a solid ring of support to her, as she in turn, molded herself into a ring of support for the complexity of newly differentiated feelings, as represented by the cluster of nested eggs.

### El Duende One Canvas Process Painting (EDOCPP)

El Duende One Canvas Process Painting (EDOCPP; Miller, 2012) was initially developed for use in graduate art therapy training programs; however, its focus to aesthetic and relational awareness, including attention to intrapersonal and professional development, make it ideal for supervision of pregnant art therapists. EDOCPP involves engagement in spontaneous painting and mixed media assemblage on one surface—

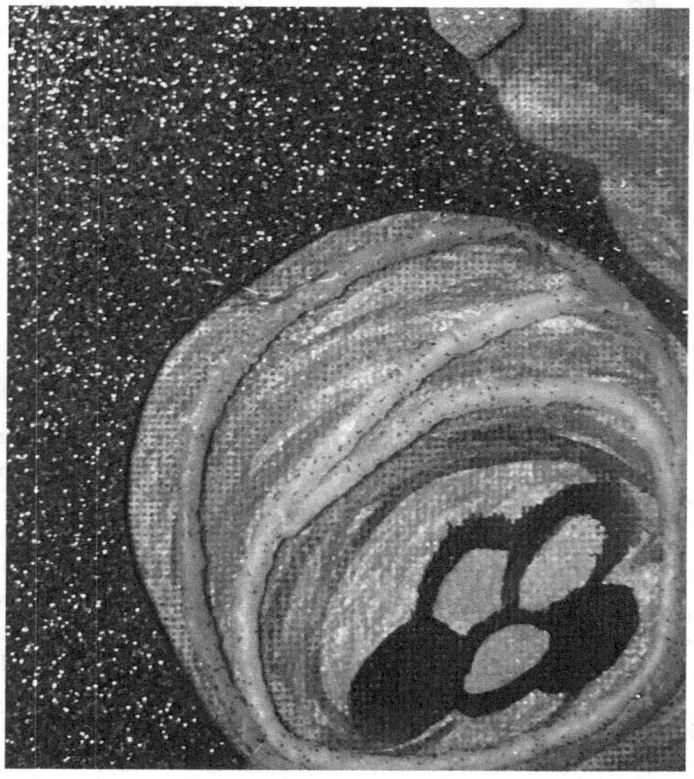

*Figure 4.5* Reflective visual journaling, supervisor's response.

typically an 18″ × 24″ sized canvas—over an extended period of time. The developing artwork becomes a focal point for intentional reflection and processing of emergent symbolic, metaphoric, and archetypal imagery that illuminates tensions related to the clinical work. Sequential layering and delayering is an integral part of the process, which can be enhanced by journaling, imaginal dialogue, or sequential photography to record and preserve the supervisee's transformational progression (Miller, 2012; Miller & Robb, 2017). Aesthetically and relationally attuned supervisor feedback (and peer feedback, if used within groups) is also an important part of this approach. EDOCPP used in group supervision was found to elicit supervisee self-disclosure and self-reflexivity towards the goals of increased cognitive and emotional awareness, self-resiliency and self-efficacy (Miller & Robb, 2017; Robb & Miller, 2017).

Grounded in a framework of transformational learning (Miller & Robb, 2017), the appreciation of complexity inherent to EDOCPP synchronizes well with the rapid changes and transformation experienced in the third and final trimester of pregnancy. The supervisory focus must necessarily shift to planning for closure and saying goodbyes as the end of the supervisee's pregnancy draws near. Although the art therapist may fully intend to resume practice post-pregnancy, setting an end date with no promise of return has been advised given the uncertainties of childbirth and the post-adjustment period (Dyson & King, 2008; Miller & Giffin, 2019). The intersection of personal and professional becomes especially salient, as the supervisee faces decisions about how to maneuver her career path with emergence into new (or additional, if not the first pregnancy) responsibilities of motherhood.

EDOCPP allows for exploration of these issues in a natural and spontaneous way, but still within a defined boundary. Similar to RVJ, it allows for broader scope of supervisory focus than does visual case processing; however, in contrast to RVJ where artwork created on separate pages can remain intact, the process of layering and delayering is a unique characteristic of EDOCPP that evokes the progressive and transformational nature of the pregnancy journey itself. Moreover, whereas pages can be closed and obscured from view in RVJ, whatever is created from week to week in EDOCPP remains visible and on view in a manner akin to the increasing prominence of pregnancy as it moves towards a new transition phase. One potential limitation is that the large size of the canvas (combined with physical fatigue or difficulties often prevalent in the third trimester) may mean that, unless the size of the canvas is reduced, it is most tenable as an in-session supervisory approach. Although supervisors who prefer spontaneity or work from a Jungian framework may find this ABS approach most resonant, EDOCPP has been flexibly paired with several conceptual frameworks (Miller, Miller, & Lindemann, 2013).

Figures 4.6 and 4.7 show the weekly progression in a process painting created by Kendra, an art therapy supervisee expecting her first child who I worked with in individual supervision. In Figure 4.6, the image of a flower that she identified as reflecting her blossoming identity as an artist-therapist is being crowded out by decals of numbers and letters, symbolic of the early days of childhood. The flower had been prominent in previous stages of the painting, but as Kendra moved closer to her due date, the flower became increasingly obscured (Figure 4.7).

Kendra indicated that the visual transformation reflected feelings of sadness and fears that becoming a mother would mean losing touch with a vital part of herself—particularly her artist–therapist identity—and uncertainties around how she would continue to work and develop professionally. Kendra also exhibited guilt for feelings that she surmised as "socially unacceptable" given difficulties she had experienced when trying to conceive. Swan-Foster (2012) remarked on the paradoxical psychological space that may be encountered when pregnant women experience feelings akin to a psychic loss of self. Getting in touch with and accepting the reality of her own complex, and at times contradictory feelings, enabled Kendra to remain attuned to the various and complex ways that her clients expressed loss as she moved towards separation and

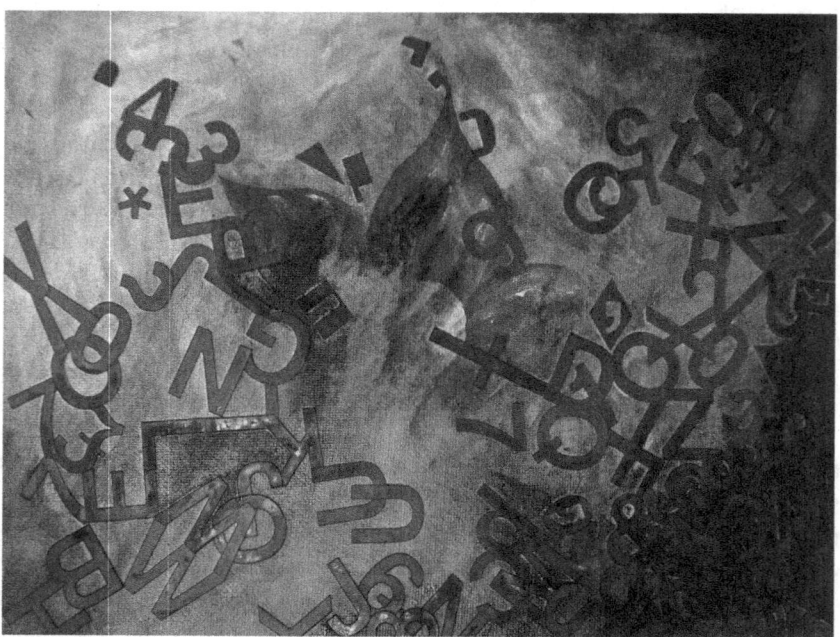

*Figure 4.6* EDOCPP, Kendra's painting #1.

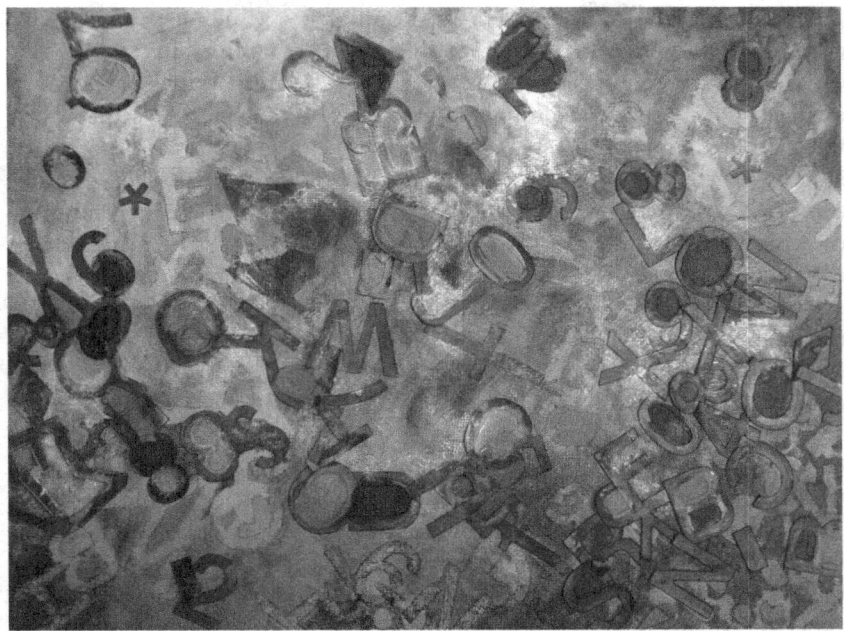

*Figure 4.7* EDOCPP, Kendra's painting #2.

closure with each of them. Use of EDOCPP in supervision helped facilitate Kendra's reflection to important clinical and professional identity themes as she prepared for closure in the final stages of her work at the setting.

## Practical and Ethical Considerations

Supervisors who wish to utilize these or other ABS approaches with pregnant art therapy supervisees should be aware of a number of different practical and ethical considerations. In general, supervisors should heed the recommendations set forth by Deaver and Shiflett (2011) that would be applied when using ABS with any supervisee, whether pregnant or not. In brief, these include practicing within the scope of one's training and competence; being knowledgeable about the properties of media, their potential hazards, and the range of affective responses that might be elicited; and engaging in an informed consent process around use of ABS with the supervisee. All of these recommendations are intended to ensure and safeguard the overall well-being of the supervisee. It is worth highlighting several additional caveats extending from these points with regards to common needs or concerns that may arise for pregnant supervisees.

First, considerations of media should expand beyond supervisors' competence and comfort to ensure nontoxicity, while also considering contraindication of some materials due to sensory sensitivity or physical discomfort issues experienced in pregnancy. Materials that are large in size, heavy or otherwise cumbersome may pose challenges as the supervisee's pregnancy progresses. Both for ethical and safety reasons, the supervisee should have complete control over material usage, with the option of declining media at any point. The same is true concerning use of ABS methods overall, as second, the supervisor must be mindful that experiential processes are likely to tap into personal content experienced as inseparable from professional and clinical content. Although often this will be perceived as welcome from the perspective of the supervisee, it may also be experienced as unfamiliar, uncomfortable or threatening, and consequently, amplify feelings of vulnerability.

Supervisors should be aware that pregnant supervisees may already be feeling higher levels of vulnerability on average than other supervisees due to a combination of individual, supervisory and sociocultural factors. These include heightened vulnerability associated with physical and hormonal changes; keen awareness and attention to the power differential in the supervisory relationship; and a wide range of social issues frequently experienced by pregnant women that give rise to professional insecurities, including the reality of pregnancy discrimination, uncertainties concerning maternity leave, fear of professional retaliation or loss of career opportunities, and various other reasons that cause women to feel unsupported and leave the workforce at higher rates than men (Collins, 2019; NPWF, 2016). Without the necessary caution, ABS approaches could highlight these feelings in a way that is experienced as anxiety provoking or even invasive rather than helpful, particularly given power differences in the supervisory relationship. This may be especially so when the supervisor holds decision-making power that directly impacts the supervisee's job.

For these and other reasons, it is of utmost importance that the supervisor engages in a sound informed consent process before utilizing any approaches that have the potential to prompt emotionally laden material pertaining to the supervisee's personal life. Informed consent should contain discussion of the risks, benefits, and limits of ABS approaches under consideration; rationale for using these approaches and what they would involve; and an open and transparent discussion about power dimensions in the supervisory relationship (Batten & Santanello, 2009; Deaver & Shiflett, 2011). Further, using ABS approaches with any directive invoking the art therapist's pregnancy should *always* be the supervisee's choice, as doing so otherwise may constitute an abuse of the supervisor's position of power and authority. Moreover, if mutually agreed upon, focus to the supervisee's pregnancy should only be for purposes of increasing understanding of how the pregnancy impacts client treatment or the therapist's self-determined exploration of the intersection of personal and professional roles and identity development.

## Conclusion

In conclusion, clinical supervision has an undeniably important role to play in supporting pregnant art therapy practitioners at an especially momentous time, both personally and professionally. Arts-based supervision approaches that promote supervisee reflectivity towards development of case conceptualization skills, as well as aid in exploration of transference, countertransference and inseparably experienced personal and professional identity issues, may be especially useful in work with pregnant art therapy supervisees. The art therapy supervisor is encouraged to consider use of the ABS approaches described and illustrated in this chapter—visual case processing, reflective visual journaling, and El Duende One Canvas Process Painting—with mindful attention to practical, ethical, and sociocultural concerns as highlighted, as a valuable place to start.

## References

Amundson, N. E. (1988). The use of metaphor and drawings in case conceptualization. *Journal of Counseling and Development, 66*, 391–393.

Anekstein, A. M., Hoskins, W. J., Astramovich, R. L., Garner, D., & Terry, J. (2014). "Sandtray supervision": Integrating supervision models and sandtray therapy. *Journal of Creativity in Mental Health, 9*, 122–134. doi:10.1080/15401383.2014.876885

Batten, S. V., & Santanello, A. P. (2009). A contextual behavioral approach to the role of emotion in psychotherapy supervision. *Training and Education in Professional Psychology, 3*(3), 148–156.

Baum, N. (2009). Supervisors' responses to pregnant supervisees. *The Clinical Supervisor, 28*, 3–19.

Bernard, J. M., & Goodyear, R. K. (2019). *Fundamentals of clinical supervision* (6th ed.). New York, NY: Pearson.

Borders, L. D., & Brown, L. L. (2005). *The new handbook of counseling supervision.* Mahway: NJ: Lahaska Press.

Calvert, F. L., Crowe, T. P., & Grenyer, B. F. S. (2017). An investigation of supervisory practices to develop reflective competence in psychologists. *Australian Psychologist, 52*, 467–479. doi:10.1111/ap.12261

Capacchione, L. (2002). *The creative journal (2nd ed.).* Franklin Lakes, NJ: New Page Books.

Cheng, A., LaDonna, K., Cristancho, S., & Ng, S. (2017). Navigating difficult conversations: The role of self-monitoring and reflection-in-action. *Medical Education, 51*, 1220–1231. doi:10.1111/medu.13448

Collins, C. (2019). *Making motherhood work: How women manage careers and caregiving.* Princeton, NJ: Princeton University Press.

Deaver, S. P., & McAuliffe, G. (2009). Reflective visual journaling during art therapy and counselling internships: A qualitative study. *Reflective Practice, 10*, 615–632. doi:10.1080/14623940903290687

Deaver, S. P., & Shiflett, C. L. (2011). Art-based supervision techniques. *The Clinical Supervisor, 30*, 257–276. doi:10.1080/07325223.2011.619456

Dewey, J. (1933). *How we think: A restatement of the relation of reflective thinking to the educative process.* Boston, MA: Houghton Mifflin.

Durkin, J., Perach, D., Ramseyer, J., & Sontag, E. (1989). A model for art therapy supervision enhanced through art making and journal writing. In H. Wadeson, J. Durkin, & D. Perach (Eds.), *Advances in art therapy* (pp. 376–389). New York, NY: Wiley.

Dyson, E., & King, G. (2008). The pregnant therapist. *Psychodynamic Practice, 14*(1), 27–42. doi:10.1080/14753630701768958

Elkins, D. E., & Deaver, S. P. (2015). American Art Therapy Association, Inc.: 2013 membership survey report. *Art Therapy: Journal of the American Art Therapy Association, 32,* 60–69. doi:https://doi.org/10.1080/07421656.2015.1028313

Fish, B. J. (2017). *Art-based supervision: Cultivating therapeutic insight through imagery.* New York & London: Routledge.

Fouad, N., Grus, C. L., Hatcher, R. L., Kaslow, N. J., Hutchings, P. S., Madson, M. B., & Crossman, R. E. (2009). Competency benchmarks: A model for understanding and measuring competence in professional psychology across training levels. *Training and Education in Professional Psychology, 3*(4, Suppl.), S5–S26.

Frawley O'Dea, M. G., & Sarnat, J. E. (2001). *The supervisory relationship: A contemporary psychodynamic approach.* New York, NY: Guilford Press.

Frolund, L., & Nielsen, J. (2009). The reflective meta-dialogue in psychodynamic supervision. *Nordic Psychology, 61,* 85–105. doi:10.1027/1901-2276.61.3.85

Ganim, B., & Fox, S. (1999). *Visual journaling: Going deeper than words.* Wheaton, IL: Quest Books.

Goldberger, M., Gillman, R., Levinson, N., Notman, M., Seelig, B., & Shaw, R. (2003). On supervising the pregnant psychoanalytic candidate. *Psychoanalytic Quarterly, 72,* 439–463.

Graham, M. A., Scholl, M. B., Smith-Adcock, S., & Wittman, E. (2014). Three creative approaches to counseling supervision. *Journal of Creativity in Mental Health, 9,* 415–426. doi:10.1080/15401383.2014.899482

Guiffrida, D. A., Jordan, R., Saiz, S., & Barnes, K. L. (2007). The use of metaphor in clinical supervision. *Journal of Counseling & Development, 85,* 393–400.

Gunja, M. Z., Tikkanen, R., Seervai, S., & Collins, S. R. (2018). What is the status of women's health and health care in the U.S. compared to ten other countries? *The Commonwealth Fund.* Retrieved from https://doi.org/10.26099/wy8a-7w13

Hart, G. M., & Nance, D. (2003). Styles of counselor supervision as perceived by supervisors and supervisees. *Counselor Education & Supervision, 43,* 146–158.

Health and Care Professions Council [HCPC]. (2019). *Registration snapshot- April 2019.* Retrieved from www.hpc-uk.org/resources/data/2019/registrant-snapshot—april-2019/

Holloway, E. L. (2016). *Supervision essentials for a systems approach to psychotherapy.* Washington, DC: American Psychological Association.

Holloway, E. L., & Carroll, M. (1999). *Training counseling supervisors.* London: Sage.

Hurdman, C. M. (1999). Clinical issues and client reactions arising from the art therapist's pregnancy. *The Arts in Psychotherapy, 26*(4), 233–246.

Imber, R. R. (1995). The role of the supervisor and the pregnant analyst. *Psychoanalytic Psychology, 12*(2), 281–296.

Ishyima, F. I. (1988). A model of visual case processing using metaphors and drawings. *Counselor Education and Supervision, 28*, 153–161.

Jenkins, S. (2010). Relationships. In J. C. Thomas & M. Hershen (Eds.), *The handbook of clinical psychology competencies* (pp. 123–152). New York, NY: Springer.

Kagan, N. (1980). Influencing human interaction-Eighteen years with IPR. In A. K. Hess (Ed.), *Psychotherapy supervision: Theory, research, and practice* (pp. 262–283). New York, NY: Wiley.

Kolb, D. A. (1984). *Experiential learning: Experience as a source of learning and development.* Englewood Cliffs, NJ: Prentice Hall.

Ladany, N., Friedlander, M. L., & Nelson, M. L. (2005). *Critical events in psychotherapy supervision: An interpersonal approach.* Washington, DC: American Psychological Association.

Lee, A. C. Y. (2010). The 2009-2010 National survey of art therapists in Canada. *Canadian Art Therapy Association Journal, 23*, 36–50. doi:10/1080/08322473.2010. 11432336

Loganbill, C., Hardy, E., & Delworth, U. (1982). Supervision: A conceptual model. *The Counseling Psychologist, 10*, 3–42. doi:10.1177/0011000082101002

Malchiodi, C. A., & Riley, S. (1996). *Supervision and related issues.* Chicago, IL: Magnolia.

Miller, A. (2012). Inspired by El Duende: One-canvas process painting in art therapy supervision. *Art Therapy: Journal of the American Art Therapy Association, 29*, 166–173. doi:10.1080/07421656.2013.730024

Miller, A., Miller, R. D., & Lindemann, Y. (2013). *Three variations on one-canvas process painting.* Paper presented at the American Art Therapy Association annual conference, Seattle, WA.

Miller, A., & Robb, M. (2017). Transformative phases in *el duende* process painting art-based supervision. *Arts in Psychotherapy, 54*, 15–27. doi:10.1016/j. aip.2017.02.009

Miller, R. D., & Giffin, J. A. (2019). Parallel pregnancies: The impact on the supervisory relationship and art therapy. *Arts in Psychotherapy.* doi:10.1016/j. aip.2018.12.007

Moffett, L. A. (2009). Directed self-reflection protocols in supervision. *Training and Education in Professional Psychology, 3*(2), 78–83.

National Partnership for Women & Families [NPWF]. (2016). *By the numbers: Women continue to face pregnancy discrimination in the workplace.* [Data brief]. Retrieved from www.nationalpartnership.org/our-work/resources/economic-jus tice/pregnancy-discrimination/by-the-numbers-women-continue-to-face-preg nancy-discrimination-in-the-workplace.pdf

Neimeyer, R. A., Woodward, M., Pickover, A., & Smigelsky, M. (2016). Questioning our questions: A constructivist technique for clinical supervision. *Journal of Constructivist Psychology, 29*, 100–111. doi:10.1080/10720537.2015.1038406

Neufeldt, S. A. (1999). Training in reflective processes in supervision. In M. Carroll & E. L. Holloway (Eds.), *Education of clinical supervisors* (pp. 92–105). London, UK: Sage.

Neufeldt, S. A., Karno, M. P., & Nelson, M. L. (1996). A qualitative study of experts conceptualization of supervisee reflectivity. *Journal of Counseling Psychology, 43*, 3–9.

Orchowski, L., Evangelista, N. M., & Probst, D. R. (2010). Enhancing supervisee reflectivity in clinical supervision: A case study illustration. *Psychotherapy Theory, Research, Practice, & Training, 47*(1), 51–67.

Robb, M., & Miller, A. (2017). Supervisee art based disclosure in *El Duende* process painting. *Art Therapy: Journal of the American Art Therapy Association, 34*, 192–200. doi:10.1080/07421656.2017.1398576

Ronnestad, M. H., & Skovholt, T. M. (2013). *The developing practitioner: Growth and stagnation of therapists and counselors*. New York & London: Routledge.

Ross, E. J. (2015). 'I think it's self-preservation:' risk perception and secrecy in early pregnancy. *Health, Risk & Society, 17*, 329–348. doi:10.1080/13698575.2015.1091922

Schon, D. (1983). *The reflective practitioner*. New York, NY: Basic Books.

Shiflett, C. L., & Remley, T. P., Jr. (2014). Incorporating case conceptualization drawing in counseling group supervision: A grounded theory study. *Journal of Creativity in Mental Health, 9*, 33–52. doi:10.1080/15401383.2013.878680

Skaife, S. (2012). The pregnant art therapist's countertransference. In S. Hogan (Ed.), *Revisiting feminist approaches to art therapy* (pp. 237–254). New York & Oxford: Berghahn Books.

Stoltenberg, C. D., & McNeill, B. W. (2010). *IDM supervision: An integrated developmental model for supervising counselors and therapists* (3rd ed.). San Francisco: Jossey-Bass.

Swan-Foster, N. (2012). Pregnancy as a feminine initiation. *Journal of Prenatal and Perinatal Psychology and Health, 26*(4), 207–235.

Tangen, J. L. (2017). Attending to nuanced emotions: Fostering supervisees' emotional awareness and complexity. *Counselor Education and Supervision, 56*, 65–78. doi:10.1002/ceas.12060

ter Maat, M., & Vandersyde, A. (1995). The pregnant art therapist. *American Journal of Art Therapy, 33*(3), 74–83.

Usher, C. H., & Borders, L. D. (1993). Practicing counselors' preferences for supervisory style and supervisory emphasis. *Counselor Education & Supervision, 33*, 66–79.

# 5   Using Art to Prepare for Births as a Doula-Grandmother[1]

*Jane Margaret Hunt*

## Coming to Art as a Personal Practice

I did not grow up in a family of artists, but in a family of doctors. Art was a rote childhood activity for me, until I discovered art museums and began to make my own art along with my children. Once I gave myself permission to experiment with a wide range of materials, I began to experience the healing nature of art.

When I returned to school, at midlife, to earn a social work degree and become a psychotherapist, a graduate art therapy program was just starting up alongside the existing Master's in Social Work (MSW) program. In my second year, the art therapist Bruce Moon, chair of that new department, served as my advisor on a qualitative research project—I offered weekly art sessions as an adjunct to weekly talk therapy for patients at a county mental health clinic. I remember feeling moved, each time I walked into his office, that he had an oil painting—in process—on an easel there.

It's important to say that I am not a certified art therapist. During my Jungian training, the art therapist and Jungian analyst Ethné Gray taught us classes on using art as a personal practice, inviting patients to use art, and gently interpreting patients' art in a symbolic way, similar to a Jungian interpretation of dreams. I continue to paint and to encourage patients to make art.

## Preparing to Attend a Birth

I started researching birth in early 2012, when my daughter, who lives in Chile, asked me to be the doula for her births with midwives. I agreed, reread my own birth stories, and met with a local doula in my home community in the United States, who talked me through the normal birth process and how a doula, at each stage, might be supportive. This activated my body memory of giving birth and began to give me confidence that I might be helpful. I read several contemporary books on childbirth, but I was still nervous about understanding enough Spanish to follow what was happening in labor. Brigitte Jordan's book,

*Birth in Four Cultures*, added a different, anthropological framework for how birth unfolds. Jordan's (1993) cross-cultural perspective suggested ways I might watch and infer behavioral communication and power dynamics, rather than rely only on verbal communication.

Then, I dreamed an image and painted it (Figure 5.1).

The image shows, on the right side of the painting, what was already known in conscious life between myself and my daughter, so I will call this the ego position because I'm identified with it. But, what about the left-side image of me and the pregnant black woman, who stands even closer to me and grips my arm in a non-mutual way? This might be a communication from the unconscious. The cane reflects real life because I had injured my right foot some months before and was still walking with difficulty. But, the cane might also indicate a weakness, a wounded quality in my central ego position, especially on the left—unconscious—side, where the black woman has taken hold of me.

I also imagine the image might be related to a much earlier dream, from the start of my psychoanalytic training. That dream takes place in Harlem, during a time when my daughters, in real life, were involved in an African American dance form, and the little girl reminds me of a white, female dancer whose last name is "Palm":

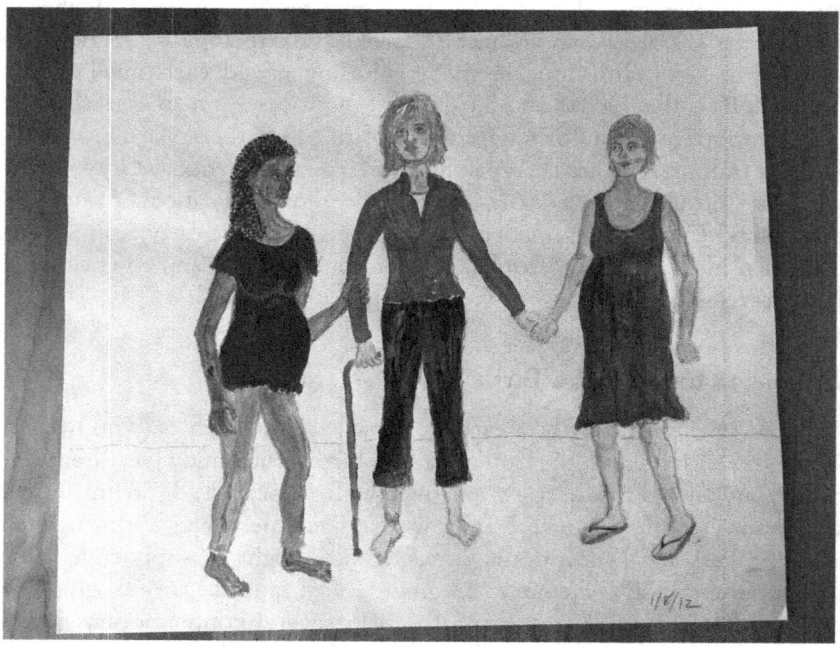

*Figure 5.1* "Three Pregnant Women" acrylics.

I am heading out through a hallway that is narrow, narrow, then up, steeply, to a tiny opening. I can't possibly fit through here, I think, but a voice encourages me—a little black girl. I press on—up—and there's a metal hand contraption that now opens, first in one direction, then on a hinge in another. My head just fits into the palm of the hand—but now what? I press up with my feet against the walls, and the hand then lifts my head automatically, forcing me through the small opening, and I pop out onto the asphalt—toenails scraped, splotched with blood, crying hard. The little girl stands on the pavement nodding to me.

I shared the dream in class, and another of the training candidates, a midwife, suggested that I was likely born by forceps. I asked my mother, again, about my birth, but she remembered only that I was born forehead first, after a lot of back labor.

Now, I also wonder if the adult, pregnant, black woman in my painting might be a more grown-up version of the friendly black girl in my dream, who helped me imagine surviving initiation—being born anew—as a Jungian analyst. And this black woman is pregnant, facing, with me, another birth. Bruce Moon wrote about making art as similar to giving birth, as "being laid open by art." He added, "May we all connect with the joy, pain, and 'awfully hard work' of being born" (2009, p. xv).

C. G. Jung developed the concept of "shadow" as a way of understanding parts of our psyches that we haven't yet integrated, parts that we may have actively repressed or just never known. These parts can show up in dreams as unfamiliar figures, often of the same sex as the dreamer. Becoming conscious of the shadow, he explained, "involves recognizing the dark aspects of the personality as present and real." He recommended "closer examination of the dark characteristics—that is, the inferiorities constituting the shadow" (1948/1970, p. 8).

The black analyst Fanny Brewster criticized Jung's use of language: "The initial understanding of shadow was that it was negative, dark, and primitive and belonged to that of the primitive," that is, to people of color themselves (2017, p. 5). I hear in her writing a call for us to carefully question this racist association and work to tease apart which aspects of, say, a black character in a white person's dream might have to do with *personal* shadow qualities versus the *impersonal* suffering and active oppression from white culture itself.

The actual first birth went like this: my daughter's water broke in the middle of the night, and a few hours later we drove to a small hospital in Talagante, outside Santiago. One of the midwives led us into a tiny examining room, where she attached an electronic fetal monitor and noted the irregular pattern of short, infrequent contractions. But, then, she set the device aside and described her conversation with the obstetrician on call: "I told him your water broke," she said, "and he asked if I was going to induce you. I told him, 'No, we'll wait and see.'" As my daughter translated the story, I noted with relief this important communication about the space we were entering, in which the midwife was in charge of her own cases, a peer to the obstetrician, not his underling,

My worry about understanding enough Spanish turned out to be irrelevant because the two midwives *modeled* the behavior they wanted to encourage in us, speaking primarily with their bodies, through gesture and tone of voice, rather than relying on words. They poured lotion into their own hands and massaged my daughter's shoulders, neck, hips, and then held the lotion out to our hands, inviting us to massage with them, doing as they were doing. The midwives spoke—only and always—in quiet, calm voices, repeating, "E-so, e-so, e-so" [That's it, that's it]. These soft, low, chanting words became the soundtrack of the labor and birth, the ceremonial songs creating and maintaining the ritual space.

At one point when both midwives were absent, a floor nurse walked into the room and rattled off a question. I thought perhaps I didn't understand because of her rapid Spanish, but then I could see that my Chilean son-in-law didn't understand, either. After a pause, he responded, simply, "Estamos con las matronas" [We're with the midwives], and the nurse turned on her heel and left. I could see, then, that there were two separate systems functioning within the hospital, and we were on the non-medical, midwifery side.

In some second- and third-world countries, where births take place in simple homes, the sounds and activities of a birth cannot be effectively separated from the rest of the household. Brigitte Jordan described how there may be no more than a cloth curtain separating the laboring woman and her attendants from others in the family. But, she found that, when asked about birth, those who are not yet socially allowed to attend—children, for example—respond by insisting that they know *nothing* about birth, even though they may be standing right next to it (1993, p. 24). I understand this to mean that the dividing line between conscious, ceremonially created initiation spaces and ordinary, everyday spaces—or between two different types of initiatory spaces, like medical and non-medical—can be visible, temporary, or even invisible boundaries that are nonetheless felt and respected as "real."

The midwives acted like elders, for me, with their slow repetition of "E-so, e-so, e-so, tran-qu-ilo, e-so." Whenever I got worried or anxious, I would look at their faces—they were always calm and untroubled. Even in the strangely empty pause right before birth, at ten centimeters of dilation, when the contractions stalled for a tough 20 minutes or so, their faces looked only tired, never worried, and never, ever anxious. So, I didn't need to be worried or anxious, either. I could be calm for my daughter because the midwives were radiating calm into the contained space for all of us.

When it was time for the pushing stage, the midwives gestured toward the various positions and locations my daughter might try out—an upright birthing stool, a bar to hold onto, a semi-reclined birthing chair. Then, they truly "rotated" around her, slowly picking up the small, stainless steel tray with a few instruments on it, along with a white cloth, and literally following her to each new location, setting down the tray and spreading the white cloth on the floor, then patiently moving the tray and spreading the cloth in another position, and yet another, until my daughter was settled, had chosen for herself where she would give birth. The phrase Brigitte Jordan learned in the Yucatan for this is *buscar la forma* [to find one's way or what feels right] (1993, p. 33).

There was no episiotomy. Rather, one of the midwives continuously massaged my daughter's perineum with liquid petroleum jelly. She gently rubbed the tightened flesh between her left index finger, on the inside, and a thumb, on the outside. Then, she poured more oil and massaged more, then more oil and more rubbing, over many minutes.

When my grandson was born, the midwife moved in one slow, curving, continuous gesture, first bending to receive him and then, without pause or any hurry, arcing him in her arms upward, slowly, until she completed a full circle and set the new baby gently back down on his mother's belly—on the outside of her body, this time. There was no suctioning, no wiping or washing, no intervention at all, at that moment, simply a returning of the newborn baby to his mother's belly, to the place he came from.

Initiation ceremonies are gestural rites—they *show* us what's happening rather than tell us. Birth anthropologist Robbie Davis-Floyd wrote, "Rituals work to align the belief system of the individual with that of the social group conducting the ritual" (2003, p. 10). In this birth, the belief system of my daughter was upheld. She intuitively trusted the midwives and their system, and through her choice I was able to experience and join and feel securely held within a birthing tradition that is a mostly absent counterpart in the United States.

Minutes after the birth, I walked into a hallway to retrieve my things and, from there, could see into a smaller, adjacent labor room. Unlike the fading natural light I had just left, bright fluorescent bulbs illuminated this room, revealing a fixed scene, like a still life: two stern-faced men in knee-length, white coats stood over a seated woman in a thin hospital gown, dejected-looking and slumped like a rag doll over her full, rounded belly. No one talked or moved. A feeling of stasis and defeat washed over me. Of course, this was only a snapshot of another woman's labor. But, to me it looked and *felt* like a labor inside the patriarchal, medical birthing system. I imagine I was seeing, again, across the invisible curtain between the two.

Then, I stepped back into the *matronas'* space where my grandson was born—where my daughter became a mother, my son-in-law a father, and where I became a grandmother. This was my initiation into a birthing world outside the strictly medical. By allowing the birthing woman to take up the center, we could all be initiated—re-membered—into the holding environment that fosters birth in both a literal, physical way and a psychological, emotional way at the same time.

## Processing the Birth

My father was an obstetrician, so I heard birth stories from before I can remember. I come from the medical model, a family with seven male physicians over four generations. My paternal grandfather founded a hospital in southern Minnesota but also attended homebirths for 30 years. He practiced much like his medical ancestors—both in the midwifery tradition and as a physician. The birth stories in his memoir show that he knew how to allow a birth to unfold, with the woman as the center, *and* how to step into a central role and offer chloroform or use forceps. My paternal grandmother, who grew up in a sod house on the prairie, gave birth four times at home (Hunt, 1961).

My father completed his OB-GYN residency at the Mayo Clinic. I know that he was beloved by many of his patients because mothers of friends would put a hand on my shoulder and say, "Your father is such a kind man." His career, though, spanned the decades of the most highly medicated births in the United States. He never attended a homebirth, to my knowledge, and most of the natural births under his care were not planned—they simply went too fast for anesthesia. That's a lot of change in childbirth practices in just one generation.

My own birth—this is the one birth we have all attended—took place at St. Mary's, the teaching hospital for the Mayo Clinic, and my father was likely present. My mother said he gave her a copy of Grantly Dick-Read's book, *Childbirth Without Fear*, and that it helped her relax during contractions. But, I find this story painfully ironic. She had very little memory of her births—I suspect mine was a twilight sleep birth—and she gave birth in a hospital setting that was closed to the midwifery approach. She also said that my father was not able to provide the continuous emotional support the book described "because that's not the way he was." But, continuous emotional support *is* the heart of the midwifery model (Dick-Read, 1959).

My next experience of birth was at 19, when my father invited me to attend a delivery at a teaching hospital in Pennsylvania. The laboring woman lay sprawled in a prone position with knees splayed and strapped into stirrups. She was fortyish and obese. Her eyes fluttered, half-closed and unseeing. She moaned loudly, intermittently. There were no words.

My father, as the attending physician, stood back, watching. I stood and watched with him. But, I began to feel, gradually, coldly alone, without language, myself, for what I was seeing. After a time of the moaning and fluttering, some slow but agitated movement, and then louder groaning, someone said the baby might be coming, now, look, you can see its head.

The resident, sitting on a stool and bending down toward the level of the woman's vulva, reached over and picked up a pair of blunt, stainless steel scissors, with bent blades. We had a pair of these bandage scissors at home when I was a child, and I used them to cut out paper dolls under the desk in my father's den. The resident slipped a gloved finger inside the woman's perineum, gripped the skin between middle- and forefinger, and began to snip, snip, snip, an inch or so toward her anus. Blood jumped from the bright, cut edges. I knew this was an episiotomy and felt less startled by the cutting itself than by the use of such a homely and familiar tool on flesh.

Then, the baby's head slid into view, along with a gush of blood and fluid. I don't remember if anyone was telling the woman to push. I don't remember anyone talking to her at all. Perhaps the shoulders slipped out. There were strange, metallic smells. I began to see dark spots on the periphery of my vision and knew I was about to faint, so I stepped into the hallway. A nurse followed, led me to an empty labor room, and helped me crawl onto a bed until the dizziness subsided. I rested there, horizontal, empty of words.

The way this event made its way into story, in my family, was like this: that the smell of blood made me dizzy, made me pass out, was too much for me. Perhaps I said this. It was the smell of the blood. And that part is true. What I couldn't say at that time was: Who was that man, that man who used to be my admired, heroic father, standing there quietly, seemingly himself but obviously not, not anyone I ever knew before? While that woman, not herself at all, not any kind of a someone, at the moment, was cut and emptied and wiped without a glance or a word from anyone. There was no conscious new mother present to exclaim over or to hold her new baby. And, perhaps this mother, too, would have no birth story to tell.

I understand this story, now, as a kind of initiation for me. What is it that I was initiated into? "Ritual's primary purpose," according to Davis-Floyd, "is to symbolically enact and thereby to transmit a group's belief system into the psyches of its participants" (2003, p. 10). An initiation ritual is a primarily nonverbal process, an enacted one. Davis-Floyd goes on:

> The single factor that most influences how a woman responds to her socialization process is the degree of correspondence between the technocratic model dominant in the hospital and the belief system she herself holds when she enters the hospital. This belief system may be upheld, or overthrown, by the rituals of hospital birth. When it is upheld, she will generally perceive her birth experience as positive and joyful; when overthrown, as negative and traumatic.
>
> (2003, pp. 6–7)

My mother's belief system was upheld; I never heard her question the rituals of her births. But, *my* belief system—in my father as heroic provider of good care and in the medical system he represented—was fractured. I suspect part of what shook me was witnessing a birth so similar to my own: my father was again physically present but emotionally absent; the mother again unconscious, but this time I was conscious and awake. The experience turned out to be protective for me because I understood that I would not be able to trust entirely in my father's medical system.

Jungian analyst Claire Douglas, who worked for ten years as a childbirth educator and doula, wrote of "an odd, wordless sense of betrayal" experienced by daughters of mothers who "came from a lineage of women who mistrusted their own natures and adapted themselves almost completely to the world of the fathers and to masculine values" because that's what they understood as "right" (2006, p. 91).

I first gave birth seven years later, but the natural birth movement had flexed the medical model, just in that short time, so I opted to stay inside it and use my sense of betrayal to push for what I wanted. Although I knew midwives existed, I didn't yet understand that they work within a separate and equally reliable birthing model, only that they functioned outside my known world. Nevertheless, I did manage to have three natural births. It would be hard to overstate the differences between my own births and the one I witnessed: I felt myself as the main actor, each time, as much in the center as I could manage. Along with a sense of accomplishment, though, I also experienced, each time, brief but painful intrusions from the medical surround.

In the mid-1990s, I read Laurel Thatcher Ulrich's book, *A Midwife's Tale*, and learned about the history of the repression of midwifery in the United States (1990). Many, many others have written about this history—midwives like Ina May Gaskin, Peggy Armstrong, and Claudine Smith; anthropologists like Margaret Mead, Brigitte Jordan, Robbie Davis-Floyd, Sheila Kitzinger, and Cynthia Gabriel; historians like Ulrich and Susan Smith; doula Penny Simkin; even the poet Adrienne Rich—but the significance of this information still has not made it into mainstream understanding of birth in the United States.

As a daughter of the medical model, I also struggled to let it in. I kept hearing a critical voice in my head that insisted, *These female writers are telling a different history of birth because they're midwives or they're aligned with midwives*, as if this made them illegitimate. But, I kept reading and by the fifth or sixth book began to notice, as if out of the corner of my eye, that they all referenced the same historic medical articles. When I finally tracked down and read the articles, I could hear, with my own ears, the misogyny and racism expressed there.

Much of the anti-midwife propaganda was aimed at recent immigrants, poor women, black women moving up from the Deep South, and Asian women out West. It used racially coded language to discredit midwives' expertise and birth rituals, even though many midwives trained at reputable schools or in sturdy lay-midwifery traditions. American doctors and obstetricians wanted their patients—or "obstetric material," as Dr. Charles

Ziegler referred to birthing women in the most famous of these articles, "The Elimination of the Midwife" (1913, p. 33). Zeigler proposed a baldly strategic and ultimately successful takeover of birth by the medical model, which resulted in 30 years of worse birth outcomes and, I would add, an unconscious, collective, psychic wound that we still carry.

Claire Douglas elaborated on the "folk healers, granny women, and midwives" that Ziegler disparaged:

> These positive role models were discarded as primitive and shamefully ignorant. Great progress was made in the growing sophistication of medicine and its ability to save lives, but, in the process, the old native wisdom was lost. We ceded our wisdom to the experts' theories.
>
> (2006, pp. 22–23)

What I call the "Red Face Painting" is a dream image that arrived a few months after the amazing, ecstatic, surprising and healing experience of attending my first grandson's birth in the midwifery model (Figure 5.2).

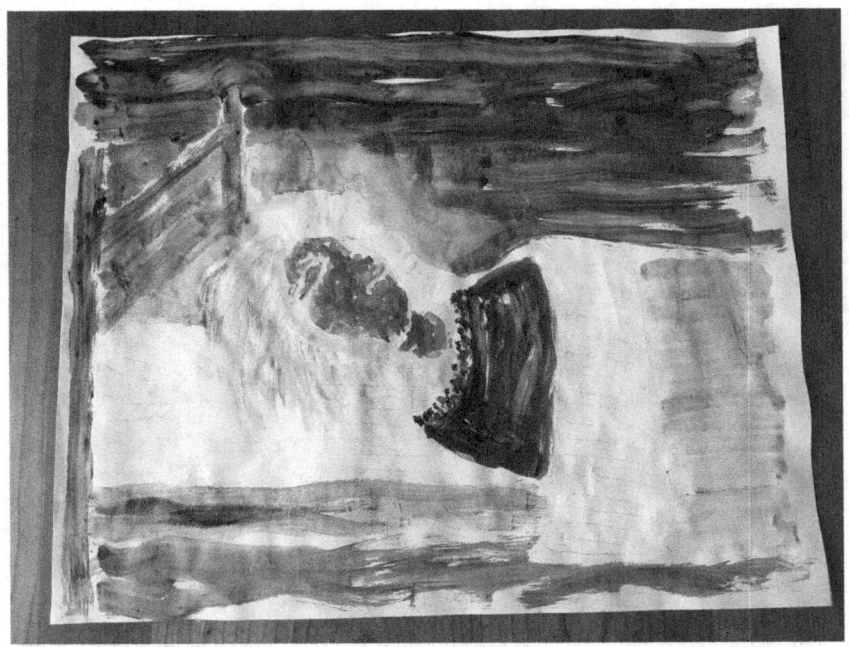

*Figure 5.2* "Red Face Painting" acrylics.

*In the dream, I am horizontal, tucked into a single bed. As a child, I slept in a green-painted, steel bed from Hunt Hospital, but this dream bed is made of wood, a natural rather than "man"-made material. My face and neck are bright red, the color of fresh blood.* The image communicates, to me, feelings of deep shame and passivity—shame about my inherited, dec-ades-long, unconscious acceptance of the patriarchal medical model as the only safe, reliable model of childbirth, a passive, incurious "lying-down" that sacrifices the more active and individual *buscando la forma* of the midwifery model. Only after experiencing midwifery from the inside can I now fully feel this shame, which is both personal and cultural.

The next painting (Figure 5.3) was stimulated by D. W. Winnicott's poignant description of how a tiny baby might experience emotional abandonment:

If left for too long (hours, minutes) without familiar and human contact, they have experiences that we can only describe with such words as:

> going to pieces
> falling forever
> dying and dying and dying
> losing all vestige of hope of the renewal of contacts. (1987, p. 86)

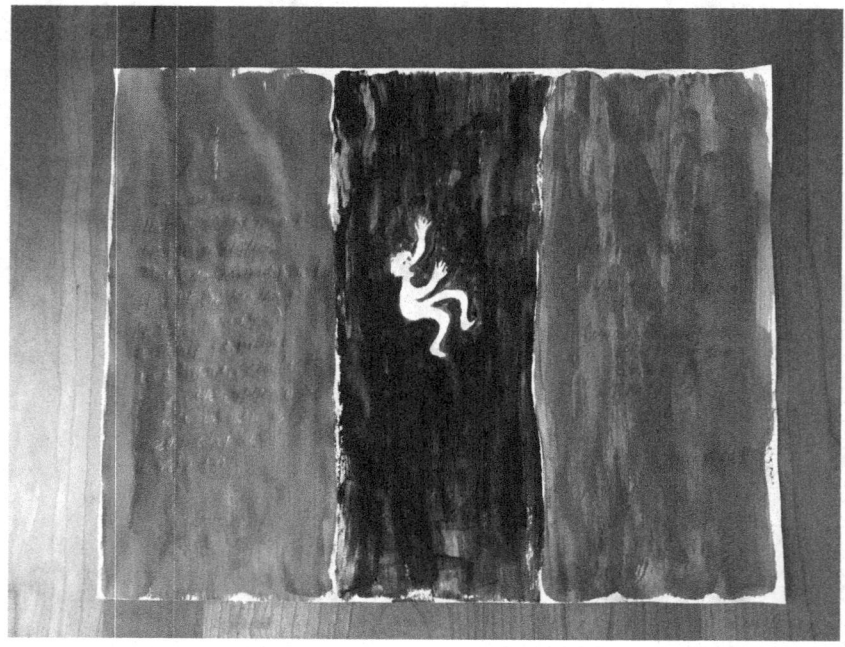

*Figure 5.3* "Falling Through Space" acrylics.

After participating in a warmly held birth, I can now identify that part of me feels utterly abandoned by the dramatic contrast in body memory between (1) intensely medical births, like my own birth and the one my father shared with me at 19, and (2) the warmly collaborative midwifery births of my grandsons.

What do I mean by a "warmly held" experience? Winnicott wrote that "the individual's maturational processes ... require a facilitating environment" (1958/1992, p. 134). This "held" quality arises, he said, when "the environment is holding the individual, and *at the same time* the individual knows of no environment and is at one with it" (p. 283).

## Preparing to Attend a Second Birth

My daughter visited the United States near the end of her second pregnancy. One day, I was playing a game with my then three-year-old grandson that we had invented together. I had just been looking at images of the Egyptian goddess Nut, a sky goddess who shelters the earth with her long, starry body. As we played, I was pondering the birth experience to come, for myself as a doula-grandmother and for a three-year-old about to be re-born as a big brother. It was "as if" I briefly felt the presence of Nut, and "as if" my grandson briefly experienced me as both an ordinary grandmother and as a Great Mother at the same time. I painted this image (Figure 5.4) and wrote a story next to it:

> My grandson says, "Memé, make a bridge," so I do. He rides under me, then stops, gets off the tricycle, pauses. I ask, "What's up?" He says, "I have to fix my tricycle, the wheel is broken." He climbs off and works on it for a while. I have just been looking at images of the goddess Nut. I think, he's just starting to explore outside the Mother, working on his vehicle, but needs to return often for fixing. We all need to return when it's time for more repair.

Winnicott described a new mother's experience when he wrote, "*Ordinarily* the woman enters into a phase, a phase from which she *ordinarily* recovers in the weeks and months after the baby's birth, in which to a large extent she is the baby and the baby is her" (1987, p. 6). I would call this a necessary "taking over" of a new mother's—or grandmother's —everyday ego function, a kind of inflation, even, as if she can know and do things out of the ordinary, "as if" like a goddess, temporarily, bridging conscious and unconscious. Winnicott added that the "facilitating environment" provides an "experience of omnipotence ... more than magical control ... the creative aspect of experience. Adaptation to the reality principle arises naturally out of the experience of omnipotence" (1958/1992, p. 179). Even though he is writing about infants, I would

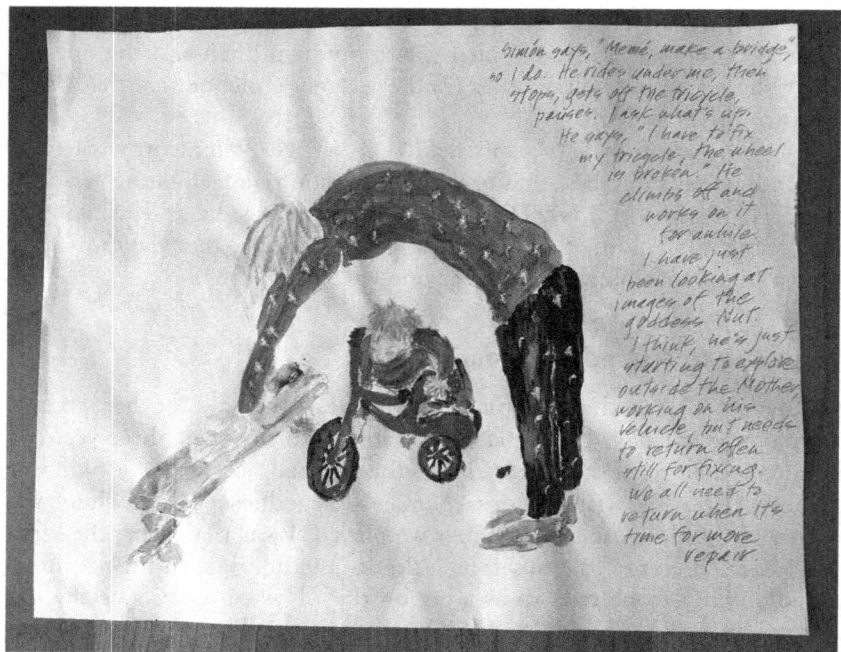

*Figure 5.4* "Becoming a Bridge" acrylics.

argue that his words apply to birthing and new mothers, as well as everyone in close proximity to a birth.

In the final painting I made to prepare for a second birth, I wanted to re-activate my body memory of attending birth, particularly the experience of feeling emotionally "held" in the presence of the Chilean midwives and passing that "holding" on to my daughter.

I found myself particularly moved by Leonardo da Vinci's painting, *The Virgin and Child with Saint Anne*, from about 1503, which shows Mary sitting on her mother Anne's wide lap. Anne's body is literally much larger than Mary's and accentuates the symbolic difference in their capacity to "hold" emotionally; Saint Anne draws on three generations of experience and body memory, which means her image can contain— or hold—more.

After studying this Renaissance masterpiece, I began to sense an image that I wanted to paint. In one way, I am embarrassed to share this painting because it is messy, incomplete, and not very well executed. In another, the image itself is impossible—how can I show myself sitting on two midwives' laps at the same time? But, it felt important to try. The goal was not a perfect work of art but rather a deepening into myself, and the painting did its job very well (Figure 5.5). And, it reflects my personal experience of becoming a grandmother, of living within—and holding—three perspectives at the same time: (1) the body memory of being a baby or child, (2) conscious memories of being a mother, and (3) becoming a supportive witness in the present as a grandmother.

In this image, I am sitting on the laps of the *matronas*, holding my pregnant daughter on my lap as she releases her young son from her own lap, letting him move on from baby to big brother. My birth task is to rest securely on the laps of the midwifery tradition, as modeled and expressed by these individual midwives, and add my strength to the shared project of holding the coming birth. (It's important to note that the view of this painting privileges *my* task, not my daughter's—her image would no doubt place her in direct contact with the midwives, her primary supports.)

I am most moved by the hands in the image. Not by how well I've painted them because they appear awkward and unnatural, but by what they recall: the naturalness of the midwives' use of hands, both literally, through constant massage, and symbolically, through warm, steady relatedness. In *Of Woman Born*, the poet Adrienne Rich (1986/1995) used an old phrase, "Hands of Flesh, Hands of Iron," as the title of

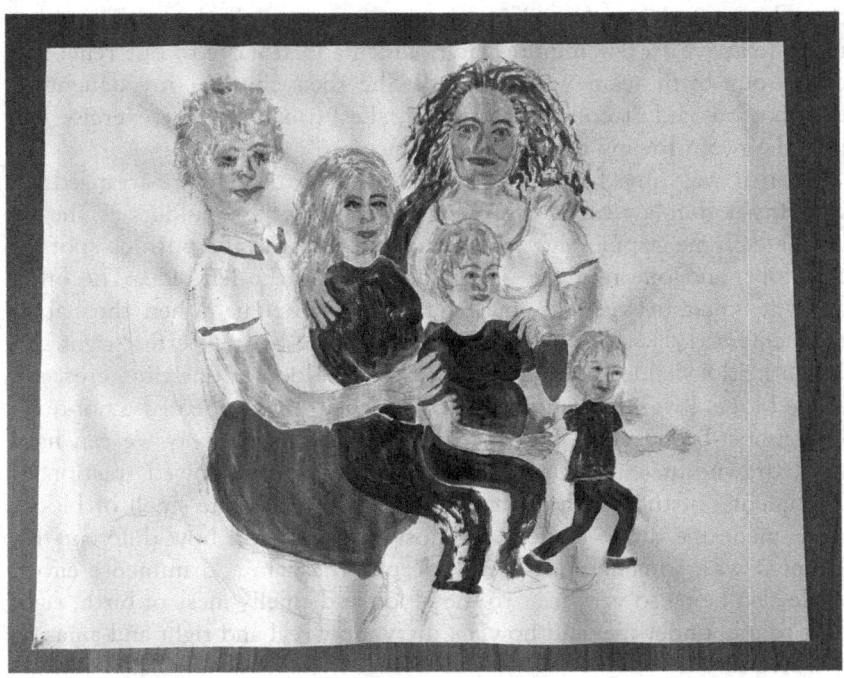

*Figure 5.5* "Sitting on the Laps of the *Matronas*" acrylics.

a chapter on the history of childbirth. Hands of flesh symbolize the midwifery model; the hands of iron are forceps, symbolizing the use of technology.

I also include, in this painting, the richly symbolic uniform of the midwives at Talagante: a white blouse with red skirt and red shoes—white, above, for the virginal girl, and red, below, for the blood of menstruation, sex, and childbirth. One midwife wore red sandals and the other low red heels—so powerful!

## Attending a Second Birth

My daughter's second birth started, again, with her water breaking in the middle of the night and progressed very quickly. I worried that the drive to the hospital might slow things down, but that didn't happen. Just as we stepped inside the hospital, there was one of the midwives, opening her arms wide. I saw my daughter slump into her, and they strode together, then, a kind of two-person unit, already, toward the labor rooms, and I followed.

The midwife's actions of efficiently arranging the room and immediately sending me to fetch the suitcase with paperwork and baby clothes in it, rather than waiting the few minutes until my son-in-law arrived, confirmed my guess that we were well into active labor. It also showed that she trusted her "read" of where we were in the labor. The other midwife arrived a few minutes later, which added more to our relief and calm—our birth team was reunited. She then checked my daughter's dilation, but didn't comment; instead, she brought a large exercise ball into the room for my daughter to bounce on.

Soon it was time for her to push, and the midwives re-arranged us, with my son-in-law behind, holding my daughter's shoulders as she sat on the ball, me gripping her right hand and acting as the pushing spot for that foot, and one midwife doing the same on the left side. The other midwife knelt between us, massaging the perineum. When the baby's head emerged, I watched, only inches from the baby's perfect right ear, which held a slender puddle of pink, watery blood in one tiny, crescent-shaped lobe. I was flooded with memory, then—enthralled by a not-quite -but-almost-born baby's bloody ear, enthralled in the way we can have long, drawn-out, elaborated thoughts even within a slowed fraction of a moment—of that birth I attended at age 19. How the smell of blood, then, made me dizzy, made me almost pass out, and how different this moment was, so calm and easeful, despite the pain and immense effort, while also being so very near to the blood and smelly mess of birth, right next to me, under me, and how *not* dizzy, how real and right and amazing this felt.

Davis-Floyd wrote, "Ritual works by sending messages to those who perform and those who receive or observe it" (2003, p. 9). In other words, ritual works mutually; it transforms both the initiates and those who hold and tend the initiatory process.

We learned only after the birth that my daughter was already seven centimeters dilated when we arrived, and that the baby was in the forehead-first position, so this was the reason for the exercise ball—to turn the baby. The midwives made a strategic decision *not* to intrude with left-brain, medical data and instead communicate nonverbally, with their bodies, right brain to right brain. Simple, positional baby-turning methods like the exercise ball were not available to my own mother because they had temporarily fallen out of the pool of birth knowledge, and because they wouldn't work with an anesthetized woman.

When I searched for an image of a woman giving birth on an exercise ball, the closest I could find was a wood engraving from 1887: this is clearly not a new position for birth but quite an old one. We also learned that this was the first time one of the midwives' patients gave birth actually on the ball—another instance of midwives improvising, allowing a woman *buscar la forma*.

## Processing Birth Experiences

I keep a handful of slots in my psychoanalytic practice open for pre- and postpartum women. For many, a traumatic birth feels like a personal failure, so we work together to tease apart what portion of that responsibility rightly belongs to them, and what might belong to the medical system that served as the cultural container for the birth. We can all practice holding birth stories as mutual, ritual experiences with our patients, mothers, and daughters, and help provide what might have been missing—informed emotional presence and consciousness. Art can help with this process, both before and after a birth.

## Note

1 Portions of this chapter were previously published as an article, "Childbirth as Initiation: *Dar a Luz*," in *Psychological Perspectives*, Vol. 63(1).

## References

Brewster, F. (2017). *African Americans and Jungian psychology: Leaving the shadows.* London: Routledge.

Davis-Floyd, R. E. (2003). *Birth as an American rite of passage* (2nd ed.). Berkeley, CA: University of California Press.

Dick-Read, G. (1959). *Childbirth without fear: The principles and practice of natural childbirth* (4th ed.). London: Pinter & Martin.

Douglas, C. (2006). *The old woman's daughter: Transformative wisdom for men and women.* College Station, TX: Texas A&M University Press.

Hunt, R. C. (1961). *Incidents in a doctor's life.* Publisher: Author.

Jordan, B. (1993). *Birth in four cultures: A crosscultural investigation of childbirth in Yucatan, Holland, Sweden, and the United States* (4th ed.). Long Grove, IL: Waveland Press.

Jung, C. G. (1970). The shadow (R. F. C. Hull, Trans.). In H. Read, M. Fordham, G. Adler, & W. McGuire (Series Ed.), *The collected works of C. G. Jung* (Vol. 9ii, 2nd ed., pp. 8–10). Princeton, NJ: Princeton University Press. (Original work published 1948)).

Moon, B. L. (2009). *Existential art therapy: The canvas mirror* (3rd ed.). Springfield, IL: Charles C Thomas.

Rich, A. (1995). *Of woman born: Motherhood as experience and institution.* (Original work published 1986). New York, NY: W. W. Norton.

Ulrich, L. T. (1990). *A midwife's tale: The life of Martha Ballard, based on her diary, 1785–1812.* New York, NY: Vintage Books.

Winnicott, D. W. (1987). *Babies and their mothers.* Reading, MA: Addison-Wesley.

Winnicott, D. W. (1992). *Through pediatrics to psycho-analysis: Collected papers.* London: Routledge. (Original work published 1958).

Ziegler, C. E. (1913). The elimination of the midwife. *JAMA, 60*(1), 32–38. doi:10.1001/jama.1913.04340010034013

# Part II

# Art Therapy

## Postpartum

# 6 Going on Being

## Losing and Finding a New Identity in the Early Phases of Treatment with Postpartum Mothers

*Linda Siegel*

Freud (1926) recognized a continuity between intra-uterine life and earliest infancy, suggesting that "the child's biological situation as a foetus is replaced by a psychical object relation to its mother" (p. 138). A continuation and a transformation of the sensory *feeling* of being inside the mother's body, a tangible feeling of being held safely and securely within the mother's womb is transformed into the feeling of being held in the postnatal womb of the mother's mind for some babies. But for the less fortunate neonates, there may be a sensory experience of a prenatal disturbance, which is tantamount to a catastrophic psychological birth (Tustin, 1983) which is likely to elicit the most primitive forms of anxiety. Thus, unbearable physiological sensations may produce the endless bodily agony of spilling, falling, dissolving, and evaporating into nothingness. A nameless dread (Bion, 1967), provoking unthinkable anxieties (Winnicott, 1960a), threatens what Winnicott refers to as *the infants' sense of "going on being"* (1960b, p. 591), and the rhythm of safety necessary for the establishment of normal object relations (Mitrani, 1995).

The transition to becoming a mother is a process that follows the primitive and profound event of giving birth, and awakens pre-oedipal conflicts. For some women, pregnancy may be one of the most enriching stages of the life cycle, if, for example, a woman's experience with her own mother has been "good enough." But for other women, the inevitable regression occasioned by pregnancy and motherhood may be a painful and frightening experience. The infantile wish to merge with the mother and the opposing fear of it, with a partial failure of self/object differentiation may be revived. Fantasies about the primary unity of mother and baby cannot be successfully integrated with adult reality where such differentiation is paramount (Bibring, Dwyer, Huntington, & Valenstein, 1961).

This focuses on the inevitable challenges of forming the new identity of mother, and respectfully acknowledges the importance of assisting women with this transition, with the goal of helping them find a self that was previously experienced as lost.

## Infant–Parent Psychotherapy

Postpartum reactions are increasingly a known and serious concern among mental health providers and a special treatment for these mothers has risen as a critical need among art therapists; more research about the use of art therapy with postpartum reactions is welcomed.

The goal of infant–parent psychotherapy, generally, is to assist the infant or toddler under age three, to achieve satisfactory socio-emotional functioning through improvement in the parent–child relationship (Lieberman, Pawl, 2008) and is conceptualized as the effort to free the baby from parental conflict. Questions of what baby, what kind of baby, and to whom are we treating is often asked. Although not self-evident, we are often treating both parent and baby. Still, the inclination is to focus on the parent as the primary patient, particularly if the parent seems significantly disturbed or distressed. Fraiberg (1961) explained that in the earliest months of life, when the infant is under the full impact of her needs, in terms of mental functioning, completely dominated by the pleasure principle, she demands one thing only from the object: that is immediate satisfaction.

## The Experience of Giving Birth

Many women experience a smooth pregnancy until just prior to birth, when the pregnant woman may be confused about whether the foetus inside her is a part of her body or something separate, and her reaction to the impending birth may include being afraid and unwilling to face the next stage of separation that birth implies .

(Daws, 1989, p. 104)

A woman's representations of her pregnancy reflect current social expectations, environmental conditions, life events, and interpretations of her own day-to-day somatic experiences, and may include residues from her past childhood identifications about her mother's procreativity, unconscious imagery of "the dark womb," and its powers of expansion and creation (Rafael-Leff, 2015, p. 4). When the transition to becoming a mother begins to set in, these pregnant women may begin to anticipate their own ways of future mothering, and is contingent on how they have "digested" and processed her own past experiences of being parented (Rafael-Leff, 2015, p. 4). These women may feel anxious and isolated. They may imagine an ideal birth, and may prepare to ensure this ideal is realized through securing birth classes, a doula, a midwife, and a lactation specialist. But, once childbirth begins, and if they have had limited emotional support during pregnancy or do not have an encouraging mother to look to for support and to discuss their anxiety and fears of childbirth, the surprising event ends in profound disappointment, often directed at themselves. Some women cling to the idea that their mother will show up as a supportive person, but when this doesn't happen, the task of the therapist then, must be to facilitate a mourning process related to an ambivalence about their relationship with their own mother. As Balint (1959) further elucidated:

> Lastly, the real aim can never be achieved by clinging. The real aim is to be held by the object and not cling desperately to it; this being held should happen without even the need to express any wish for it. It is the most cherished aim for every one of us that our environ-ment should meet our wishes, especially our wish for security, without even asking for it. To ask for security and still more, to move our object to grant us security, i.e., to cling to it, is always humiliating and inherently only a very poor second. This kind of relationship cannot but lead inevitably to ambivalence.
>
> (pp. 33–34)

I do recognize that many of these mothers have a deep longing for an ideal loving mother, a mother with whom will need to be mourned, although confronting an internal mother figure can result in intense anxiety, struggle, and pain in the first few days.

## Struggles for a Sense of Self Constancy

According to Jacobson (1964) the "self" is an abstraction used to describe our sense of identity, and is a mental phenomenon that has continuity in time and a location in space, synonymous with the special representation of our body. Many feelings, urges, and impulses are connected in our inner experience to our sense of self, so that it does not feel like an abstraction. As Sheldon Bach (2001) aptly described:

> A crucial element in the ability to evoke good enough and reliable images of self and object in times of stress underlies not only self and object constancy, but also the development of memory and the symbolic processes. This ability is crucial in the mother's ability to retain a vivid, cohesive, and reliable memory of her child, and to engage, in a multitude of ways, in a process of mutual holding. And, where this process is deficient, the child and later the adult may experience discontinuities of the self, which find expression in profound anxieties, phobias, and problems of memory and learning. And as these discontinuities are revived in the transference and the countertransference, both patient and therapist must work together to keep each other reliably alive in memory.
>
> (p. 437)

With Bach's idea in mind, "the therapist must also constantly bear the anxiety of the unknown" (Lombardi, 2017, p. 168) that sometimes floods the dyad; transitory states of confusion in the therapeutic relationship, according to Lombardi, "should be considered an actual tool, which can facilitate in-depth communication so that we can utilize our *reverie*" (p. 142). The confusion process of giving birth and transitioning into becoming a new mother can stir memories of one's early years with her own mother and various childhood experiences. Discontinuities in self-experience, possibly resulting in an anxiety related to a fear of disappearing, are exacerbated by the birth. Ogden (Ogden, 1999) wrote that "in a psychological field in which the individual has little if any sense of internal space, the concept of internalization becomes virtually meaningless" (p. 72). On the other hand, "it is possible to create a place in which the patient can feel, through bodily sensations, that she exists" (p. 130).

Art therapy has much to offer. The art therapist can detect the verbal and nonverbal cues, which can be examined within the artistic parameters of sight, sound and motion, specifically rhythms, and in color, texture, and form. "Our work is about making the inanimate animate, giving form to diffuse energy or ideas, in essence, breathing life into sterile communications" (Robbins, 1989, p. 44), and keeping the session and the memories of one another alive. My work focuses on and utilizes many senses, as I will discuss in the next section that I refer to as "Kinesthetic Holding."

## Kinesthetic Holding

Much has been written about how creating art in the presence of an art therapist is a valuable tool, particularly because artmaking engages both the mind and the body. Robbins (1998) reminded us that for the therapist to be present with our patients, we must be open and receptive to both primary and secondary modes of the communication process, including being able to shift ego states. Furthermore, "we must be comfortable with a holistic, intuitive, and receptive orientation that is essentially spatial" (p. 19). Engaging the mind and body in this work is critical. When thinking about Cane (1951), who wrote, "Because the need to 'shape everything without,' the artist in each of us comes into being," (p. 21) so too, can the mother "come into being" through the process of engaging in kinesthetic artmaking.

I observe the interactions between mother and baby and look for a connection between them. I may encourage the mother to stay with the bodily sensations if I detect stress or tension. As Davis (2015) outlined: Being able to notice and be present with what a strong emotion feels like—fear, for example, can interrupt the cycle before it runs rampant. This entails the development of reflexive skills (p. 43).

An intervention with image forming or artmaking can be useful in accessing an "embodied" experience. Embodiment, as stated by Kossak (2015), "includes an awareness of breath, movement impulses, sensation and associative emotions and can be directly linked to psychological states of being" (p. 37). Sometimes I encourage intentional breathing in sessions. Breathing can be used as a technique for bringing a person into the present moment, and later as a starting point for optimizing engagement in the creative process (Kossak, 2015).

> Breathing is inherently connected to a rhythm, which influenced our first experiences of human creativity. The practice of breathing with artmaking can increase expression and promote the experience of connecting mind and body in a more fluid way, and gives us a multimodal experience of integration.
>
> (Siegel, 2019, pp. 252–253)

I have come to refer to what I describe previously as "the rhythm of art therapy." I may instruct my clients to find form in the breath, for example, and draw that. It may be difficult to find a form, but a few tries helps the woman find a form that reminds her of her life with the breath. I encourage exploration of quick breath to feel a restriction, and long, deep breath to feel more expansion. I also incorporate other senses, such as sound, and instruct her to restrict her throat on the out-breath, so that the breath sounds like an ocean, an AAHHH like sound, so she can "hear" her breath (2019, p. 264). These variations give the woman an opportunity to feel differences in expansion and contraction, and most importantly, as is related to psychological states, she can and does breathe. She can notice differences throughout her day and be with those experiences.

Images of being held, pressed to a mother's warm body, sensing its smell and movements, and of being carried, rocked, and caressed, sometimes fill my own mind and stimulate my imagination when the mother is breast feeding in session, and I become aware of the hungry baby in me. Lombardi (2017) explained that the primacy of sensory pressure comes to light from working though, and creates a connection with bodily experience. The therapist, then, must operate on the same unorganized levels. Lombardi referred to this as "somatic countertransference." The therapist may be containing in her own body, the pre-symbolic sensory manifestations that predate mental phenomena. "The somatic countertransference is the therapist's transference into her own body, and is a prerequisite for the therapist's working through" (p. 35). The "breast" is the term commonly used by therapists to identify the total reality experienced by an infant. The breast is, on the one hand, a source of nourishment, and, on the other, an object that fills; its skin is warm and soft to the touch and it is also an active, stimulating receptacle. The mother's breast is the "earliest mental object" (Anzieu, 2016, p. 42).

In his early writings, Bion emphasized what the mother does for the infant: the infant evacuates an internal emotional experience (1962, 1967), into the mother, who digests what has been projected, and gives it back to the baby in a more palatable state, not unlike a mother bird pre-masticating food for her newly hatched offspring (in Brown, 2011). When I introduce artmaking, I can also be the mother who "pre-chews" and makes more absorbable something creative, on her behalf. The therapist and the mother feed each other.

## Holding States of Mind

When the baby is present in the session, it is important that the role of the mother not be taken away. Yet, the mother can be both the baby and the mother, these two things co-exist. The therapist must remain sensitive to the fact that she is a mother and a baby, that she can be both with the therapist, although, it is not always clear as to who is who. The oscillating movement of losing and finding the mother state of mind and the baby state of mind need careful holding respectfully, and can be both the challenge and the focus of the work.

The idea of a "holding" and a "containing" state of mind are drawn from infant observation. Pam Sorenson (1997) distinguished "containing process," from containment, thus emphasizing that the containing process, "which is observed in regular mother-baby interactions, is active rather than passive in nature and is a complex, subtle, and lively mental activity that contributes to the work of a containing mind" (p. 13). The various ways I "hold" the mother, while in the presence of the baby, or otherwise, functions as a modeling for the mother. Incorporating art into the session requires a "transition into" new ways of feeling and expression, and it is through artistic expression that we can hope to keep in touch with our primitive selves. I work bit by bit, staying aware of what the mother can "metabolize," in some ways, like an infant. My thinking is that we do not feed baby solid foods because her system cannot digest those foods. And thus, with the mother, my inclination is to introduce artmaking slowly, so she can metabolize the experience.

I offer different types of materials that have texture, and I have her make "rubbings." When paper is placed over the textured item, she rubs the surface of the paper with charcoal or chalk pastels. What is emerging? What are the patterns? This offers a kinesthetic experience, and she can add to it, and also change the patterns. "Holding" with materials and "holding" directives is familiar to art therapists. I use Model Magic, a soft, pliable material for shaping into containers or for embedding objects that are "held" in the material or for making imprints, and I have her think about the imprint as a fossil, something that has existed a very long time. I also have on hand, chenille pipe cleaners that are colorful, bendable, sensuous, and fluffy. She can bend the pipe cleaners into some type of container, and easily change the shape, expand it or shrink it down. The pipe cleaners are bended and twisted together, creating a basket-like shape. What is intertwined? What can be held in the form?

Many women like to make books from a variety of collage materials and sometimes personal photographs: Before and After themes. These are a few examples of ways to incorporate art into the sessions with this work. More kinesthetic artmaking suggestions will follow in another section.

## Do I Exist?

Some women may be plagued with wondering whether they still exist after the birth. This anxiety seems to be related to a fear of annihilation, and I became aware that this is often related to the temporary feeling of being lost. This is a big part of prenatal anxiety—adjusting to wandering/lost/annihilation anxiety. As Swan-Foster (2012) wrote, "Her need to create a 'home' or 'nest' for *other* may constellate a wandering" (p. 229). Klein (1946) considered the death instinct the source of annihilation, as the basis for anxiety, and posited that the infant's central problem comes from the presence within the infant of the "death instinct," a genetically constituted endowment. Fairbairn (1963), on the other hand, did not believe there is a death instinct, and that aggression is a reaction to frustration and deprivation. Additionally, he reminded us that the earliest and original form of anxiety, as experienced by the child, is separation anxiety. Some women experience an anxiety related to a fear of dying, resulting in sleeplessness. I use the sound of my voice to decrease anxiety, help with grounding, and as a reminder that she exists, and would, in fact, go on living. I also sometimes sing a lullaby to the mother, as this may awaken the baby (in the mother) and the baby (in the room), if it is sleeping.

## While Baby Sleeps

Fears of losing oneself can happen while the baby is sleeping. Considering the idea of regulation brings me to the relevance of Beebe and Lachman (2002) in this context, who refers to three similar terms of regulation: mutual regulation, bidirectonal regulation, and co-constructed regulation. Beebe and Lachman explained that these terms mean that contingencies flow in both directions between partners, in other words, the behavior of each partner is contingent on, "influenced" by, or "predicted" by that of the other (p. 27). Clinically, it is interesting for us to consider that the physical space between mother and baby exacerbates, in the mother, an experience of not being real, perhaps related to a missing of this mutual regulation Beebe carefully researched and wrote about. Or perhaps the baby in the mother, in this context, struggles with differentiating between what is inside and what is outside, like babies, and therefore what is real and what is not real. The space in-between the two of them can be felt as too vast, and is a place where forgetting where she is and who she is (as though she was still suspended in the timelessness of giving birth—an experience she has not yet reconciled) triggers the symbiotic orbit that is wished for. The sleeping baby causes the mother to feel "left" and lost, and even one's maternal pre-occupation with the sleeping baby cannot help the mother feel contained in her body or mind. Bach (2001) wrote:

> It can be a burden and a worrisome responsibility for a parent and a child to hold each other closely in mind, witness the presence, not only of pain, but also mutual liberation when children finally leave home. While there is a need and desire to be remembered by the parent, there is also a need to forget and be forgotten, to be released from the bonds of memory, to soar to freedom, or to sink into the oblivion of sleep.
>
> (p. 11)

Still, for the mothers I refer to in this chapter, my hypothesis is that, while awake, that is to say, not sleeping, the physical contact between mother and baby, and the mother's experience of love and reverie becomes a mutual, co-created regulation, which keeps both mother and baby alive. And more so, while baby sleeps, my contact with the mother becomes the mutual regulation that keeps her alive while baby sleeps.

## Going on Being

I recognize my focus on maintaining a regulating, rhythmic presence in this work, and that the frequency and constancy of my contact in the early weeks, can enable the mother to survive each day and to experience "the going on being." Establishing a rhythm in the early weeks and months of the treatment is important, much like the mother-baby rhythms that Winnicott (1960b) so eloquently described. I understand rhythms to include nonverbal communications, including where I position myself, the tone of my voice, and my keeping the baby in mind. This can actually be considered a technique, which Ogden (1999) described as an "implicit (rather than explicit, sic) presentation of countertransference" (p. 129). Damasio (1994) indicated "the dynamic role that the sensory flow plays in the body-mind relationship in establishing mental activity and self-awareness, with the result that the mind is not conceivable without some sort of embodiment" (p. 234). Lombardi (2017) suggested that we must consider what the music of our bodies generate or the unheard melodies (2017) of our proto-sensory states (p. 19).

Robbins (1989) wrote that the movement and music of treatment is woven into our work, as we tune into our sensitivity and become alert to the patient's intonations, emotional resonance, and the responsiveness, as well as their bodily expressions. He continued, "The nonverbal nuances congeal into an image and organize this very complex structure of form, space, and time. These images then become the core language of our senses and emotions that filters into the transitional space of treatment" (p. 198).

The mother's and the therapist's role in safeguarding the continuity of the infant's or child's experience of being and becoming over time is well known and at the core of Winnicott's (1960a) concept of "holding," and that psychological development is a process in which the infant or child increasingly takes on the mother's function of maintaining the continuity of her experience of being alive. Maturation, from this perspective, entails the development of the infant or child's capacity to generate and maintain for herself a sense of the continuity of her being over time, a time that increasingly reflects a rhythm that is experienced by the infant or child as outside of her control (Ogden, 2004).

Establishing a rhythm through these processes of holding helps construct a cohesive representation of me, as the therapist, and also helped me as the therapist, to construct a cohesive representation of the mother. The frequency of sessions over time helps to create a visual sense of continuity that is essential in establishing a deep transference. It is also evident that providing the mother with these early experiences of being and becoming over time is essential so that the mother can provide this for her baby. So, therefore, the therapist must keep both mother and baby in mind, while the mother "holds" onto baby is a regularly re-visited phenomena as I have addressed from different perspectives.

## Losing and Finding/Separating and Re-Uniting

Repetitive separating and reuniting of the mother and baby, is a reminder of the *Hide and Seek* game, a more elaborate form of peek-a-boo, and, of course, a variant of the Fort Da game played by Freud's 18-month-old grandson (Freud, 1915). This game is understood as

> a common childhood creation that usually begins in the second year of life (Kaplan, 1995), when the child is becoming accustomed to the mother's comings and goings, and the game becomes a way for the child to both express and master this potential threat to their identity.
>
> (Bergman, 1999, p. 419)

As the peek-a-boo games develop into more elaborate games of hiding and finding, certain characteristics remain constant; the need to repeat the game over and over again, the excitement with which the game is played, the manageable amount of anxiety about being found and not being found, or about finding or not finding, the surprise that exists even if the result is well known and repeated over and over again, and finally, the joy of reunion to master the object loss that is entailed in the process of separation-individuation and the achievement of self-object differentiation (Bergman, 1999).

Another game that is understood as a sophisticated game of hide and seek is Winnicott's own Squiggle Game, which is described (1963) as "a child's establishing a private self that is not communicating and at the same time wanting to communicate and to be found" (p. 86). Winnicott believed that this search for a private self, that is to say, the searching and the hiding, is the tension of opposites that formed the life-and-death struggle of the work in which we may, as therapists, be asked to help find what the patient is looking for. On the other hand, and possibly referring to Winnicott, Kahn (1989) wrote, "Only the genius finds what he is looking for, the rest of us have to be content with re-discovering the discovered" (p. 13). There is an element of surprise in being found and surprise is central to Winnicott's conceptualization of playing. Winnicott (1971) stressed that "it is in playing and only playing that the child or adult is able to be creative and use the whole personality, and it is only in being creative that the individual discovers the self" (p. 54).

## Kinesthetic Artmaking

This section provides suggestions for what I am calling kinesthetic artmaking in the early stages of treatment with postpartum mothers. There are likely many other possibilities.

1.  Seiden's (2001) activity of scribbling, or spilling, drawing or painting, as if you are a child, is a powerful and playful way for the woman to experience her child self, and to develop empathy for herself and to assist her in imaging her baby growing into a child.
2.  Model Magic is a soft, pliable material that is easy to use. Color can be added with markers and for a marbling effect, and it dries hard for painting. You can ask the woman to "sculpt the baby you" or make a fossil from an object that is imprinted in the material, or form into a shape where you can embed objects that can be "held", or sculpt a bowl or container
3.  Utilizing Winnicott's Squiggle Game idea, an example of play.
4.  I have on hand a variety of pipe cleaners, specifically the thick chenille pipe cleaners that are soft and sensuous.

5. Drawing Breath—this exercise combines breathing exercises with drawing. Adding the senses to include sound, movement, use of space by turning the 2D drawings into 3D sculpture using tissue paper or pipe cleaners, adds dimension. Bubbles can also be added for another sense experience of "catching the breath" (Siegel, 2019).

6. Collage and picture journal book—have on hand a variety of materials for book and collage making. The book can be kept with the therapist or taken home to work on if requested. This exercise gives the woman time to reflect on her daily and weekly experiences and to keep as a memento.

7. Any kind of artmaking that address Before and After themes is useful.

## Conclusion

Re-enacting needs to be found and when discovered can be utilized in treatment to facilitate the ability to carry or hold a memory or representation of a woman's self in a connected way, and the art functions as a transitional object. Wishes to be found as both a mother and a woman with her own identity may bring these women to therapy, but fears and terrors of not being found, and not finding her "new self," results in an inability to form a constant self. The hiding and seeking, so to say, of the therapeutic relationship enables a process of mastery in life, which includes a dawning awareness of the object loss, and continues into her new identity. Through the experience of finding a new object from the therapeutic relationship, and utilizing the creative process with the use of images and artmaking, results in a feeling of a more constant self within her, because, as Winnicott's writes, (1988) "she had found me, used me, forgotten me repeatedly, lost me, and over time, found herself" (p. 103). And as Michael Eigen writes (2013), "one is not found until lost. The other is not discovered until vanished."

Life is ever changing, but love provides a constancy. When we love our work, feel a love for our patients that translates into love and caring for them, and believe in creativity, we give ourselves a constancy, which enables us to "go on being" in our lives and as therapists.

## References

Anzieu, D. (2016). *The skin ego: A new translation by Naomi Segal*. London, England: Karnac.

Bach, S. (2001). On being forgotten and forgetting one's self. *Psychoanalytic Quarterly, 70,* 739–756.

Balint, M. (1959). *Thrills and regressions*. London, England: Maresfield Library.

Beebe, B., & Lachman, F. (2002). *Infant research and adult treatment*. Atlantic City, NJ: The Analytic Press.

Bergman, A. (1999). *Ours, yours, mine: Mutuality and the emergence of the separate self.* Lanham, MD: Jason Aronson.

Bibring, G. I., Dwyer, T. F., Huntington, D. S., & Valenstein, A. F. (1961). A study of the psychological processes in pregnancy and the of the earliest mother-child relationship. *Psychoanalytic Study of the Child, 16,* 9–24.

Bion, W. R. (1967). *Second thoughts.* London, England: Karnac.

Bion, W.R. (1962). *Learning from experience.* New York: Basic Books.

Brown, L. (2011). *Intersubjective process and the unconscious: An integration of Freudian, Kleinian and Bionian perspectives.* London, England: Routledge.

Cane, F. (1951). *The artist in each of us.* Washington, DC: Baker-Webster Printing Company.

Damasio, A. (1994). *Decarte's error: Emotion, reason, and the human brain.* New York: G.P. Putnam's Sons.

Davis, B. J. (2015). *Mindful art therapy: A foundation for practice.* London, England: Jessica Kingsley.

Daws, D. (1989). *Through the night: Helping parents and sleepless infants.* London, England: Free Association Books.

Eigen, M. (2013). Meigenworkshop. Retrieved from www.yahoogroups.com

Fairbairn, W. D. (1963). Synopsis of an object relating theory of the personality. *International Journal of Psychoanalysis, 44,* 224–225.

Fraiberg, S. (1961). *The magic years.* New York, NY: Charles Scribner's Sons.

Freud, S. (1915). Instincts and Their Vicissitudes. *Standard Edition, 14,* 111–140.

Freud, S. (1926). Inhibitions, symptoms and anxiety. *Standard Edition, 20,* pp. 77–174.

Jacobson, E. (1964). *The self and the object world.* New York, NY: International Universities Press.

Kahn, M. M. R. (1989). *Alienation and perversions.* London, England: Karnac.

Kaplan, L. (1995). *No voice is ever wholly lost.* New York, NY: Simon & Schuster.

Klein, M. (1946). Notes of some shizoid mechanisms. *International Journal of Psychoanalysis, 27,* 99–110.

Kossak, M. (2015). *Attunement in expressive arts therapy: Toward an understanding of embodied empathy.* Springfield, IL: Charles C. Thomas Publisher.

Lieberman, A., & Van Horn, P. (2008). *Psychotherapy with infants and young children: Repairing the effects of stress and trauma on early attachment.* New York, NY: Guilford Press.

Lombardi, R. (2017). *Body-mind dissociation in psychoanalysis.* London, England: Routledge.

Mitrani, J. L. (1995). Toward an understanding of unmentalized experience. *Psychoanalytic Quarterly, 64,* 68–112.

Ogden, T. H. (1999). *Reverie and interpretation: Sensing something human.* London: Karnac.

Ogden, T. H. (2004). On holding and containing, being and dreaming. *International Journal of Psychoanalysis, 85,* 1349–1364.

Rafael-Leff, J. (2015). *The dark side of the womb: Pregnancy, parenting, & persecutory anxieties.* London, England: The Anna Freud Centre.

Robbins, A. (1989). *The psychoaesthetic experience: An approach to depth-oriented treatment.* New York, NY: Human Sciences Press.

Robbins, A. (1998). *Therapeutic presence: Bridging expression and form.* London, England: Jessica Kingsley Publishers.

Seiden, D. (2001). *Mind over matter: The uses of materials in art, education and therapy*. Chicago, IL: Magnolia Street Publishers.

Siegel, L. (2019). Drawing breath: Breathing into the rhythm and form of art therapy. *American Imago, 76,* 251–267.

Sorenson, P. (1997). Thoughts on the containing process from the perspective of infant/mother relations. In S. Reid (Ed.), *Developments in infant observation: The Tavistock model* (pp. 113–122). London, England: Routledge.

Swan-Foster, N. (2012). Pregnancy as a feminine initiation. *Journal of Prenatal and Perinatal Psychology and Health, 26*(4), 207–236.

Tustin, F. (1983). *Autistic states in children*. London, England: Routledge.

Winnicott, D. W. (1960a). Ego distortion in terms of true and false self. In *The maturational processes and the facilitating environment* (pp. 139–152). London, England: Karnac.

Winnicott, D. W. (1960b). The theory of the parent-infant relationship. *International Journal of Psychoanalysis, 41,* 585–595.

Winnicott, D. W. (1963). Communicating and not communicating leading to a study of certain opposites. In *Maturational processes and the facilitating environment* (pp. 178–192). London: Hogarth. 1965. Reprint. London: Karnac, 1990.

Winnicott, D. W. (1971). *Therapeutic Consultations in Child Psychiatry*. London: Hogarth. Reprint. London: Karnac, 1996.

Winnicott, D. W. (1988). *Babies and their mothers*. London, England: Free Association.

# 7 Perinatal Mood and Anxiety Disorder

## Processing Trauma through Couples' Art Therapy

*Alison Silver*

At the peri/postpartum mood and anxiety center where I have worked for over five years, I offer creative arts therapy to individuals, couples, and groups. This program is a part of maternal health and wellness within a larger hospital system but held within a local hospital at the Jersey Shore. I was brought on during the induction of the program as the Trauma Specialist and Creative Arts Therapist to assist mothers in processing their new identities and roles. This, in turn, led to the exploration of how the mothers may have felt compromised during the birth of their child, and at times, during conception. One of my roles is to find a unique art therapy method for each individual, group or couple so they might gain insight into and process the trauma that has occurred during the birth process.

Although I am extensively trained in trauma work, my own experience with a traumatic personal hospitalization gave me greater insight into how mothers were storing and holding on to their own traumas and why. In this chapter I will refer to one couple with whom I have worked for over two and half years. The couple has a unique history and is laden with complex childhood trauma. I will refer to this couple as "Joe and Melissa" and will disguise certain details to maintain confidentiality

## Current Status of Perinatal Mental Health

Before we look at clinical examples or how the center is organized, let's examine how peri/postpartum is defined in our current mental health field. According to the *DSM-V*, "Postpartum" has been categorized as an "Other Specified Depressive Disorder":

Major Depressive Disorder with postpartum onset:
    Presentations in which symptoms characteristics of a depressive disorder that causes clinically significant distress or impairment in social, occupational, or other important areas of functioning. Due to the predominate criteria being met the unspecified category affords the

clinician to not specify and includes presentations that may have insufficient information for a more specified diagnosis.

With peripartum onset: This specifier can be applied to the current or, if full criteria are not currently met for a major depressive episode, most recent episode of major depression if onset of mood symptoms occurs during pregnancy or in the 4 week following delivery.

(American Psychiatric Association, 2013, pp. 184–187)

By this definition, I ponder the criteria used in the specification of maternal wellness and have a feeling that my population is being viewed as an afterthought or an addendum to an umbrella term of "Depression." My clients, who undergo an antenatal disturbance, often experience these symptoms as a form of humiliation and shame. If they are somehow not experiencing an idealistic "glow" of becoming a mother and adapting instantaneously to the new identity that motherhood has thrust upon them, then they are left feeling "less than" and cannot complete the conceptual image in their heads of what motherhood should be.

The common themes that I witness when working with clients are control (or lack of control), identity, intimacy, and boundaries, which have all been compromised during the transition into motherhood. I often express to the mothers that these themes have been problematic prior to having their child but have since been magnified. Due to these disjointed ideals, my clients often feel like they are alone in a less-than-suitable medical and insurance system, and are fighting for their sanity within the confines and parameters of society. I believe this realm of women's mental healthcare continues to personify and magnify the holes in our capacity as a system to treat proactively rather than reactively. Our society as a whole holds a myopic view to healthcare compared to other countries, such as Sweden, Norway, and Denmark. These Nordic countries provide longer paid leave, and some countries provide new mothers with an at-home nurse for the first few weeks of the newborns' life to assist with medical care, nightly duties, and education.

## Program Structure

To address some of these issues, the peri/postpartum program, led by Lisa Tremayne, RN, and Pat Vena, LCSW, is a labor of love that is determined to attain services for women and families who are undergoing the symptoms of peri/postpartum depression, anxiety and mood disorders. The center provides a yearlong program (approximately) that begins at the birth of the child; sometimes the program begins at conception if persistent symptoms are inhibiting the day-to-day activities for the mother-to-be. If a mother comes to the program during pregnancy, the timeline for services still remains in place and the program will continue for that family for one year, postpartum, or until the child's first birthday. The program includes a multidisciplinary approach to assist the whole family system rather than just the individual or the identified patient. The center offers numerous services including but not limited to: lactation support groups, peer-to-peer support groups, infant CPR, introduction to first foods classes, trauma support groups, and individual sessions. Other services include baby care basics, mother/infant bonding sessions/classes, infant massage, creative arts therapy (individual, couples and group), DBT coping skills group, sleep training, medication evaluation, and management, psychiatric evaluations, and referrals to supportive services.

The large pool of skilled clinicians ranges from APNs, RNs, and Social Workers to Licensed Massage Therapists (pregnancy and infant specialized) and a Lactation Specialist. I provide creative arts therapy within the program's holistic model. The peri/postpartum program is the first within the United States to attain the Platinum Level Maternal Mental Health Friendly Certification (MMHF), a new criteria for standard of care that has been based upon the Ten Canons of Care (Figure 7.1).

In addition, as one of 23 facilities across the United States with a postpartum Maternal Mental Health program (ranging from Inpatient Perinatal Psychiatric Programs to Outpatient Perinatal Mental Health programs), our hospital has the only program that offers the latest FDA approved infusion to combat the symptoms of Postpartum Depression. The hormone infusion of brexanolone—a neuroactive steroid gamma-aminobutyric acid (GABA) and a receptor positive modulator—that is administered for 60 continuous hours. Eight of our postpartum mothers (after the center underwent a rigorous sequence of discussions with their insurance providers) were cleared to participate in an inpatient medical infusion process. These eight mothers were utilizing the PMADs program, but had seen little to no improvement in their mental well-being since the beginning of the outpatient program, even after approximately two to six months of individual and group facilitations. As such, they were introduced to the latest intervention through family discussions and an infusion information series. All eight women have seen a dramatic difference in their mental health as soon as 12 hours from the start of the infusion. The change has been extraordinary. From the onset, these mothers presented flat and apathetic and now have transformed to bright and passionate about life, love, and their new identities as mothers.

## The Group Dynamic and Melissa

One of the ways I work with mothers is to explore, in a group dynamic, how they might be storing and holding on to their own traumas and why. I first met with Melissa for two hours twice a week (on Mondays and Wednesdays) for a few months within a group setting. The group

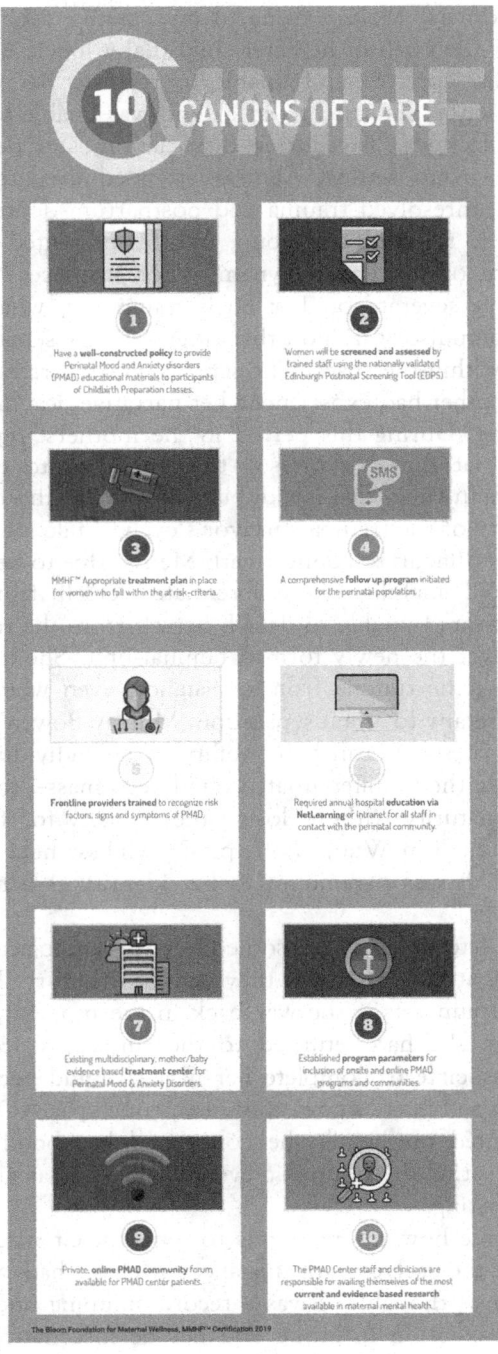

*Figure 7.1* "The Ten Canons of Care."

consisted of 12 women who utilized art therapy to process their new identities as mothers. Melissa came to my creative arts therapy group just weeks after the birth of her first child (Baby Joey). At first, Melissa presented as disassociated and unable to regulate her emotions. She would cry as soon as she tried to speak and was unable to maintain eye contact. Her affect was flat during dissociation, and depressed when present in the group setting. Melissa attended the group for many weeks, but her unresolved trauma and postpartum depression made it difficult for her to fully use the group, and this presented challenges due to the structure of the group dynamic. For instance, Melissa would unconsciously perseverate on her birth trauma in, what appeared to present as, a compulsory fashion that often left her separated from the other mothers within the space. The separation occurred due to the fact that no other mother had experienced her narrative, leaving no space for empathy to exist. During this period in the mothers' reparative thera-peutic work, I, at times, witnessed their inability to expel empathy toward another. In time, this is exhibited slowly, as though the partici-pants grew weary of the trauma survivor's cyclical tale.

It was initially difficult to connect with Melissa due to her unconscious identification and inability to differentiate herself from the (birth) trauma. She appeared unable to detach herself from the trauma and the effects it held over the newly formed familial unit. She definitely had difficulty viewing the trauma from a distance, even when utilizing the process of art therapy to attain separation. Murray Bowen explained that "differentiation of self [means] the ability of an individual to separate emotionally from the undifferentiated family ego mass—to achieve inde-pendence and maturity without losing the capacity for free emotional connection" (as cited in Wiley, 1991, p. 32). Melissa held her trauma so close, as though it was paramount to her identity as a mother and as a wife.

One way to determine where someone is psychologically with their trauma is to pay attention to how they convey the story. Melissa would talk about her trauma as if she was back in the moment, reliving each detail as though she had returned to the surgical space. She would immediately dissociate to complete her narrative and become mentally distant, seeming to "float" above the therapeutic space. Once her beha-viors were pointed out while she considered her bodily and mental reactions to revisiting the traumatic events, Melissa was able to identify the feeling of floating.

We can also see how trauma tends to replay itself when reoccurring themes present themselves. For instance, Melissa had a tendency to repeat her story as though she was a record skipping under the stylus. Due to her presentation in group and her defense mechanism of dis-sociation, I was not surprised to learn that Melissa also had complex childhood trauma(s). She grew up in a home with physical and emotional abuse, an alcoholic father, and a mother who had her boyfriend living (alongside her father) within the family/marital home. Throughout her youth and young adulthood, Melissa endured physical assaults from her mother and sexual assaults from her own boyfriend; she underwent an abortion at a young age, and had three significant head traumas that necessitated hospitalizations.

As Melissa moved through life, she continued to preserve the complex trauma of parental alcoholism and emotional and physical abuse that she endured during her childhood close to her. When she graduated from college, Melissa met her now husband, Joe, dated him exclusively, and then moved into his condo. After she moved in with Joe, Melissa recognized signs of alcohol abuse but ignored Joe's incessant inebriation because "it did not look like her father's drinking." Joe was also able to provide for Melissa economically and exist within societal norms; both of these were qualities that Melissa's father could never withstand for long durations. Joe and Melissa got married and after years of repeated overindulgences with alcohol, Melissa gave Joe an ultimatum, "Our marriage, our love, our future together … or drinking." Joe gave up alcohol cold turkey, immediately joined AA, and established a sober life style that he continues to this day.

## Melissa's Birth Story

When Melissa came to the center, like many of the moms I work with, she had a detailed birth plan that included every last element the couple could imagine. However, Melissa was overly identified with the plan and could not entertain any divergent possibilities should her childbirth take a different path, revealing a habitual way of defending against the unknown or uncertainty in life. According to Simkin (2011),

> The propensity to develop post birth PTSD has to do with how women felt they were treated in labor, whether they felt in control, whether they panicked or felt angry during labor, whether they dissociated, and whether they suffered 'mental defeat' (i.e., they gave up, [felt] overwhelmed, hopeless, and as if they could not go on) .
>
> (p. 168)

Melissa was the first to tell the group that her "birth went terribly wrong and I was completely out of control." All of the mothers could connect and empathize with Melissa's acknowledgement because, even though they did not undergo a traumatic birth experience, their birth plans also did not go as designed.

As Melissa was giving birth, she was unable to proceed with a vaginal delivery as Baby Joey was not progressing through the birth canal. Baby Joey was in duress/distress and the medical team deemed a cesarean section to be the best option for the safety of both mother and child. But the next moments went quickly and there was no time for Melissa or Joe to process what was happening or decide on their own what the next steps should be in the birth of their child.

After the cesarean section, Melissa had a postpartum hemorrhage. The emergency happened quickly and the room filled with doctors and medical staff. The medical staff went into hyper drive to keep Melissa alive. Melissa recalls the moment with clarity and acuity of thought: "At this moment I knew I was going to die and I was at peace with it." Joe and Baby Joey were rushed into a triage room that had multiple beds separated by a curtain. This was the room where families who had just given birth stayed until they could go to their individual rooms. In no uncertain terms Joe referred to the room as a "cold and isolating space" where he was continually overwhelmed by "the sounds of new parents just beyond the flimsy curtains that encased [him]."

As Joe sat with his new son on his chest, skin to skin, as Melissa had requested in their birth plan, he was alone in shock and awaited any news of the health and well-being of his wife. Stramrood et al. (2013) explained that "witnesses of traumatic birth, such as partners and health care providers, also have a risk of developing PTSD and depression" (p. 3). Joe recalled feeling terribly upset as he could hear the families on either side having the experience he had dreamed of: the idealized image of the mother in bed with the child on her chest and the partner cooing over them both in utter awe over the miraculous event that had transpired. Joe continued to witness the experiences that he resented and grew jealous of as he sat and waited ... waited ... waited to hear anything from the hospital staff.

While Joe waited, he heard the final words of his wife resounding through his head, "Goodbye, I love you!" As we understand from his self-reports, he remained in shock from his experience and this traumatic state isolated him from family or any source of normalcy. According to Scheepstra, van Steijn, Dijksman, and van Pampus (2017), "Traumatic birth may not only have major consequences for the patient, but also for their partners" (p. 3). As Joe remained in the triage room, the medical team worked diligently to stabilize Melissa. She received multiple blood transfusions due to extensive blood loss from the postpartum hemorrhage. Melissa retained no memory from this point forward and had only spotty recollection of what transpired prior to being anesthetized. However, this is not uncommon as "anesthesia causes unconsciousness by suppressing neural mechanisms mediating arousal and awareness. It also causes amnesia by disrupting mechanisms of memory consolidation" (Glannon, 2014, p. 651).

## Identity, Control, Motherhood, and Loss of Voice

Once Melissa became a client of the PMADs center, I became witness to her repeated efforts to fill in the pieces of lost time and gaps due to the anesthesia. Dunning, Harris, and Sandall (2016) said that "women who had experienced a severe PPH had tried to make sense of the emergency once back home. Some adopted information seeking behaviors afterwards" (p. 5). During an individual art therapy session, Melissa and I attempted cognitive memory retrieval by creating a structured timeline that would make sense to her.

Yet, when Melissa sat in the group, she would repeatedly recall her birth trauma and rigidly hold on to it, even if the conversation was focused on concepts of identity, control, motherhood, or loss of voice. Looking back over her birth narrative, we can see where each of these concepts lies heavy upon her recollection and why she was unable to separate any of these thoughts that transgressed as she moved from birth to postpartum or peripartum. Melissa *had no voice* due to the circumstances surrounding her birth story; she was unable to experience the beginning of *motherhood* as she was unconscious during that period. She lost *control* of the birth experience as soon as she and the baby became distressed, and her *identity* had been stripped from her as she repeatedly disassociated from her body. The disassociation made her unable to understand who she was as an individual. I understood this to be a developmental impedance due to the complex trauma of parental alcoholism and emotional and physical abuse that she endured during her childhood. In other words, the triggering effects that occurred as she gave birth reenacted some aspects of and fit into the concepts of the complex traumas Melissa had undergone throughout her life.

## Individual Art Therapy

After months of group work, Melissa started individual art therapy where we focused on her trauma history. First, we verbally reviewed her traumatic history and together explored what details she held on to and why. In particular, we considered what she gained by holding on to certain memories and what she might imagine she'd gain if she did not identify so closely to these trauma memories.

Melissa then began to create a visual timeline as a map of her life that allowed her to see the progression of events. In this directive, by International Association of Trauma Professionals Family Trauma certification, the individual begins to see where the holes and trauma triggers exist. The timeline also affords the client a tangible piece of evidence to concretize events and receive instrumental validation from the witness. After reviewing her initial timeline, I witnessed that Melissa only marked or represented moments that she clarified and deemed as negative moments in her life. We explored why she received the directive as a representation of negative moments and why she did not choose to represent positive moments in her life. After processing and exploring the necessity to validate her experiences through a negative lens, Melissa remade the timeline. This new visual representation became the first evidence of positive, as well as the known negative, moments/attributes that were sprinkled throughout her lifetime (Figure 7.2).

We utilized this new timeline to attach important patterns of behaviors, responses, and attain bodily awareness of significant memories within the piece. We then drew connections to historical patterns of behaviors that were being repeated in the PTSD from the birth of her son. Melissa would dissociate throughout these moments of connections, as evidenced by loss of eye contact, lapse in bodily posture, and a glaze that would form over her eyes. When I witnessed these behaviors, I carefully pointed them out and asked for her to acknowledge where she went and to find a place in her body that she felt safe upon returning to the space.

Melissa and I worked diligently to explore and process the events throughout her life. This was the first moment that a therapist had given witness to *all* of Melissa's past, including the good and the bad. I made sure to validate each step of her timeline, as no one in her life was able to provide that piece for her; I found that this was an extremely important part of the trauma work that Melissa and I were embarking on. In order to attain bodily awareness, especially where trauma was being stored, Melissa and I explored connections from one piece of her timeline to another. van der Kolk (2005) explained that "unless the tendency to repeat the trauma is recognized, the response to the environment is likely to replay the original traumatizing, abusive, but familiar, relationships" (p. 407). Throughout Melissa's development, she had lost her voice, her identity, and her boundaries due to the complex traumas she had

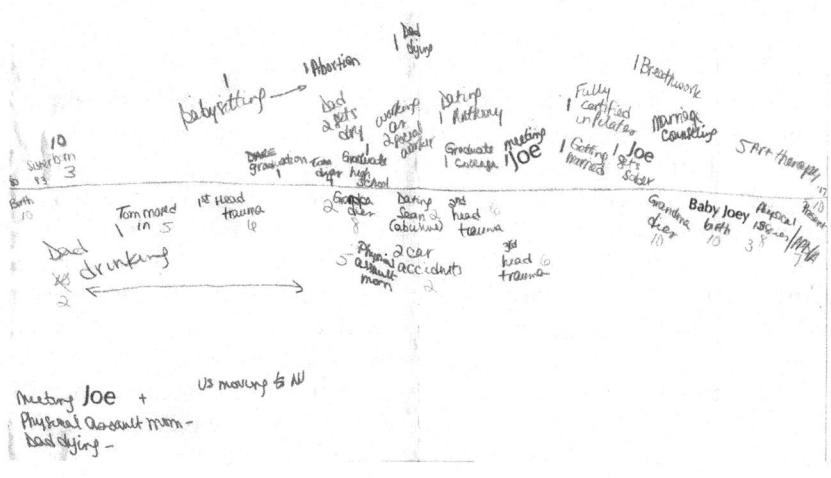

*Figure 7.2* "Drawing #1."

endured. The birth trauma once again triggered these responses from her childhood and early adulthood, which often left her feeling powerless.

## Melissa and Joe: Couples' Work for Postpartum

At this point, Joe needed to be brought into Melissa's therapy process as he carried some of the positive aspects of her life. When Melissa and I explored her experience in relationship to Joe, she could consciously remember this being a time where she had gained control, was validated by an adult, and found a solution that had been attained by all parties within the relationship. She realized that this was the *first time* her voice had been heard! At that moment, I deemed it necessary to begin work with the couple to further explore their relationship and follow the patterns that were being exhibited by both entities within the relationship. I invited Melissa and Joe to my couples' creative art therapy group sessions.

### Couples' Group Art Therapy Session

In the group couples' sessions that I led at the center, it became clear that families who were utilizing the center found comfort with their peers and recognized that they were not alone in their worries, struggles, or conflicts. Melissa and Joe's first group session centered around intimacy—emotional as well as physical—during the postpartum period. The women in the group all had similar feelings regarding physical intimacy with their partners and felt that they didn't have the same drive as they had experienced prior to giving birth. Several different reasons/issues for not feeling intimately connected came up: body image; feeling as though their bodies were utilitarian due to breastfeeding their children; feeling "touched out"; having a loss of identity because they could not embrace the new role as mother; and recognizing that their boundaries were being challenged post birth. The partners uniformly expressed frustration surrounding the loss of physicality as well as the emotional disconnection they felt from their wives.

The directive was set around intimacy and Joe went straight to drawing. Upon processing his drawing, Joe repeatedly expressed that he was just making shapes and was unaware what it was or what he was thinking (Figure 7.3). However, through the processing portion of group, the collective, including Melissa and Joe, arrived at the realization that Joe was drawing the head of his penis entering his wife.

Joe expressed that they had always had an intimate sexual connection and since the birth of their son, he felt as though they had some distance between them that he was unable to navigate effectively. The two partners processed that due to the traumatic events of Baby Joey's birth, Melissa appeared to be exhibiting secondary trauma that was related to her abusive past. Melissa was able to recognize and identify that she had been holding the sexual trauma of her past and it was

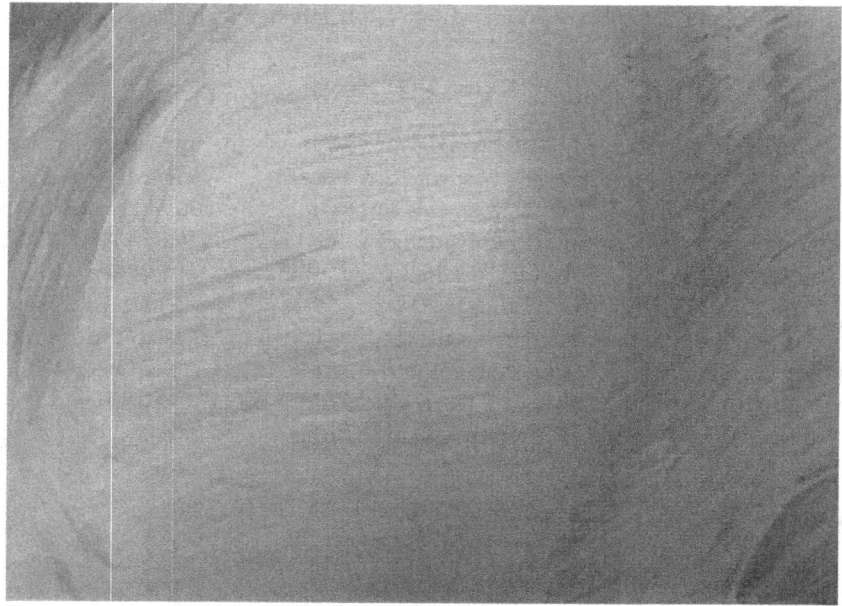

*Figure 7.3* "Drawing #2."

revisiting her through the birth trauma of her son, especially as her body was continuously being challenged with blurred boundaries. Melissa's physical pain caused by the C-section, breastfeeding, and postpartum hemorrhage continuously and repeatedly traumatized her by triggering the feelings of bodily pain and discomfort she had felt during the traumas of her past.

Shortly after this session, I had a major medical trauma experience of my own. I was diagnosed with a cervical spine infection that had disintegrated my C5-C7 vertebrae within my cervical spine. I was admitted to the hospital and immediately scheduled for an emergency surgery the following day. My last lucid memory is of getting an MRI on my spine; after that, my memory was clouded by the extensive doses of pain medication that I had been administered once I was at the hospital. I underwent the spinal surgery, and then, according to my husband, I was in the hospital for approximately five days. I have limited recollection of this time frame. Once I came home, I repeatedly asked my husband to go through the events of the week. I begged him to make a timeline with me so that I could piece together my missing days. This became a repeated request that my husband grew tired of until we finally created a tangible representation that I could review over and over again, unassisted. It was during this time that I realized that Melissa could not release her trauma because she did not have a tangible piece of evidence to review to recreate those missing days after the birth of Baby Joey. My own personal hospitalization had allowed me to better understand Melissa's relationship to her traumatic birth experience.

### Individual Couple Session

Once my doctors cleared me to go back to work and I was reinstated to the PMADs program, I immediately made an appointment with Joe and Melissa. I stated that we needed to do an intervention that would chronicle the birth from both of their perspectives. This directive is a "draw it out"[1] idea to afford traumatic memory processing. The graphic narrative exercise allows the family as a whole to process the events as they remember them.

**Directive:** Fold a piece of paper until it has nine squares. The center square is the traumatic event (the worst possible moment). The client will go backwards from the middle square and delineate the moments prior to the event (the first square will be a moment in time prior to any knowledge that something horrific was going to occur) and then move forward from the traumatic event until you are at the last box, which will represent when the fear(s) is/are over or manageable (Figures 7.4 and 7.5).

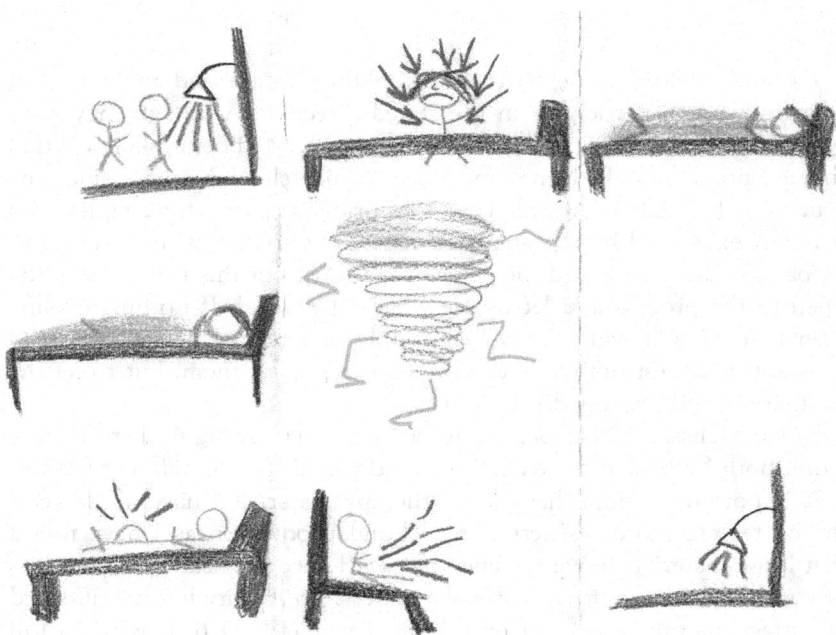

*Figure 7.4* "Drawing #3."

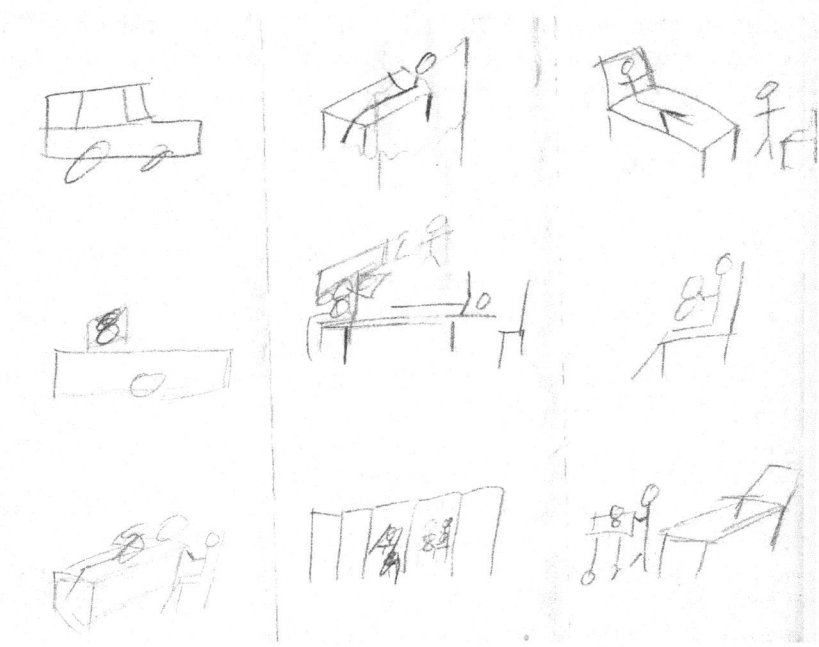

*Figure 7.5* "Drawing #4."

Joe and Melissa came to the session fully aware and in a state of preparedness to participate in the stated directive. Although they were open to processing the traumatic events, Joe reported being skeptical that this art process could bring any peace to himself or his wife since the trauma had already occurred. This is a normal response for couples who may feel exhausted by repeatedly reviewing the trauma while learning to be parents. Joe challenged me in prior sessions, but this time I said, "Be open to the process and let us see what will unfold. If nothing occurs, then that is what will be." When couples are feeling demoralized and resistant, it is best not to enter into a struggle with them, but to let the art therapy and process do the work.

I gave Melissa and Joe paper with an array of drawing tools to choose from. Both Melissa and Joe chose colored pencils but of different brands. It is important to note that the art therapy materials I have available at the center are more restrictive in feel and production as I have found that loose materials move the clients toward decompensation due to loss of control. The inability to control a material in totality has not afforded advantageous outcomes so I have limited materials of (this is not a full list): Play-Doh, colored pencils, pastels, oil pastels, gel pens, magic markers, tissue paper, decorative paper, and glue sticks.

Melissa and Joe worked diligently. Joe giggled throughout his creative time and repeatedly stated, "I don't even know what I am drawing." This response is a common statement that I have heard time and time again at the center. I have come to realize that it is a declaration that alleviates expectation of self, judgment from others, and appears to utilize an unconscious coping strategy to assuage anxiety when working within the constraints of trauma. Melissa moved through her drawings with ease, but became stuck at points, such as the open/blank box due to loss of memory. Joe was more contemplative in each box he came across. It appeared as though he was unsure of how to depict each moment. I encouraged Joe to move through the drawings without too much consideration as we would verbally go through each moment together during processing.

The processing of Melissa's drawings began to open a dialogue between me, as the facilitator, and the couple. The themes that became apparent throughout Melissa's drawings were loss of control, loss of voice, loss of physical capabilities due to the administering of medications, loss of memory, and, finally, entrapment or loss of freedom. If we look at these themes, we can recognize the same struggles and challenges Melissa faced in her postpartum experience and her symptoms associated to PMADs. In addition, an acknowledgement of a real, life-threatening endangerment throughout Melissa's lifetime is apparent in both sets of drawings as a repetitive pattern that we were threading together through the use of the timeline. The last frame of Melissa's drawing, as processed by Melissa, is an image of trying to cleanse herself of the trauma. Once again, this is a repetitive behavior that she remembered as the final stage of the traumatic experiences in her life; she was only able to recognize this after concretizing and establishing tangible evidence of events in her life through the establishment of the timeline.

After listening to Melissa's recollection of events, it appeared that her memories were fragmented and required further assistance from Joe's drawings, so we began to process the same story from Joe's view point. Joe's drawings afforded the ability for Melissa to now fill in the moments that she had lost during the birth. However, a repetitive leitmotif within Joe's remembrance was astonishing. Joe had either deleted himself from the drawings or was separate from Melissa, sitting as a spectator of the unfolding events. As we processed this evidentiary piece of information, Joe started to become emotional and appeared to be unable to process what was being pointed out. At this time, Joe tried to continue with his narrative until he got to Box 5, which represented the traumatic event, and broke down into tears. Joe reported that he was terrified at the thought of having to raise the baby alone. Joe stated, "This was not the plan. I never agreed to live without Melissa." Joe reported feeling resentful toward Melissa for admitting that she was ready to die and abandon him.

At this moment, both Melissa and Joe became emotionally dysregulated and required assistance in regaining control of their sensations.
I assisted the couple to work together to ground themselves by reaching
out for one another—instead of retreating from each other—and to
utilize breathing techniques that they could employ as tools today and
in the future. For the first time, this moment provided Melissa an
opportunity to understand exactly what had happened during the birth
of her son; it also allowed her to not feel alone in her trauma as she
realized that Joe had experienced his own trauma. This was an opportunity to validate both partners' occurrences and afford the space for Joe
and Melissa to understand that they each had faced significant traumas.

Melissa expressed, "I am not alone; this is the first time since Baby
Joey was born that I do not feel isolated in my trauma. I no longer feel
alone to repeat the moments in isolation." Joe reiterated the sentiment
and was able to go back to his isolation within the drawings. At this
time, Joe was able to recognize and process his feelings of loneliness
during the crisis and the birth experience in its entirety. Melissa conveyed feeling empowered by the knowledge that she was not alone, and
Joe resounded the feelings as well. At this moment, a levity seemed to
appear within the therapeutic space that afforded the couple to gain
distance from their experience, now that they both felt that they were
not unaccompanied in their memories.

This was the last time Melissa would speak of her trauma in the same
way that she had prior to this session; she had finally attained emotional
distance from the experience. The trauma could no longer consume,
define, or identify her. This was the last time that the couple was asked
to review their traumatic experience and the more time I spent with
Melissa and Joe over the year, the more I recognized that the trauma was
still able to hold a place in their lives, but they were now able to move
around it without constraints, and were no longer tethered to it.

## Conclusion

Melissa finished out her year at the center and continued to attend
creative art therapy groups twice a week. She and Joe also met with me
as an individual couple a few more times to, as Melissa referred to the
work, "oil the wheels" of their relationship when moments as parents
became overwhelming. She had worked to attain self-awareness and to
recognize triggers of her prior traumas. She ascertained information and
learned where they (traumas) were being stored within her body. The
skills she established while working with me afforded her the ability to
remain present within the world, with her son, and with her partner as
well as more frequently recognize and circumvent her defense mechanism of dissociation. She no longer appeared to be a passive passenger to

her trauma, but rather was an active avenger to understand and thwart the power her trauma once held over her.

Melissa has since come back into the center to work with me as she has become pregnant again and is expecting her next son in February 2020. We are continuing the journey of self-awareness and bodily awareness, and we continue to explore the traumas she has gone through, as they attempt to regain strength and power over her. However, at the moment, she maintains a confident position in the relationship of Melissa vs. Trauma, and I believe she will remain the victor again and again.

## Note

1 The "Draw it Out" Directive was introduced by Robert Rhoton, PsyD, LPC, DAAETS and Vice President of International Association of Trauma Professionals (IATP) during my training to become a Certified Family Trauma Specialist.

## References

American Psychiatric Association. (2013). *Diagnostic and statistical manual of mental disorders* (5th ed.). Arlington, VA: American Psychiatric Association. Retrieved from https://doi.org/10.1176/appi.books.9780890425596

Dunning, T., Harris, J. M., & Sandall, J. (2016). Women and their birth partners' experiences following a primary postpartum hemorrhage: A qualitative study. *BMC Pregnancy and Childbirth, 16*, 80. doi:10.1186/s12884-016-0870-7

Glannon, W. (2014). Anesthesia, amnesia and harm. *Journal of Medical Ethics, 40*, 651–657.

Scheepstra, K. W. F., van Steijn, M. E., Dijksman, L. M., & van Pampus, M. G. (2017). Post-traumatic stress disorder in women and their partners, following severe post-partum hemorrhage: A study protocol for a prospective cohort study. *Cogent Medicine, 4*, 1. doi:10.1080/2331205X.2017.1278840

Simkin, P. (2011). Pain, suffering, and trauma in labor and prevention of subsequent posttraumatic stress disorder. *The Journal of Perinatal Education, 20*(3), 166–176. doi:10.1891/1058-1243.20.3.166

Stramrood, C. I., Doornbos, B., Wessel, I., van Geenen, M., Aarnoudse, J. G., van den Berg, P. P., ... van Pampus, M. G. (2013, April). Fathers with PTSD and depression in pregnancies complicated by preterm preeclampsia or PPROM. *Archives of Gynecology and Obstetrics, 287*, 653–661. Retrieved from. http://dx.doi.org/10.1007/s00404-012-2611-0

van der Kolk, B. A. (2005). Developmental trauma disorder: Toward a rational diagnosis for children with complex trauma histories. *Psychiatric Annals, 35*, 401–408.

Wylie, M. S. (1991). Family therapy's neglected prophet. In *The Family Therapy Networker 15*, 25–37, 77.

# Part III

# Art Therapy

Grief and Loss

# 8 Cultivating Aliveness after Pregnancy Loss

## Somatic Art Therapy, Ritual, and Grief Work

*Merryl E. Rothaus*

The loss of a wanted pregnancy can be one of the most devastating, dissonant life passages for a woman. Most women form an affection and sense of attachment to the specific being growing inside of them from the moment they learn they are pregnant. Expecting new life, a woman is confronted with death (Kohn & Moffit, 2000). Additionally, she is faced with the loss of a dream and trajectory that was centralized around the life growing inside of her (Rothert, 2019). The loss is further complicated in that it is both somatic, since pregnancy and the loss are experienced physically, as well as being emotionally heart-wrenching. Despite the fact that approximately one in four pregnancies in the United States end in miscarriage, in Western culture, which is largely grief-adverse, most women suffer alone silently. Such a loss is a "grief without a shape" (Seftel, 2006) that goes unseen and unrecognized, and as a result this cohort of women is not supported in talking about their losses let alone grieving them. Grief and memory are held in the body and therefore, women who have lost life from within their bodies need expressive forms in which to move and process the layers of somatic grief and trauma. Additionally, they need sacred witnessing and honoring of their experience by others so that they are not suffering alone in the margins.

While birth and death are largely honored through ritual, in Western culture, rituals to honor the loss of a pregnancy are not. Bringing ritual to women who have endured babylosses honors their stories, and through such a sacred, initiatory threshold, she may be transformed into a generative version of herself and a type of understanding and movement toward acceptance and integration of her loss. Supporting women who lose wanted pregnancies through somatically oriented art therapy, grief work, and ritual can transform a loss that exists within the shadows, into societal awareness. Art making, which transcends words and holds strong emotions, can be a ritualistic venue for the inexpressible nuances of grief, as we "turn to art in challenging times to experience the transformation of difficulties into affirmations of life" (McNiff, 2019, p. 163). Inspired by art therapy pioneer Florence Cane who noted that the engagement of the body was necessary for true artistic expression (1951), this chapter discusses my methodology of what I call, *somatic art therapy*, which integrates awareness and engagement of the soma into art therapy prior to, during gestation of an image and its creation and into the process of working with it upon its completion. Through somatic art therapy, the textures of grief can be articulated, expressed and sequenced from the body through attention to the soma before, during, and in working with the created image upon its completion. Ritualizing the process of art making allows the grief to be honored and brought into sacred territory where as Dissanayake noted, we "make [it] special" (1992). The art object then becomes a talisman (Schaverien, 1992) that holds and tells the sacred story of the woman's journey, thus helping her to further transform and befriend her grief.

As the etymology of the word Miscarriage (n.d.) means mistake, error, or "misbehavior" and therefore suggests blame onto the mother, the terms "babyloss" and "pregnancy loss" as more humane terms will henceforth be used. This chapter will begin with a discussion of grief, followed by the inclusion of ritual in art therapy and the efficacy of somatic art therapy in working with babyloss. Two case examples of somatic art therapy within the frame of grief work and ritual with women who endured pregnancy losses—one being the author—will be shared.

In 2011, 13 weeks into a planned and most wanted pregnancy, I began to bleed. A pregnant mother's worst reality ensued, and over the course of the next 16 hours, in my home, I labored through physically and wretched contractions, copious amounts of blood, and eventually gave birth to my dead daughter. Two years later, at my ten-week ultrasound, my doctor informed me that my second baby would not live and I shockingly endured another babyloss. My third loss, at six weeks pregnant, came and went when I began to bleed, amidst my emotional numbness. The complex grief of multiple babylosses brought me to the most despairing point I had ever known. I experienced a destruction and desolation of my spirit, faith, and a belief in the benevolence and fairness of life.

Living within a tragic story of unsuccessfully trying to become a mom over the course of seven years, it became clear that I needed to surrender to and befriend the dark terrain of grief that lived in my body, and allow it to "sequence," from the body, a term used in somatic psychotherapies, so that I would walk in the world of the living again. With faith in myself and in the terrain of this dark night of the soul, I began, as Mr. Rogers taught, to "look for the helpers." This came through my love of ritual and the life affirming experience of making, both of which could hold my grief. As art therapist Shaun McNiff (1992) wrote, "Whenever illness is associated with loss of soul, the arts emerge spontaneously as remedies, soul medicine" (p. 1).

# On Grief

Rarely in this culture is grief considered a somatic experience. However, the etymology of the word Grief (n.d.) is "Hardship, pain, suffering and bodily affliction. Physical pain. Make heavy (gavis)." It is derived from the old French words of "burden," "oppression," and to "make heavy."

This physiological reality of grief, often referred to as "broken heart syndrome," explains why we feel heavy in our bodies when in the midst of grief (Peck, 2019). Therein lies a broken heart. Grief is a universal phenomenon, across cultures all over the world. However, *how* people grieve and how it is thought about differs amongst cultures.

## Literature

Most well known and recognized in Western culture is Elisabeth Kubler-Ross's five-stage theory of grief (1969). She identified denial, anger, bargaining, depression, and acceptance as stages through which a griever moves. Worden's model (1991) addressed the four tasks of grief, including accepting the reality of the loss, working through the pain of grief, learning to adjust to life without the deceased and continuing with life while also keeping a connection to the deceased. Stroebe and Schut (1999) developed a dual process model of bereavement, suggesting that people shuttle back and forth between loss-oriented activities and stressors as well as restoration-oriented activities and stressors that are related with secondary losses. These Western models place grief-work into a formulaic, intellectual process.

But what about the inclusion of the body in grief work? In the Burkino Faso area of West Africa, 40 tribes hold grief rituals daily. Dagara Tribe Elder and teacher Malidoma Some (2019) explained that in these rituals, the work is "to be in the presence of grief and grieve fully. To get inside of grief and let it move ... with community." The body, in its need for expression is always part of grief, as he emphasized, "The hurt that a person feels should be taken as a language spoken by the body" (Some, 1993, back cover). Similarly, "keening," a grieving practice most well known in Ireland, is about "giving voice to the madness ... singing a lament" and includes "wails with rage and heartbreak" (Burns, 2018, p. 2). A collective practice, its roots date back to 2600 BC in Egypt, with Isis as the first keener following the death of her beloved Osiris (Burns, 2018). While the soma is inherent in these grieving practices, grief in Western culture, as we see above, is not viewed or encouraged to be a somatic experience. Westerners are perhaps enculturated to beliefs that to "be strong" means to be stoic, and expressive crying or wailing is unsanctioned or weak. Therefore, a griever is most often socialized to suppress its true nature and maintain an indifferent, "strong" presence, which disallows grief to *move*. The intelligence of the soma is that it is *wanting* to release stress and tension and to be included in the grief process. As Francis Weller (2015) wrote:

> Grief is subversive, undermining the quiet agreement to behave and be in control of our emotions. It is an act of protest that declares our refusal to live numb and small. There is something feral about grief, something essentially outside the ordained and sanctioned behaviors of our culture ... Contrary to our fears, grief is suffused with life-force. It is riddled with energy. It is not a state of deadness or emotional flatness. Grief is alive, wild, untamed and cannot be domesticated. It resists the demands to remain passive and still. We move in jangled, unsettled and riotous ways when grief takes hold of us.
>
> (p. 9)

The Western cultural experiences of repressed grief are even more true with pregnancy loss because it is a loss that happens alone and is rarely seen or expressed. For many women, it remains a secret held within the body. Given opportunities to have the grief acknowledged and expressed, as can happen through ritual and somatic art therapy, women who have lost pregnancies may have an opportunity to follow the intuitive movements of the soma's intelligence. This creates more freedom and lightness in their body, and in so doing, providing a more spacious view into their stories being made of sacred triumph and aliveness.

## Ritual and Art Therapy

Malidoma Some defines ritual as a conversation with the sacred that goes beyond words—a way to bypass the psyche—through entering into sacred space with total self and presence (verbal communication, October, 2019). Rituals exist in all cultures as symbolic behaviors that we do before, during, and after meaningful life events (Gino & Norton, 2013). To create ritual is to create a "unique social space" (Schirch, as cited in Najarian, 2007, p. 17). Ritual is about making meaning and marking initiation into a significant life event through action. One establishes a sacred relationship with the ineffable, or numinous. As Martin Buber (1923) named, an "I-thou" relationship is created and becomes known between the person and the numinous.

How do we bring ritual into an art therapy space? First, the therapist holds a ritual context and intention through which a sacred environment is created. In this co-created space between therapist and client, the environment, creative process, *and* the art object can become the sacred "thou." As ritual involves doing, the creation of imagery can be paired with an intention to mark a significant life event that results in "art in action" (Wasilewska, 1992, p. 198). Adaptable to Some's aforementioned definition of ritual, the creative process can bypass the psyche. As expression rises from the unconscious or numinous, the art process in and of itself *is* ritual. When held with such intention, the completed art object can then become imbued as a sacred talisman capable of providing the person a degree of resolution and meaning in their life (Schaverien, 1992).

For a woman who is grieving a pregnancy loss and is surrounded by this kind of venerable presence, deep witnessing and compassionate attention can offer her comfort. Such a humane experience can shift her orientation from solo suffering to one that is seen, validated, held in sacred space, and revered as an initiation. Ritualized art therapy space serves to uplift and dignify her, and leaving with a symbolic art object, she may feel more empowered to also see her loss as a rite of passage that, within its grief, has also seasoned and changed her in valuable ways.

## Somatic Art Therapy

Art therapy is recognized as a safe therapeutic venue through which to process painful or traumatic experiences and memories. Art therapy can gently access the images that are tucked away in the body and psyche and give voice to their rising toward a degree of healing. Through art, our sensory (visual, auditory, kinesthetic, and tactile) memories can be contacted and processed (Malchiodi, 2011). For babyloss, a sensory experience, this is especially true. Regarding art therapy and babyloss, Seftel (2006), wrote

> The arts provide a powerful way to express stories that are otherwise hidden or whitewashed. Rather than seeking out simplified and sanitized points of view, the arts offer a range of experiences—as messy, contrary, and unpredictable as they need to be in order to capture authentic reactions to these emotionally complex losses.
>
> (p. 30)

As is the nature of grief, one can get messy with art media, focusing on process-based art that is about the expression of affect (Thompson, 2009).

Our images, like memories and feelings, can be felt and sensed within our bodies (Rappaport, 2009; Rothaus, 2014) and then further excavated and explored externally. So, while the body is a repository for our images, the usage and awareness of it has been largely left out of the discourse of art therapy. Rarely is art therapy considered to be a somatic therapy. However, art therapy has significant roots in the body. Florence Cane, one of the mothers of art therapy noted that "the release of the creative faculty through the free rhythmic use of the body" was necessary to have "true art expression" (Cane, 1951, p. 37). Integrating Eugene Gendlin's "focusing" into art therapy, Rappaport developed "Focusing-Oriented Art Therapy" with an emphasis on mindfulness and the felt sense in the creative process (2009); Hakomi body-centered therapy has also been combined with art therapy (Rothaus, 2014). And, I posit that art therapy is inherently poised, as it is, to unite with somatic therapy. Somatic art therapy is about bringing awareness to and engagement with the body prior to, during, and after the creation of the imagery as well as during the exchange with the image itself. Doing so can result in the sequencing of strong emotions that both the body and images contain, which can then be unpacked in a somatic process that leads to further meaning making, insight, and integration.

While the case studies below will provide the reader with a deeper understanding of somatic art therapy, I will outline its fundamental aspects here. Integrating aspects of Hakomi psychotherapy, I begin with orienting a client into mindfulness (Kurtz, 1990) in order to access the terrain of her soma. In this exploratory state, we often discover the presence of mental imagery (Morgan, 2006). Attention to the body is also necessary in the case of helping to regulate a dysregulated nervous system through using tools from Peter Levine's Somatic Experiencing therapy (2012). Within the process of "assisted self-discovery" (Kurtz, 1990), we continue to mine and explore the images located in the body, and they are encouraged to be felt and experienced somatically in as much detail as possible. With the imagery and corresponding body awareness established, she moves into articulating the somatic imagery using art media while maintaining connection with her body throughout. I become a background voice and encourage her to the sensations in her body as well as her movements as she creates, offering considerations to augment the somatic art therapy process. What does she notice? Where and how does she feel it in her body? What feels satisfying? How? When a repetitive body movement occurs while making art, I encourage her to pay attention to her body's inclination for that movement as well as the somatic and emotional result. Often, a repetitive movement is the body's intuitive wisdom; orienting toward a need for self-soothing, pleasure or the release and sequencing of a difficult or traumatic experience. After the image is complete, it is viewed from a distance. If comfortable with closing her eyes, she is invited to "take-in" the image—embody it, feel it in her body from where it arose, and study its details, presence, and wisdom within. Opening her eyes to the now embodied image, she somatically relates to it outwardly with expressing it and/or studying it further. What follows is a practice of this back and forth oscillation. Somatic art therapy invites attention and practice to both an active and receptive exchange—a doing and a reflecting, an initiative and a surrender with the image and the entire creative practice (Cane, 1951; McNiff, 1998; Rothaus, 2014; Rubin, 2011).

As the image is often life-enhancing and generative, I assist the client to anchor it in a place in the body or with a correlating movement so that it may be regularly accessed. Working with it somatically, creating it visually, and talking about its symbolic meanings leads to its imprint as an embodied talisman and, consequently, to enduring change. Somatic art therapy and ritual in the processing of babyloss grief are elucidated in the following case studies.

### Case Study One: "R"

R sits on the couch in my office with a glazed look in her eyes and informs me that she lost her baby at ten weeks. Knowing that my losses prepared me for this day, and having arrived at a place where I am a clear vessel of support, I meet her wet eyes with mine. I identify that her body, stiff without evident breath, was in a freeze state of sympathetic nervous system arousal. Using regulation tools from my training in Somatic Experiencing (Levine, 2012) to assist her parasympathetic nervous system to initiate, I call to engage her senses through handing her two cloth balls filled with lavender. I ask her to smell them and squeeze them in her hands. She exhales. Her parasympathetic system begins to come online. I help her to orient to the present through engaging her senses by looking around the room and finding something visual that she likes. She chooses a cobalt blue bottle lit by the sun. Her shoulders relax. I ask her to place her feet on the ground and press them into the earth while describing the sensations. I lead her in simple breathing exercises and see her present moment awareness. I encourage her to follow the wants of her body. She sways back and forth, a self-soothing indicator. I mirror her movements. She is ready to tell her story.

My beloved late teacher, Sobonfu Some, from Burkino Faso, West Africa, once instructed me to have a blue glass bowl in my office, filled with fresh water, as a symbol of the flow of tears and the holding of grief. In bringing ritual into therapy, I place it in front of her on the art table, inviting her to set an intention. She wants to process some of her "stuck" grief. I bring out and invite us to light a tealight candle in honor of her baby, who she has named J.O. We pause and silently honor this moment of ritual and sacred intention. Tears come.

Knowing this client over the course of many years, I am aware that her ego strength is strong, and as such I know that inviting her into her body, and particularly to the site of trauma—her womb—is therapeutically sound. With her eyes closed, I orient her into connection with her body, to notice sensations and what is happening internally. She reports feeling "empty." I say gently, "See if it's okay to place a hand on your womb," in an effort to safely bring her in touch with somatic sensations while staying within her window of tolerance. She does, and I encourage her flowing tears. "Through your tears, see if it is okay to stay with your womb. Just be there letting your hand offer compassionate tending from you to you." I am helping her in bringing attention both to the body, as well as with the body (Csordas, 1993).

Proceeding slowly, I use my Hakomi training so that she may study her somatic experience and any accompanying imagery. "Notice what you feel or see. Perhaps an image, colors, sensations, words?" She describes emptiness again as an internalized image develops. I ask her to describe the sensations and image in detail. We take time with this, as she studies the somatic presence and the nuances of the image. Eventually, she is ready to express the image onto paper. I suggest that paint would be a helpful medium for articulating the raw messiness she describes. I know that the fluidity of paint will also assist with supporting the necessary movement of her body. She begins with a paintbrush, using upward strokes. Her breath increases. She drops the paintbrush and follows her body's cue, smearing paint with her hands in upward movements. Big tears come. I encourage her to bring body awareness into the process and to focus on "what feels satisfying" and she begins a rhythmic pushing of the paint. I notice her jaw clenching and encourage her to allow it to follow its desire to open, while encouraging the expression of any sounds that may want to emerge. Quiet moans begin and I mirror some of the sounds. As she pushes the paint, she is sequencing unexpressed grief out of her body and onto the page.

After some time, complete with art making, I tape the image on the wall so that she can be in relationship to this somatic image and unpack it further somatically (Figure 8.1).

She says, "I can feel the image in my womb" and that the art helped her to contact the "bloody sensation of death" within her body and though the release of some grief, has resulted in "relief and spaciousness" inside of her body. Before concluding and giving her homework to witness write (Allen, 1995) at home, I make sure she is in her body through leading her in gentle breathing and swaying back and forth while maintaining contact. I see that she is enlivened and regulated.

At the beginning of our next session, the ritual bowl is filled and another candle is lit for J.O. I am curious to assess where she is in the grieving process. She names that she is feeling anger, an emotion that she fears and is normally inaccessible to her. Her intention today is to welcome the medicine of her anger. I give her larger paper to express the anger spaciously. She chooses paint and again begins to smear in upward movements. Soon, she moves to using thick oil sticks. I encourage her to stay with what is happening in her body and to feel the somatic sensations. She pushes and smears and names the rising of anger as I encourage her to notice where and how she knows the anger in her body. Instead of her familiar collapse in the face of anger, the art helps her to feel her continual body sensations as does the repetitive movement of her arms using the art media. Similar to the first image, her movements emanate upward from the bottom of the page. She

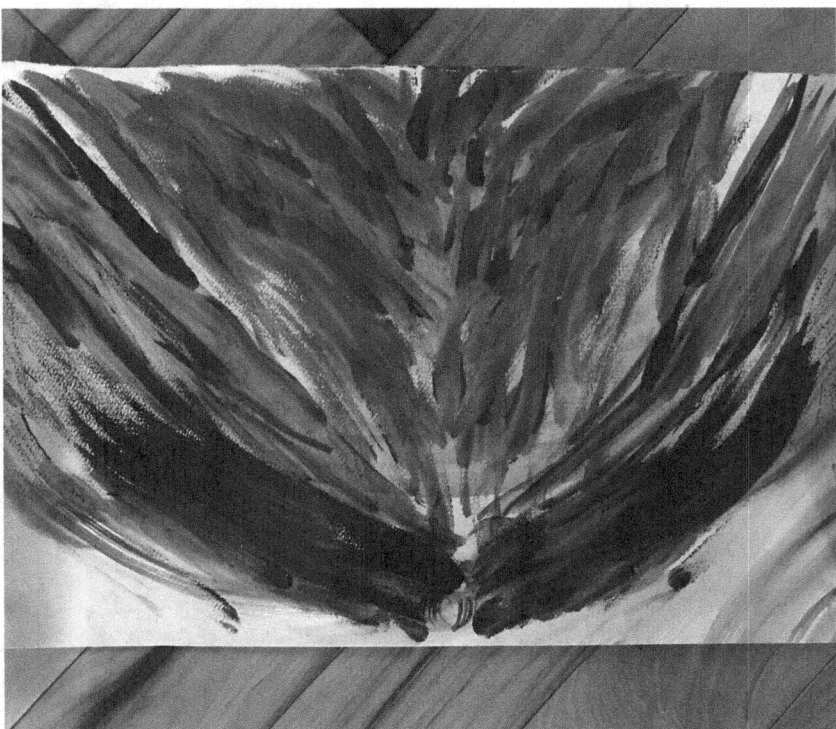

*Figure 8.1* Flow. Release. Grieve.

begins to verbally express the anger of losing J.O. As one grief often stimulates others, the loss of her baby touches the loss, pain, and anger of her maternal relationship and she becomes acutely present to the anger she has never been able to express toward her mother. I encourage her to rely on the art to keep this process moving and she follows her body's desire, increasing the push of oil sticks into the paper and smearing with her hands. Wanting to support the sequencing of her normally disassociated anger, I hand her an etching tool in the event that this might be helpful to facilitate this process. She begins to scratch into the oil sticks and smiles with satisfaction.

Her jaw opens and her breath increases. I encourage her to stay connected to the image and be present in her body while feeling this precious anger. Eventually, she feels complete with her image. Her eyes are bright and wide and she says, "I feel so alive!"

I have her stand and we tape the image to the wall to look at it from a distance. I remind her to feel her feet on the ground and to notice the movement surging through her. "Keep moving" I say, and she does, naming the "power" in her body. I ask her to oscillate between looking at the image and then going into her body with closed eyes to feel its existence internally. I have her become the image and express it through body movements. She emulates the image with sweeping arm motions that begin at her feet and rise up into the air. She is breathing quickly now, and I reflect that she is not collapsing, that her anger is moving, and that this life-giving experience ironically began with the muse that was the death of her son. As this experience and image is so generative for her, I have her again practice embodying the image through looking at it, taking it into her body, expressing it with movement and in so doing, anchoring its meaning and power (Figure 8.2).

Reflecting on these sessions, she reports,

> These sessions helped me to really solidify who I am. I can still feel that image in my body. I can touch into how full and whole I feel now. They integrated these pieces for me. I can feel the anger

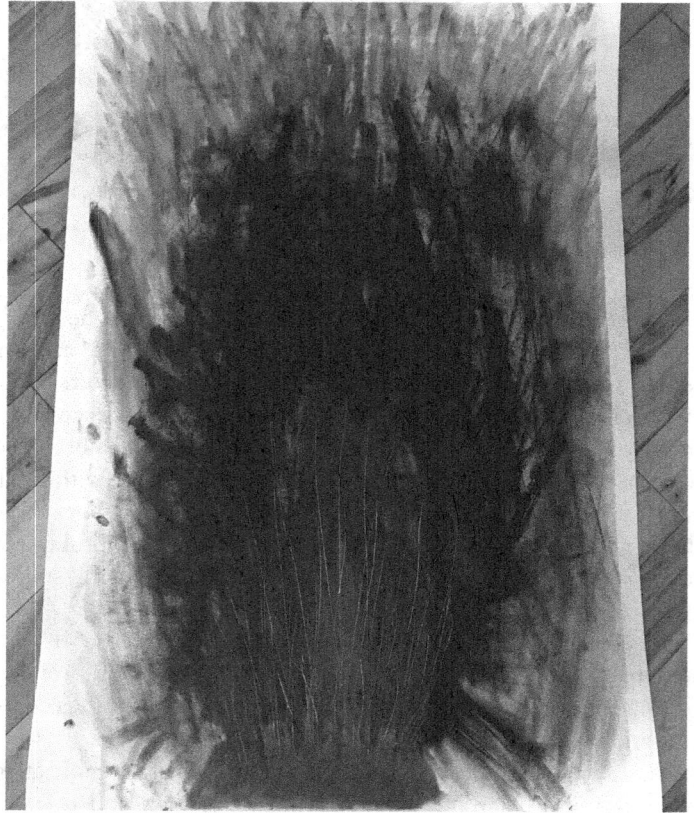

*Figure 8.2* Rage. Heal. Transform.

without collapsing. It was like I was missing the experiences of anger and grief in my life and that was a portal to fill that gap in.

She continued with the ritual of filling her own blue glass bowl with water and lighting a candle for a full year.

### Case Study Two: My Own Experience

A year and a half after losing my third baby, the grief still felt stuck in my body and I struggled to accept that I was not going to mother. I was flooded with "Whys." Why don't all women get to be mothers? Why did this happen to me? This isn't fair, I'd think over and over again. In addition to my anger and despair, myriad unanswerable questions needed release, yet my body felt too soaked with grief that doing much of anything felt laborious. I faced the realization that I needed to get a hold of my mind and its despairing thoughts. I was riding an edge of trauma that was not being moved through talking about it with my therapist, or with many well-meaning loved ones who did their best to support me. I needed to tell my story *but words could not reach the violent imagery and grief of what I had experienced in birthing death.* I leaned into the creative process of making art through choosing the medium of an altered book.

Wadeson (2011) referred to an altered book being a metaphor for an altered life and wholeheartedly articulates my experience. Altered books support the exploration of alternative narratives throughout their pages and offer the reauthorization of an existing book, and in so doing, the reauthorization of one's story (Negash & Cobb, 2010). I could open and then close the book when necessary, and therefore it was the perfect choice in which to chronicle my story.

My altered book began with my joy and elation of conceptions and pregnancies, and continues to narrate my babylosses. The journey of my grief and descent into my own "shero's journey" is told through scant words, uncensored images, and concludes with the life-saving aspects of my spiritual practices and the unknown foray into my future.

With each creative emotional dive into my grief, I fill my blue glass grief-bowl with water, and I light three tealight candles—one for each of my babies. Prior to beginning a new page, I close my eyes and turn my attention inward to listen to what my body intuitively wants. Sensations of rage, anger and indescribable grief feel stuck in my solar plexus. I ask my body what it wants and my hands claw into the air as if wanting to tear. I listen and use an exacto knife and find myself repetitively cutting and carving circles into pages of the book. It feels satisfying in my body to carve circles and I hold curiosity and wonder what I am seeking to discover here. Circle after circle cuts make it through the page. I eventually learn that they represent my aging eggs and waning fertility as well as windows into the next pages of my unknown future.

I stop at points to weep and then smear my wet tears on the pages with my fingers, adding movement to the watercolor paint. It is through the context of ritual that my tears become an offering to be sacredly and safely held within my story of this book. I pause and note the pleasure in my body from pushing like this. I continually listen to and follow what my body wants, which is to get into the messiness of my ordeal through smearing and pushing fat oil sticks with my fingers, noticing sighs and releases from deep within my body. It feels satisfying and honest, and serves to liberate some of the angst living within me internally. I contact the rage and WHYs that have no answer in my story. As I hold ritual and intention to let go of that which no longer serves me, I burn papers from one of the many appointments I had with a reproductive endocrinologist, and offer a prayer for moving forward in acceptance of my losses. I glue some of the burnt paper and ashes to a page and use some of my menstrual blood as paint (Figure 8.3).

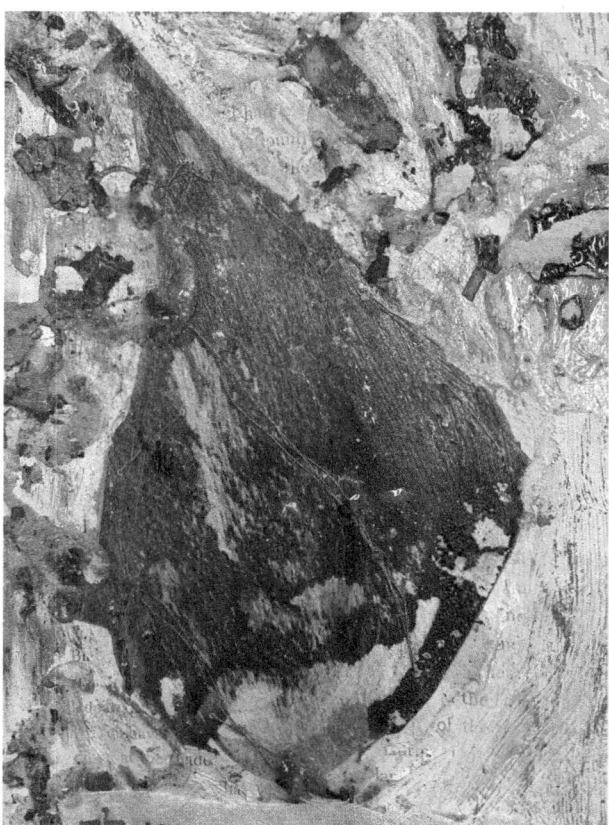

*Figure 8.3* "My Violent Descent Away From Motherhood" mixed media.

The presence of my menstrual blood represents the significant meaning of death and loss, specifically that which never came to fruition. I use a sharp etching tool and I scratch onto pages covered with layers of oil sticks, feeling the satisfaction in my body of violent slashing and ripping—metaphors that aptly articulate my internal feelings. Releasing contractions of strong affect through engaging intentionally with my body and the art, I create pockets of acceptance that I am not to become a mother of living children in this lifetime. Eventually, after deep purging of my pain into the book, my refuge of my Buddhist spiritual life presences itself, and from the gentle presences in my body, I find my way toward a sobered, softer acceptance represented in pages painted with bright colors (Figure 8.4).

I plaster medical bandages that I paint gold to the hard front and back covers of the book, gilding, enveloping, and honoring the sanctity of my painful, yet illuminating, shero's journey initiation.

As part of my desire to use art as social action and bring awareness of pregnancy loss to the public, my book eventually is displayed in two art shows, bearing its raw truth (Figure 8.5).

I choose an uncensored title: "Because Not All Women Get to Birth Live Babies." Showing my book to the public and posting images and words about it on social media, I begin to accrue followers. My story is no longer

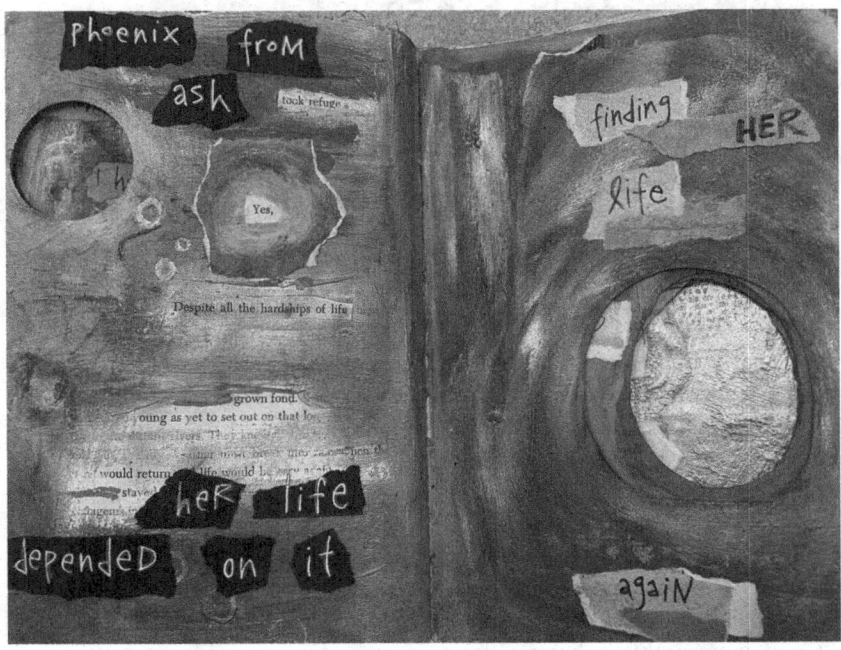

*Figure 8.4* "Let the 10,000 Things Rest: Learning Surrender" mixed media.

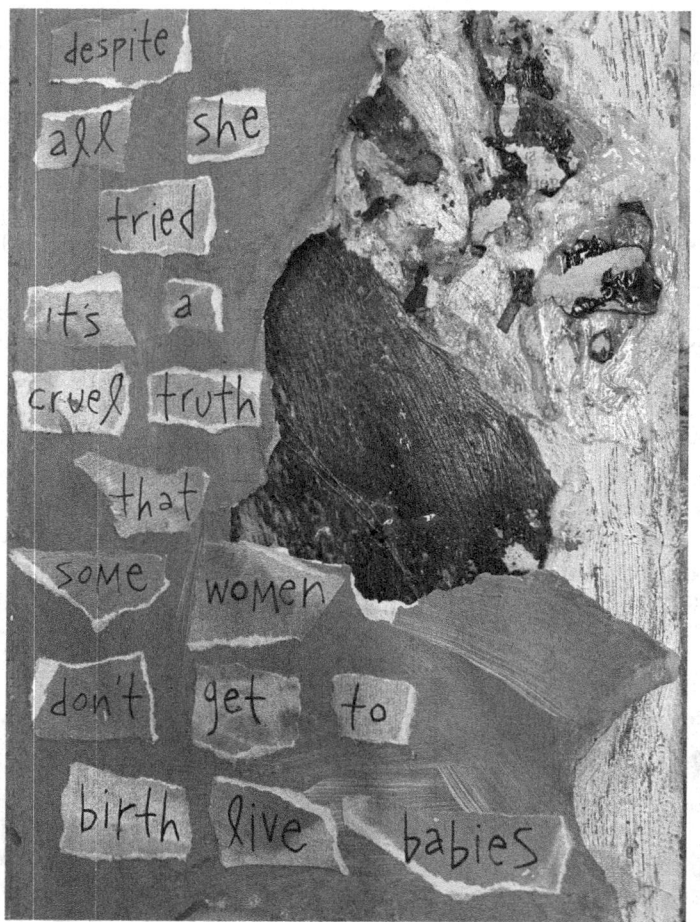

*Figure 8.5* Because Not All Women Get to Birth Live Babies.

hidden, and therefore I am able to "defy grief's isolation" (Seftel, 2006, p. 114) and bring babyloss into the awareness of the larger community.

While therapists may face the dilemma of self-disclosure, I intentionally chose to share my story, knowing that as the saying goes, "Silence is the voice of complicity." I am passionately committed to being an example of a woman who shares her story versus contributing to the norm of women who suffer silently. My choice to "out" myself has resulted in many clients who have experienced babyloss/pregnancy loss being able to find me so that I can help them therapeutically.

Grief is something that we carry in our stories versus something we relinquish. The act of truly listening to grief as my muse, following how it wanted to move in my body and authentically expressing it through art led me to create something beautiful out of destruction and to lighten heaviness in my body. My book and the entire process of its intentional, ritualistic creation felt life-giving, and beautiful. My book holds court as an embodied work to be openly shared. Through this process, I've come to know grief as a sacred wound, bestowing gifts to serve and support other women with this loss.

## Conclusion

As these case studies illustrate, somatic art therapy is an effective modality in supporting the grieving process for women who have endured baby-losses. Creating a sacred context of ritual supports meaning making (Schirch, 2005) through relationship with the art, and provides a venue through which the depths of grief can be sequenced from the body. For a cohort of women whose losses are greatly unseen, the witnessing of this process allows this loss to be honored and recognized, which further supports a woman's healing. As art therapists, we are poised to shift the paradigm of this particular loss from one that occurs silently in the margins to one that becomes visible and supported. As McNiff explained, "Do the work within the context of your specific community and in your distinctive way, with an openness to how it is integrally connected to the whole human experience" (McNiff, 2019, p. 162). In so doing, we may support a cultural shift that moves toward awareness of women who are grieving pregnancy losses and their inclusivity and visibility within community.

## References

Allen, P. (1995). *Art is a way of knowing*. Boston, MA: Shambhala.

Buber, M. (1923). *I and thou*. New York, NY: Touchstone.

Burns, J. (2018, March 7). Our unspent grief: The lost art of keening [article]. Retrieved from https://shamanicpractice.org/

Cane, F. (1951). *The artist in each of us*. London, England: Thames and Hudson.

Csordas, T. (1993). Somatic modes of attention. *Cultural Anthropology, 8*(2), 135–156.

Dissanayake, E. (1992). Art for life's sake. *American Journal of Art Therapy, 9*(4), 169–178.

Gino, F., & Norton, M. (2013, May 14). Why rituals work. *Scientific American*. Retrieved from www.scientificamerican.com/article/why-rituals-work/

Grief. (n.d.). In *Online etymology dictionary*. Retrieved from www.etymonline.com/search?q=grief

Kohn, I., & Moffit, P. A. (2000). *A silent sorrow*. New York, NY: Routledge.

Kubler-Ross, E. (1969). *On death and dying*. New York, NY: Scribner.

Kurtz, R. (1990). *Body-centered psychotherapy: The Hakomi method*. Mendocino, CA: LifeRhythm.

Levine, P. (2012). *In an unspoken voice. How the body releases trauma and restores goodness*. Berkeley, CA: North Atlantic Books.

Malchiodi, C. (2011, ). What art therapy learned from September 11th [blog entry]. Retrieved September 9 from www.psychologytoday.com/us/blog/arts-and-health/201109/what-art-therapy-learned-september-11th.

McNiff, S. (1992). *Art as medicine.* Boston, MA: Shambhala.

McNiff, S. (1998). *Trust the process: An artist's guide to letting go.* Boston, MA: Shambhala.

McNiff, S. (2019). AATA reflections on what 'art' does in art therapy practice and research. *American Journal Art Therapy, 29*(3), 162–165.

Miscarriage. (n.d.). In *Online etymology dictionary.* Retrieved from www.etymon line.com/search?q=miscarriage

Morgan, M. (2006). Neuroscience and psychotherapy. *Hakomi Forum 15-17,* 9–22.

Najarian, A. (2007). *Transmission of trauma, ritual and art therapy.* Graduate Projects (Non-thesis)] (Unpublished) Retrieved from https://spectrum.library.concordia.ca/view/creators/Najarian=3AAnie=3A=3A.html

Negash, S., & Cobb, R. (2010). Altered book making as a form of art therapy: A narrative approach. *Journal of Family Psychotherapy, 21*(1), 54–69.

Peck, S. (2019, Feb 4). Broken heart syndrome: When grief affects your mind and body. *Seen.* Retrieved from https://seenthemagazine.com/broken-heart-syndrome/

Rappaport, L. (2009). *Focusing-oriented art therapy: Accessing the body's wisdom and creative intelligence.* London, England: Jessica Kingsley.

Rothaus, M. (2014). Hakomi and art therapy. In L. Rappaport (Ed.), *Mindfulness and the arts therapies* (pp. 208–218). London, England: Jessica Kingsley.

Rothert, D. (2019, July 27). Pregnancy loss and infant death. (Web log post). Retrieved from http://donnarothert.com/pregnancy-and-infant-loss-resources/

Rubin, J. (2011). *The art of art therapy.* Originally published 1984. London, England: Routledge.

Schaverien, J. (1992). *The revealing image; Analytical art psychotherapy in theory and practice.* London, England: Jessica Kingsley.

Schirch, L. (2005). *Ritual and symbol in peacebuilding.* Bloomfield, CT: Kumarian Press.

Seftel, L. (2006). *Grief unseen: Healing pregnancy loss through the arts.* London, England: Jessica Kingsley.

Some, M. (1993). *Ritual: Power, healing and community.* New York, NY: Penguin.

Some, M. (2019). Personal communication.

Stroebe, M., & Schut, H. (1999). The dual process model of coping with bereavement: Rationale and description. *Death Studies, 23*(3), 197–224.

Thompson, G. (2009). Artistic sensibility in the studio and gallery model: Revisiting process and product. *American Art Therapy Journal, 26*(4), 159–166.

Wadeson, H. (2011). *Journaling cancer in words and images.* Springfield, IL: Charles C. Thomas.

Wasilewska, E. (1992). Ritual and art making. *American Art Therapy Journal, 9*(4), 198–200.

Weller, F. (2015). *The wild edge of sorrow: Rituals of renewal and the sacred work of grief.* Berkeley, CA: North Atlantic Books.

Worden, J. W. (1991). *Grief counseling and grief therapy: A handbook for the mental health practitioner.* New York, NY: Springer.

# 9 Honoring the Process

## Art Therapy with Mothers of Pediatric Palliative Care Patients

*Mary K. Kometiani and Katherine A. Holbrook*

This work often begins with the words that no mother wants to hear. When an infant is diagnosed with a life-threatening or chronic illness, clinicians struggle with heavy emotional burdens of compounded loss, extensive needs of patient and their situation, and sensitive demeanor while communicating with the family. Finding the right words to say seems impossible because there are no right words to say when a baby is dying or facing a shortened and altered life due to chronic illness.

Pediatric palliative care is an interdisciplinary, holistic, and family-centered approach that improves quality of life and provides healing to young children and their families. For those diagnosed with a life-threatening illness, palliative care aims to reduce suffering through treating the entire person (World Health Organization, 2019). This care maximizes the well-being of the child diagnosed with a serious illness including irreversible health conditions such as severe disabilities, progressive neurological disorders, and diagnoses where curative methods fail, resulting in premature death of a child (Santucci & Kang, 2017). Wide-reaching, palliative care meets not only the patient's physical, psychosocial, emotional, and spiritual needs, but also provides support to their family members, too. Within the pediatric palliative realm of healthcare, art therapy may span a child's life from birth through death and bereavement support for family members (Holley, Kometiani, & Friebert, 2017).

Palliative treatment is interdisciplinary care as this work does not occur in isolation. Palliative care extends past the healthcare setting into the home environment and the community. Palliative care teams are made of physicians, nurses, social workers, psychologists, expressive therapists, dieticians, chaplains, physical therapists, child life workers, and volunteers. Oftentimes, palliative care transitions into hospice and end-of-life care.

## Effects of Illness on Families

The patient's family has diverse and multiple needs that the palliative care team can address. The stress of a child's illness and death has many effects on a family:

- Parents may need to divide their time to care for the child at the hospital and other responsibilities at home such as work and other children; palliative care team members can provide support to the patient and family through hospitalization (for example, setting up volunteer visits if patient struggles with familial separation).
- The emotional effects from diagnosis of an illness and prognosis can be overwhelming and parents and siblings have different therapeutic needs; palliative care team members can work with various needs and meet with family members separately or in a group environment to best support them.
- Diagnosis acknowledgement can be a time of spiritual crisis when families question their faith or spirituality, and these matters can be addressed through trained palliative care clinicians.
- Financial burdens of hospitalization are numerous; palliative care can help with connecting families to resources and for assistance or medical insurance issues.
- Other hospital stressors on family members include feelings of isolation and subsequent lack of self-care, burdensome decision-making, and cumbersome communication between immediate and extended family members that can divide a family when support is needed.

The effects of a life-threatening diagnosis, lengthy and numerous hospitalizations and loss are numerous for the family members; however, palliative care is suited to address and help the patient and family navigate this time of crisis.

## Postpartum Depression

Families are especially vulnerable due to the overwhelming distress and demands; in addition, mothers who have recently given birth are even more at-risk due to the possibility of postpartum depression. The National Institute of Mental Health (n.d.) describes postpartum depression as a mood disorder for women after childbirth that results in extreme sadness and anxiety and affects one's ability to provide care. Some common symptoms include hopelessness, bouts of crying, anxiety, moodiness, difficulty eating and sleeping, trouble with focusing, somatic symptoms, loss of interest in pleasurable events, and trouble bonding with baby (National Institute of Mental Health, n.d.). Postpartum depression can be treated, but its symptoms may be similar to both depression and normal adjustment to a new baby; hence, seeking a postpartum diagnosis from a healthcare provider is crucial (National Institute of Mental Health, n.d.).

The art therapist may see indications for concern within the artwork, confirmed through verbalizations by the mother that would warrant in-depth assessment and follow-up care. Due to setting limitations, if the art therapist treats the mother for postpartum depression, the mother could alternatively be referred to a psychologist, especially if the hospital offers a neonatal intensive care unit (NICU) psychologist who could diagnose and provide the appropriate treatment to the mother. Then, the art therapist and psychologist could work together to provide consistent care to the new mother who is coping with loss, fear, and physical changes to improve symptoms and bonding between her and her child.

## Perinatal Palliative Care

Perinatal palliative care is for families who receive a prenatal life-threatening diagnosis (Silver, 2017). Perinatal palliative care utilizes a family-centered approach to plan for the birth and death of a baby; pre-planning for advance care and symptom management is done for the baby as a form of preparation (Silver, 2017). Ideally, referrals occur immediately after a diagnosis is confirmed so goals can align for families who wish to continue in pregnancy; in some cases, termination is recommended as medically necessary for a mother's health, and bereavement care can be beneficial (Silver, 2017). Memory making such as footprints, handprints, molds or artwork in addition to photographs should be offered as options for the family (Silver, 2017), and art therapy can enhance the memory-making process.

Concurrently, the art therapist and the palliative care team are integral to treatment as they offer avenues for the entire family to process their emotions surrounding the diagnosis and impending loss of the child. Support may be given for months prior to delivery and grief support following the delivery and death of the baby. When possible, grief services should be offered for the first calendar year following the death. This can include assessment of complicated grief and can be offered through home visits, bereavement groups, camps for siblings, and supportive phone calls. If this is not possible for the hospital palliative care team to provide, referrals and resources in the community should be provided to promote continued coping with severe loss.

## Case Example[1]

Art therapy benefited a family as they awaited the birth of their baby who was diagnosed with a life-threatening condition. While inpatient, the art therapist facilitated interventions for support and expression of their daily rollercoaster rides of anticipatory grief through feelings of sadness, guilt, anger, and confusion. Art therapy provided them an opportunity to share their feelings with each other when words were too threatening. The art provided a framework for the art therapist to guide their processing and as an aid for them to hear and understand how they were individually feeling and coping with the crisis and impending death of their baby.

In addition to support throughout the pregnancy, the art therapist provided daily support at bedside post-delivery. When it was clear the baby was not going to survive and the family asked to discontinue non-beneficial life-sustaining therapies, the art therapist guided them through the agonizing process of redefining their hope and future without their baby. The mother's artwork centered on her faith, incorporating scripture and colors that she found comforting. As she reflected on her painting, she could see how the use of scripture aided her decision-making and grounded her beliefs and hopes, even in death. Her art was created at bedside in the NICU and placed near the baby's crib for her to reference as a reminder to persevere through this seemingly unbearable time.

The main goals in caring for dying children are to comfort the child through death and maintain hope for parents (Greenberg, 1995). Hope may change as the child progresses through illness, and eventually hope may imply new meaning in life even through death (Limbo, Kavanaugh, & Kobler, 2017). This case example demonstrated how the art therapist helped the mother redefine hope for her child when a curative plan was no longer an option.

## Art Therapy and the Hospital Approach

Hospitals are complex bureaucratic and hierarchal systems, and families may struggle with adjusting to the new environment. The medical setting is often compared to a foreign country—there are unusual smells, the signs are confusing and it has its own language including overhead codes and medical terminology. Art therapy can normalize a hospitalization and its challenging environment. Brief stays and longer visits can be both distressing and hopeful experiences for patients and their families; however, art therapy links to life outside of the medical world and is a tangible response to this experience and instills a renewed sense of community (Councill, 2012). Art therapy not only aids with normalization, it creates a shared hope and security within the medical environment.

Medical art therapists who work within a hospital may experience various challenges that are specific to their setting. Art therapists may struggle with feeling accepted by families, certain hospital units or by other medical staff. As they are not viewed as essential medical treatments, art therapy sessions may be interrupted. Sessions may be postponed due to changes in schedule, required medical procedures that take precedence or visits from a busy physician. Art therapists are cautioned not to feel threatened by these interruptions and to remain flexible with delayed or postponed sessions by offering different times to come back. They are reminded to respect and honor the individual process and the family dynamics at all times due to the ever-changing nature of this work. Art therapists can offer interventions to promote clear communication between family members and between the family and medical team to promote trust. Finally, art therapists are always reminded to regard the patient's room as a home and respect the family's needs and personal boundaries.

Considering these challenging stressors of the work, it is important for art therapists to practice self-care to avoid burnout and workplace fatigue. Working in a medical setting—especially within palliative care—has its share of emotional burdens, personal spirituality predicaments and mental drain. Due to these demands of the field, art therapists are urged to exercise self-awareness, make art, and utilize team support and supervision when possible. As an example, Figure 9.1 is a representation of the isolation, suffering and sadness of illness.

In addition, Figure 9.2 "Resurrection" was created as a way to process the suffering of patients and redefine hope for the therapist and Figure 9.3 explains the art therapist's verbal processing following the creation of the image.

The art therapist's writing illustrates her acceptance of the gift of art therapy, her role within the relationship and its ability to heal even in death. Some hospitals have developed art therapy programs for support in the workplace, and the encouraging benefits include emotional support, processing of grief, and building team morale and community (Kometiani, 2017; Nainis, 2005).

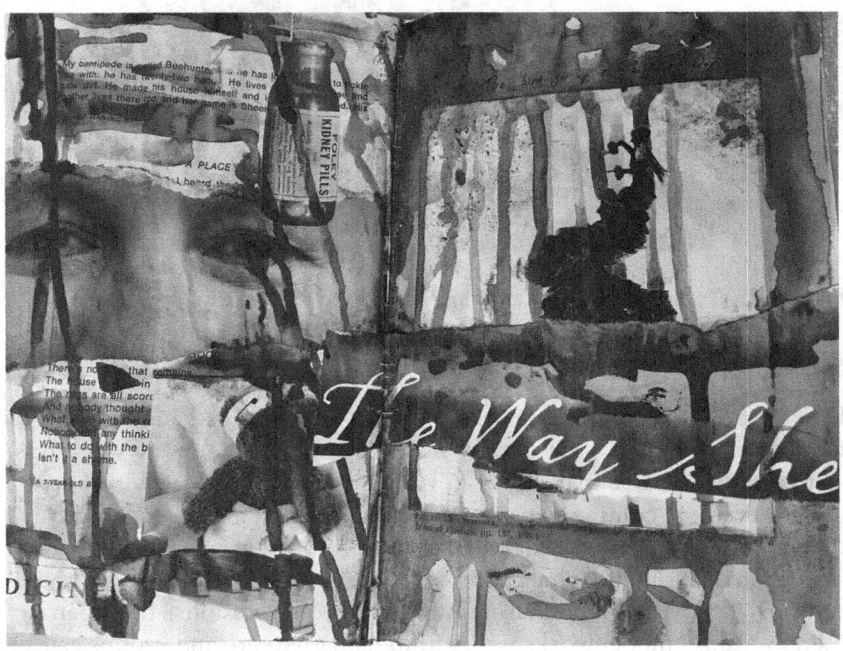

*Figure 9.1* "Untitled" by Mary, mixed media.

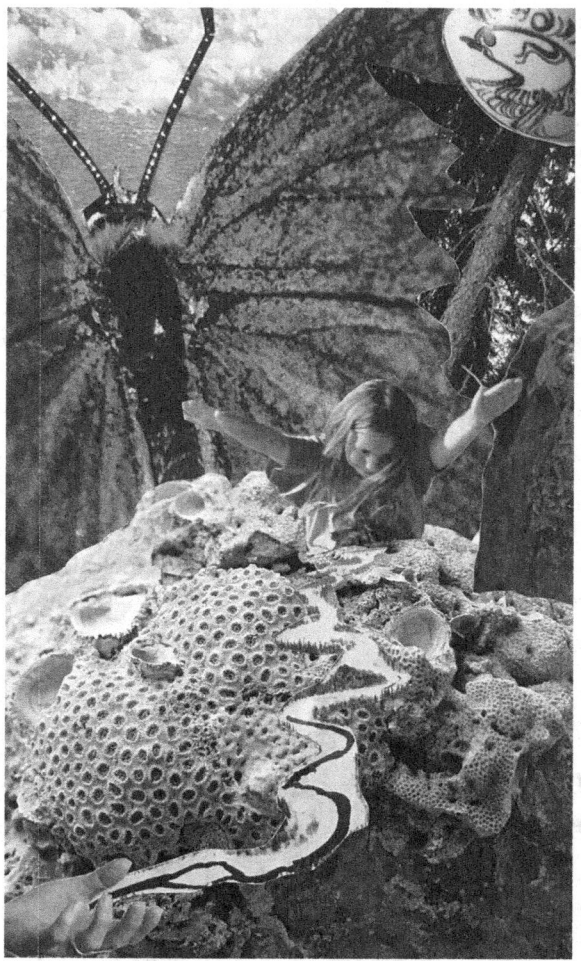

*Figure 9.2* "Resurrection" by Katherine, collage.

## Setting

Due to the flexible nature of palliative care, art therapists may meet with families at any given time of day, including evening hours or weekends. Art therapy sessions may occur in hospital rooms, home environments, waiting areas or common spaces such as an art therapy room, expressive therapy area or Ronald McDonald House (n.d.) that offer a home away from home during hospitalizations for families. Palliative care art therapists may provide individual, family, and group sessions; the open art therapy studio model works well within palliative care and groups can be attended by families and friends.

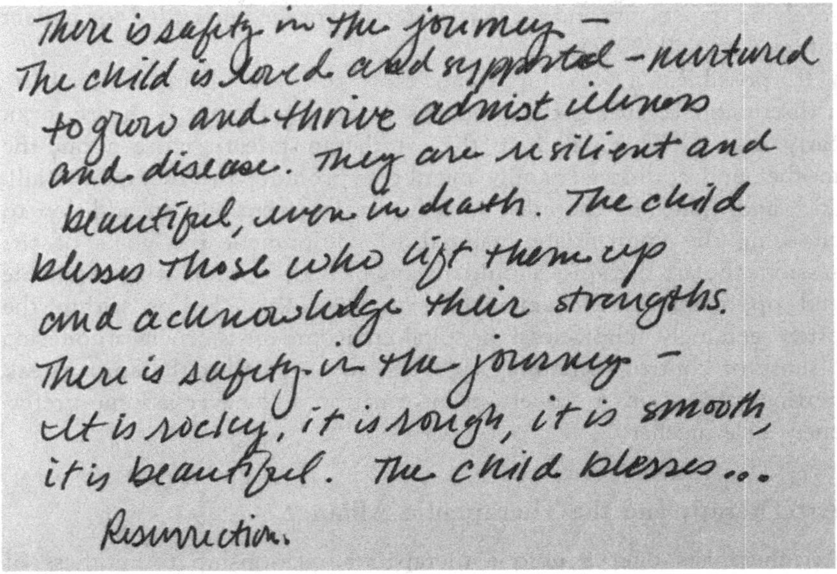

*Figure 9.3* "Untitled" by Katherine.

Art therapists may want to hold on to artwork to show progression or to use as a reflective tool in therapy; however, within this environment, this practice should be used with caution due to unforeseen health changes that occur, hospital discharges that may not leave time for a closure session, and typical lack of space for storage. It is at the discretion of the art therapist when it might be beneficial to retain artwork for future processing. For more information, see the case example in the section Grief and Loss. Art therapists may receive referrals from numerous sources including other team members, hospital staff or self-referrals. It is also appropriate for the art therapist to make referrals to any team members who may be beneficial for the family.

### Art Materials

At the bedside, the following art materials are appropriate and easy to transport: paints such as acrylic paints and watercolors; collage materials such as pre-cut images, scissors and glue sticks; scrapbooking supplies; drawing materials such as pastels and pencils; air dry and non-messy clay like model magic; and digital art or photography if available. Art therapists are cautioned against using strong-smelling materials and especially messy materials as they are working in a patient's living space.

Extreme caution with art supplies should be used with patients who are receiving transplants and new art materials are recommended for patient safety (Councill, 2012).

If possible, it is important that the art therapist facilitate a discussion regarding the mother's prior experiences with art in an early session. This will help the art therapist learn more about the mother and additional family members, promote the therapeutic alliance and guide the therapist with future interventions. In addition to choosing the appropriate material to compliment the goals of the session, the art therapist should always provide options when available and opportunities for empowerment. Providing choices within the often seemingly "choiceless" hospital environment is crucial in offering a sense of control to families. It is the job of the art therapist to ask pertinent questions to ascertain information and never assume preferences of a mother.

## Art Therapy and the Therapeutic Alliance

Art therapists offer a unique therapeutic relationship to mothers of pediatric palliative care patients. Art therapy not only offers a sense of control and opportunity to experience empowerment in palliative care, but it is also client-led (Dobbs, 2008). Art therapists provide a supportive alliance that is non-threatening and action-oriented for individuals who may have little experience with art or who do not have the words to verbalize their experience. Art therapy's focus is on the image, the creating, and the relationship with the therapist; the therapeutic relationship is of the greatest importance in art therapy (Dobbs, 2008). The results of a supportive partnership between the mother and the art therapist are powerful symbols that hold deep meaning and purpose. Within palliative care, metaphoric images that hold much meaning are often expressed (Dobbs, 2008).

### Case Example

Art therapists can promote trust building between the mother and the medical team from the therapeutic alliance that is developed between the therapist and client. When a parent has deemed a reason to mistrust medical personnel, efforts for care of the child can be undermined at critical times. For instance, art therapy improved the therapeutic alliance between a mother and an art therapist when her infant was diagnosed with the same complex disease as the infant's deceased sibling.

Following a grim conference with the medical team, the mother interpreted the medical advice to be that her baby's death was imminent. The art therapist remained with the mother for an extended period of time after the meeting, providing an outlet for her to express her deepest emotions both verbally and graphically. She was offered a choice of materials to promote her expression of loss of control. Her artwork contained abstract watercolor images. The nonrepresentational, flowing multicolored painting seemed to signify her strengths used for coping in the past and in the present. As the art therapist rotated the completed painting for her to view, the mother began to verbalize what she felt with each rotation. She voiced her understanding of how events can change rapidly and may not appear as they seem. The art was a continued reminder of the beauty that can be found, even in somber situations, and her hope was redefined for her through art therapy. The art therapist's presence throughout this crisis gave the mother reason to trust the therapeutic relationship, thus grounding future work. It should be noted that significant sessions within the palliative care framework rarely will happen in a planned manner, or will they be within a specific time frame. The nature of palliative care requires the art therapist to remain flexible and available, with a willingness to do whatever the family might need to cope with the crisis at hand.

The therapist became the main support within the hospital structure and the mediator for palliative care for this mother and art therapy continued with this mother for a few years until her baby died. The therapist provided hand and foot castings post mortem, and grief support through art therapy was utilized for the mother and family following the death of the child. It was vital to avoid an abrupt end of this relationship following the child's death to prevent an experience of abandonment for the family and add to their loss. In the case where the hospital palliative care art therapist is unable to provide continued bereavement support, a referral to another professional is recommended.

## Art Therapy Approach in Palliative Care

The main goal of palliative care is to reduce suffering whether it is physical, emotional, psychological, mental or spiritual. Although only art therapists can provide art therapy, palliative care members can collaborate and co-treat during other therapies or during treatments to address goals. The main goal of art therapy for palliative care patients and families is to improve quality of life. Palliative care is centered on living life fully, and the arts are a necessary part of this; the inclusion of art therapy in palliative care inspires, stimulates and strengthens those who face weakness, agony, death and loss (Hartley & Payne, 2008). The overarching goal of pediatric palliative care for parents is for them to feel they did the "right thing" and did not cause needless suffering to their child. The palliative care art therapist's role is to support the family through the journey.

Like palliative care, art therapy provides healing and value universally (Holley et al., 2017). An art therapist focuses on providing a supportive relationship with the family where difficulties are expressed, upsetting and unacceptable feelings are accepted, and empowering choices are offered. The palliative care art therapist can assist with interventions that allow each member to be heard and understood. Art therapists can be valuable to the medical treatment team by assisting in communication efforts so the mothers are able to voice their hopes and goals effectively, which promotes understanding and informed decision-making.

## Grief and Loss

The death of a child is perhaps the most distressing, painful event any parent may face. The death of one's child seems unnatural, and this loss encompasses loss of hope for the future and dreams for not only the child but for oneself as children represent the dreams of parents (Greenberg, 1995). Through bereavement, art therapy has been documented to help by creating visual memorials and expressing loss (Halliday, 2016; Hunter, Lewis, & Donovan, 2013; Kohut, 2011). Aiding in the multiple levels of loss and change that surround disease and mortality (Fenton, 2008), art therapy is a tangible legacy of one's life and existence (Rutenberg, 2008).

Grief is an individual process and is not orderly or predictable (James, 2017). Grief is the physical, emotional, spiritual and cognitive experience of dealing with a death of a loved one. Common feelings include shock, numbness, depression, anger, guilt, anxiety, confusion and somatic symptoms that affect eating and sleeping (James, 2017). The grief process may be obstructed by cultural beliefs such as the relationships with providers and modern medicine, the decisions that are made, intense emotional expression and communication, privacy issues between people and institutions, rituals, end-of-life meaning and beliefs, and grief expressions (James, 2017). In response, art therapy can be a part of healing grieving rituals through making a keepsake box, lighting a decorated candle, sewing a quilt from clothes or blankets, scrapbooking or creating hand castings.

## Case Example

The mother of a baby who had been diagnosed with complex medical issues from premature birth was referred to art therapy for emotional expression. The art therapist provided her with the directive to create a piece of art depicting how she felt at that particular time. Given a choice of art media, she eventually selected acrylics. The art therapist provided brief instructions for the use of the paint and remained near for guidance and processing as the art was created. The mother responded well to this approach, verbalizing her choices of colors and subject matter throughout the session.

When she had completed her painting, she and the art therapist processed the meaning of each image. The mother voiced the connection to her grief over the losses of a full-term pregnancy that coincided with the loss of her employment. These terminations were not only multifaceted, but they were also largely unresolved. Her artwork (Figure 9.4) consisted of bright colors containing a burning bush with a fire shooting from within. She included a foreground of flowers about to be engulfed by the fire.

The mother described the image as her own self-assessment of her ability to cope with her stress. The mother was overcome with emotion and asked for the therapist to remove the painting and keep it for her. This vivid painting's imagery was so strong that, without being present or referred to verbally, it became a powerful tool for the art therapist to utilize in future sessions over a period of eight months.

When it was time for the child to go home and for the therapeutic relationship to be terminated, the mother was given the same art directive she had been given in her first session with the art therapist. Unaware, the mother began to paint an almost identical image as she had painted eight months prior. The burning bush had been replaced

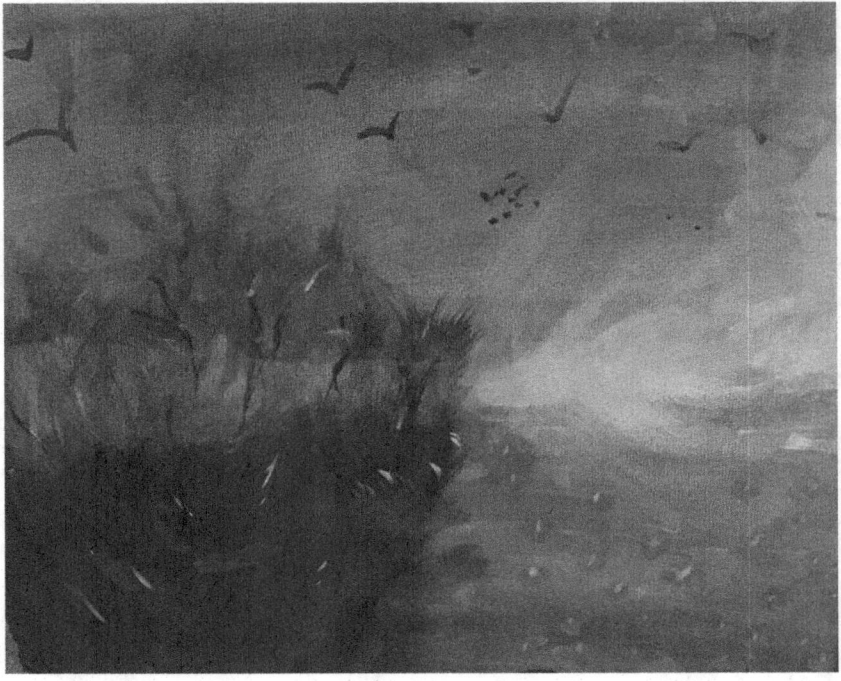

*Figure* 9.4 "Burning Bush" by mother, acrylic paint.

with a heart in the center as one of the largest shapes in the painting (Figure 9.5). However, the mother made one change to the heart—the fire had been replaced with a bright yellow light surrounding the heart. She voiced feeling loved, supported, healed, and ready to meet the challenges of care for her medically complex baby.

At that moment, the art therapist placed the original painting side by side with the new painting for further processing. The mother was speechless for several minutes before she exclaimed—with joy and awe —how far she had come in her healing from the losses and fears in her life. She noted there was no denying how hard she had worked to heal, grow, and feel more empowered for the challenges ahead of her.

### Case Example

Providing end-of-life care for a child and a family is a responsibility that requires sensitive listening and responding in a timely manner. To create legacy work, the art therapist can offer to make three-dimensional hand and foot castings, which is a tangible representation of a loved one's uniqueness that the family can cherish after death. Because creating a cast

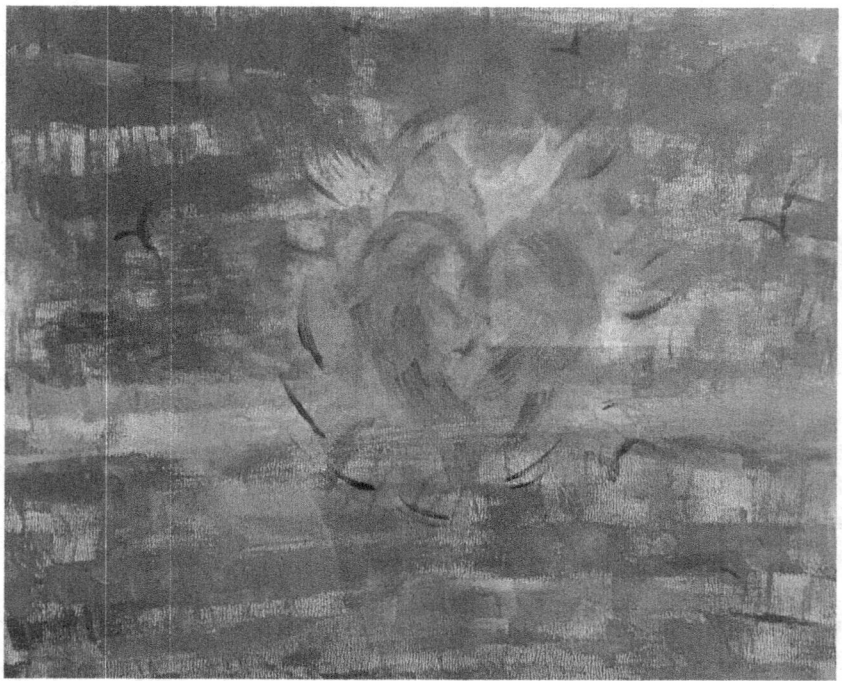

*Figure 9.5* "Heart" by mother, acrylic paint.

is truly emotional work, the offering of such an intervention should be assessed as to whether the process will impart additional emotional stress on the family. Timing is critical, and the therapist must assess when to offer the intervention and the readiness of the family to conduct the castings as this may differ widely among families. The art therapist needs to remain flexible to be prepared to facilitate the intervention at any time during impending death once the intervention has been offered. Before offering to make the castings, it is important to check with the bedside nurse if hand(s) can be placed in the casting medium and if a child's body can be moved in order to make a better casting. Nurses can help the therapist in this process by moving the child or the body into the best position for casting.

Due the emotional strain at this challenging time for the family, it is the role and responsibility of the art therapist to create a safe space for the casting to be done to promote a calm environment for the family. The therapist will want to ask the parents who they would like to be in the room, if they would like soothing music and if they would prefer to have the therapist make the castings prior to death or post mortem. The utmost respect for the child or the body of the child must be shown at all times. Permission to touch the body of the child is recommended as art therapists are not trained medical personnel. Although most parents will choose not to be present for the making of the castings, they may change their minds and participate. The therapist must make every effort to assess and respond to the parents' emotions and needs throughout the process.

As an alternative to castings, family portraits are also an option for legacy work and can improve communication between family members. A young couple was struggling with facing the discontinuation of non-beneficial life sustaining therapies for their one-week-old infant. The maternal great-grandfather of the infant struggled to accept his granddaughter's pregnancy and refused to accept the infant as his great-granddaughter, which had increased the mother's stress. As a result, the extended family had been unaware of the pregnancy and was trying to cope with acceptance of a new life in their family while also coping with the concurrent loss.

The art therapist assessed tremendous distress within the family unit and offered to create a combined family portrait of handprints. A large canvas was utilized to accommodate the number of family members. The mother of the infant chose the background color and helped to paint the canvas. Each family member was given an option for color of their handprint and asked to write their name next to their print. Tears, verbalizations of sadness, and grief were expressions released as each dipped their hands in paint and pressed on the canvas.

The great-grandfather was present for this intervention. After gentle encouragement from the art therapist to participate despite his initial resistance, he chose his color, dipped his hand into the paint, and placed his palm on the space next to her granddaughter's handprint. His hand remained on the canvas until his tears joined and mixed with the paint. The name he wrote on the canvas was "great grandfather." The art intervention facilitated a new bond among the family members and an emotional outlet that reduced their stress, relieved their sadness, fostered their acceptance of loss and reminded them of their family bonds. To receive this acknowledgement from her family was especially meaningful for the mother in her grief process. In the grief process, art therapists help individuals make peace with their life story, say good-bye in order to experience completion of a relationship, and find meaning beyond the end of life (Bertman, 1999).

## Conclusion

When a child receives an incurable diagnosis, caregivers may struggle with many different facets of stress due to familial responsibilities with other children, work obligations, financial strains of medical care, emotional havoc of physical decline, and existential concerns. Art therapy has specific appeal to mothers of palliative care patients because the active, cathartic engagement offers control over something when there is little control over so many other aspects of their lives. Art therapy helps caregivers adjust to illness and treatment (Councill, 2012) and the intrinsic connection between mothers and their children is unmistakable in the artwork (Schueler, 2015).

The different case studies presented in this chapter exemplify the range of art therapy applications in the pediatric palliative care realm; the meaningful interventions ranged from hand castings post mortem and family portraits to emotional expression and messages of faith. The purposes of art therapy within palliative care include empowerment at a time when control and choice are limited, enhanced awareness through expression, safe and cathartic containment, and opportunity for change to cope with life's adjustments (Wood, 1998). Mothers who are provided with opportunities to communicate in color and symbol reveal depth and meaning in their artwork and allow acceptance of unacceptable situations. Art therapy is way for family members to bond at a vulnerable and trying time. The art therapist facilitates connection and communication through creation. Even when families are faced with impending loss, they can focus on life and find hope.

As art therapists, we may not know what seeds are planted through our art interventions in palliative care, but it is our goal that the benefits continue to promote healing, whether it is spiritual, emotional, psychological, or overall well-being. It is our job to be present, to listen with our ears, feel with our hearts, and to holistically respond through the healing power of art therapy. Most importantly, our goal is to honor the process for the mothers and their families.

## Terms

**Pediatric palliative care** interdisciplinary and holistic care that improves quality of life and provides healing to infants, young children and their families.

**Perinatal palliative care** care for families that receive a prenatal life threatening diagnosis.

**Interdisciplinary palliative care** various professionals who work together within palliative care to achieve goals for patient and family.

**Perinatology** A specialization of obstetrics that is concerned with both at risk or ill fetus and the high risk pregnancy.

## Recommendations for Best Practice

- Art therapists are integral members of the palliative care team, and the nature of palliative care requires the art therapist to remain flexible and willing within the scope of work to meet the family's needs.
- For families, especially mothers, of pediatric palliative care patients, art therapy is a link to normalcy, a pathway for communication, and an opportunity for the family to bond, find acceptance, and feel hope again.
- This challenging work is a privilege and honor. Art therapists are encountering individuals at one of the most vulnerable times in their lives; therefore, therapists need to remember to practice self-care and find support in the workplace and beyond.

## Note

1 An amalgam of several confidential clinical situations was used to create case material so as to better illustrate art therapy and palliative care.

## References

Bertman, S. L. (1999). Grief and healing arts: Introduction. In S. L. Bertman (Ed.), *Grief and healing arts: Creativity as therapy* (pp. 1–2). Amityville, NY: Baywood Publishing Company, Inc.

Councill, T. D. (2012). Medical art therapy with children. In C. A. Malchiodi (Ed.), *Handbook of art therapy* (2nd ed., pp. 222–240). New York, NY: Guilford Press.

Dobbs, S. (2008). Art therapy. In N. Hartley & M. Payne (Eds.), *The creative arts in palliative care* (pp. 128–139). London, UK: Jessica Kingsley Publishers.

Fenton, J. F. (2008). "Finding one's way home": Reflections on art therapy in palliative care. *Art Therapy: Journal of the American Art Therapy Association*, 25(3), 137–140. doi:10.1080/07421656.2008.10129598

Greenberg, M. L. (1995). The impact of the hospital system on dying children and their families. In D. W. Adams & E. J. Deveau (Eds.), *Beyond the innocence of childhood: Helping children and adolescents cope with life-threatening illness and dying* (pp. 211–236). Amityville, NY: Baywood Publishing Company, Inc.

Halliday, J. (2016). Shifting lines: Palliative art therapy in the home. In C. Miller (Ed.), *Arts therapists in multidisciplinary settings: Working together for better outcomes* (pp. 140–152). London, UK: Jessica Kingsley.

Hartley, N., & Payne, M. (2008). Introduction—the creative arts in palliative care. In N. Hartley & M. Payne (Eds.), *The creative arts in palliative care* (pp. 11–20). London, UK: Jessica Kingsley Publishers.

Holley, L. M., Kometiani, M. K., & Friebert, S. (2017). Expressive therapy and complementary approaches in palliative care. In K. Kobler & R. Limbo (Eds.), *Conversations in perinatal, neonatal & pediatric palliative care* (pp. 87–108). Leetsdale, PA: Hospice and Palliative Nurse Association.

Hunter, H. K., Lewis, D., & Donovan, C. (2013). Young adult bereavement camp. In C. A. Malchiodi (Ed.), *Art therapy and healthcare* (pp. 291–303). New York, NY: Guilford Press.

James, K. (2017). Supporting grieving families after the death of a child. In K. Kobler & R. Limbo (Eds.), *Conversations in perinatal, neonatal & pediatric palliative care* (pp. 275–296). Leetsdale, PA: Hospice and Palliative Nurse Association.

Kohut, M. (2011). Making art from memories: Honoring deceased loved ones through a scrapbooking bereavement group. *Art Therapy: Journal of the American Art Therapy Association, 28*(3), 123–131.

Kometiani, M. K. (2017). Creating a vital healing community: Pilot study for art therapy employee support group at pediatric hospital. *The Arts in Psychotherapy.* doi:10.1016/j.aip.2017.04.012

Limbo, R., Kavanaugh, K., & Kobler, K. (2017). Honoring relationship and hope. In K. Kobler & R. Limbo (Eds.), *Conversations in perinatal, neonatal & pediatric palliative care* (pp. 35–48). Leetsdale, PA: Hospice and Palliative Nurse Association.

Nainis, N. A. (2005). Art therapy with an oncology care team. *Art Therapy: Journal of the American Art Therapy Association, 22*(3), 150–154. doi:10.1080/07421656.2005.10129491

National Institute of Mental Health. (n.d.) Postpartum depression facts. Retrieved from www.nimh.nih.gov/health/publications/postpartum-depression-facts/postpartum-depression-brochure_146657.pdf

Ronald McDonald House. (n.d.) What we do. Retrieved from www.rmhc.org

Rutenberg, M. (2008). Casting the spirit: A handmade legacy. *Art Therapy: Journal of the American Art Therapy Association, 25*(3), 108–114. doi:10.1080/07421656.2008.10129592

Santucci, G., & Kang, T. I. (2017). Introduction to pediatric palliative care. In K. Kobler & R. Limbo (Eds.), *Conversations in perinatal, neonatal & pediatric palliative care* (pp. 1–8). Leetsdale, PA: Hospice and Palliative Nurse Association.

Schueler, L. (2015, February 9). Art from the heart: Moms with hospitalized infants craft to relax. Retrieved from https://125.akronchildrens.org/art-from-the-heart-moms-with-hospitalized-infants-craft-to-relax/

Silver, H. J. (2017). Perinatal palliative care. In K. Kobler & R. Limbo (Eds.), *Conversations in perinatal, neonatal & pediatric palliative care* (pp. 141–156). Leetsdale, PA: Hospice and Palliative Nurse Association.

Wood, M. J. M. (1998). What is art therapy? In M. Pratt & M. J. M. Wood (Eds.), *Art therapy in palliative care: The creative response* (pp. 1–11). London, UK: Routledge.

World Health Organization. (2019). WHO definition of palliative care. Retrieved from www.who.int/cancer/palliative/definition/en/

# 10 Motherhood Rounds It Out[1]

## Art Therapy with Mothers Without Mothers

*Valerie Epstein-Johnson*

This chapter explores the ways art therapy can help women whose mothers have died navigate the particular difficulties they may have in decision-making around having children, pregnancy and struggles to become pregnant, the grief process, parenting, and identity integration. For motherless women, motherhood may be fraught with emotional, psychological, and behavioral challenges, yet it may also hold the promise of coming full circle on their grief and individuation journeys.

> When motherhood interfaces with the long-term mourning process, the result is exponential. Becoming a mother can give a motherless daughter access to a more enhanced, more insightful, deeper, richer, and, in some cases, ultimate phase of mourning for her mother, one that may initially be painful but eventually leads her to a more mature and peaceful acceptance of both her loss and herself.
>
> (Edelman, 2006, p. 4)

For motherhood to fulfill this promise, however, requires active engagement in birthing not just babies, but nothing less than a new sense of self that contains both Motherless Daughter and Mother parts. Expressive art making with an art therapist sensitive to these issues can be a powerful aid in this process. Supported by the attuned companioning and gentle guidance of an art therapist, images can translate the client–artist's soul experience into expression (Malchiodi, 2002), which can be profoundly healing for a motherless woman who is entering the beautiful but difficult crucible of motherhood.

In having a child and actively making meaning from her experience, a woman with a deceased mother is engaging in a process of transformation from bereft daughter to wise, compassionate mother of not just her child but her inner child. This metamorphosis can decrease suffering through the inevitable challenges of parenting and long-term grief, and promote growth in other areas of life as quoted above (Edelman, 2006).

Using case examples from art therapy with my clients (whose names have been changed to protect their anonymity) and examples of my own therapeutic art making, this chapter elucidates the psychological challenges and opportunities for growth that confront a motherless mother and makes the case for art therapy as a treatment of choice for this population. It views the therapeutic needs of motherless mother clients primarily through the lens of modern grief theory, which emphasizes identity revision, meaning reconstruction through re-storying self-narratives and tending a new relationship with the lost mother (Edelman, 2006; Neimeyer, 2001). All of these, plus techniques to cope with intense feeling states inevitably triggered by motherhood, can help women meet the practical and psycho-emotional challenges of parenting.

Such issues are largely ignored in the research literature and larger culture and often overlooked by mental health providers (Edelman, 2006); thus, they bear further attention beyond the scope of this chapter.

Lastly, it is important to address the spiritual in therapeutic work with a population engaged in multiple existential initiations simultaneously related to birth and death. For some clients, this includes a spiritual connection that bonds her mother to her and her children; for all clients, the transpersonal element of ritual in art making, which honors experience and makes it transformative, is inherent to the use of the expressive arts for depth work (Epstein, 2004).

## Theory and Practice

For our therapeutic work to be effective, we as art therapists must not only mindfully engage with our unique clients, but draw on clinical research and the wisdom of experts on loss and parenting in choosing therapeutic interventions. While personal experience varies across any population, there are typical impacts of "motherloss" of which therapists should be cognizant (Davidman, 2000). A discussion of these and interventions to address them follows below, along with case examples of each.

Not only does art therapy have the capacity to go deeper than talk therapy into the caverns of being and knowing that exist beyond the cognitive and the verbal, it is an *active* modality that engages the client's imagination, senses, and ability to physically manipulate materials into a product. This active quality aligns therapeutically with the empowerment critical to working the "tasks of mourning," developed by leading grief researcher J. William Worden. Worden (as cited in Gilbert, 2016) asserted, "Death makes you feel out of control. Being proactive makes you feel stronger. Taking steps to remember leads to empowerment, and feeling empowered is absolutely necessary for living a full, happy, and loving life" (p. xxiv). Empowerment is also critical to parenting in that we, as parents, must feel empowered to meet our children's myriad needs, yet empower them to meet their own from early on.

To heal and grow from loss and motherhood, we, as motherless mothers, must learn how and when to embrace agency and how and when to practice acceptance of the limits of our control. In my own experience, when I direct my process of mourning and make values-based parenting decisions, I do feel a degree of control that mitigates the suffering inherent to the powerlessness of loss and parenting. At the same time, when I find ways to accept the ever-changing, impermanent nature of motherhood and life itself, my suffering is also eased. Therapeutic art making has been a deeply important way to do this in my life.

When art materials are unwieldy and our envisioned images do not emerge, we experience metaphors for our own limits and imperfections. In the process, we may even come to value the serendipitous results that sometimes materialize when we exercise trust and relax attachment to preconceived outcomes. As we learn these lessons as artists, we can take them beyond therapy into our lives as mourners, mothers, and mothers-to-be. Making art with an art therapist allows that learning to be gentle. When we are held in the secure attachment experience of risk-taking with the support of a nurturing—some might say maternal—witness beside us, stretching personal limits and confronting difficult truths can be a safe and empowering experience.

## "This Isn't How It Was Supposed to Be.": Biographical Disruption

Consequences of having lost a mother for women becoming mothers typically include the experience of biographical disruption, or a sense that one's expected life trajectory has been thrown profoundly off course twice—first, through the original loss, later at a time when a mother becomes a figure of conscious identification and is particularly missed and needed (Davidman, 2000).

Davidman (2000) and others emphasized the need for creating auto-biographical narratives as a means of understanding and guiding our choices and sense of identity (Edelman, 2006 Neimeyer, 2001). Neimeyer (2001) stressed the need for honoring "cherished features" of a disrupted self-narrative and restoring a sense of coherence to it (p. 267). For instance, if celebrating holidays with certain rituals with a mother who died was an important part of a woman's life, it may be important to continue to engage in those rituals with her children as a way to honor the relationship and other beloved elements of her past.

Therapeutic activities aimed at helping motherless mother clients repair the "master narrative" (Neimeyer, 2001, p. 263) sometimes entail compassionately highlighting how unmet expectations of leading a "normal life" lead to feelings of disillusionment and isolation. One directive that may help in this is a "Shoulds" image, in which the client draws or writes all the assumptions she has had about what a "normal family" looks like. For most, this includes the presence of a mother. Picturing "shoulds" can be a powerful statement of how numerous ones expectations can be, and how predictably suffering arises when she is unable to meet them.

Other helpful interventions involve guiding clients in refashioning personal narratives into a coherent arc (Edelman, 2006). These may include sculptures, drawings, and paintings that illustrate how a mother's life before her mother's death informs her present and future and how her life story has been affected by the loss. Edelman (2006) explained that

> before motherhood, a motherless daughter's story has a distinct before-and-after quality: all that came before her mother died, and all that has come after. Motherhood, however, puts a conceptual frame around the loss. First, she had a mother, then she lost her, then she became a mother herself. The loss no longer breaks her story in two. Motherhood rounds it out.
>
> (p. 7)

In this light, motherhood may be seen as a redemptive denouement to a tragic climax.

Directives like visual timelines offer an experiential way to connect becoming a mother to having a mother and losing that mother, weaving all three into a cohesive story. If the client has felt detached from her mother, her own mother identity or loss itself, a timeline that visually unifies them may be particularly useful in cultivating a more synthesized sense of self. Experimenting with alternatives to linear motifs, such as mandalas, may help to conceptualize life in more expansive, self-affirming ways than with chronology alone.

In the spiral-shaped mandala timeline I created to represent parts of my own autobiography below (Figure 10.1), colors and shapes represent the impact of loss on my relationships and motherhood, while also conveying evolution. By using a spiral form, I was able to see my life as a story that flows from one plot point to the next, rather than the fragmented before-and-after-Mom-died narrative I had told for so long.

For my client Lena, whose mother died birthing her younger brother when she was six, art therapy has allowed her to weave the threads of her richly textured life into a self-affirming narrative that has seemed to enhance resilience, confidence, and meaning in her life. In turn, her narrative has appeared to deepen her connection to her mother as one important source of this identity. Lena's story has also been marked by other significant traumas, but as she has embraced the use of art to examine her losses and experience of motherhood, the more deeply she

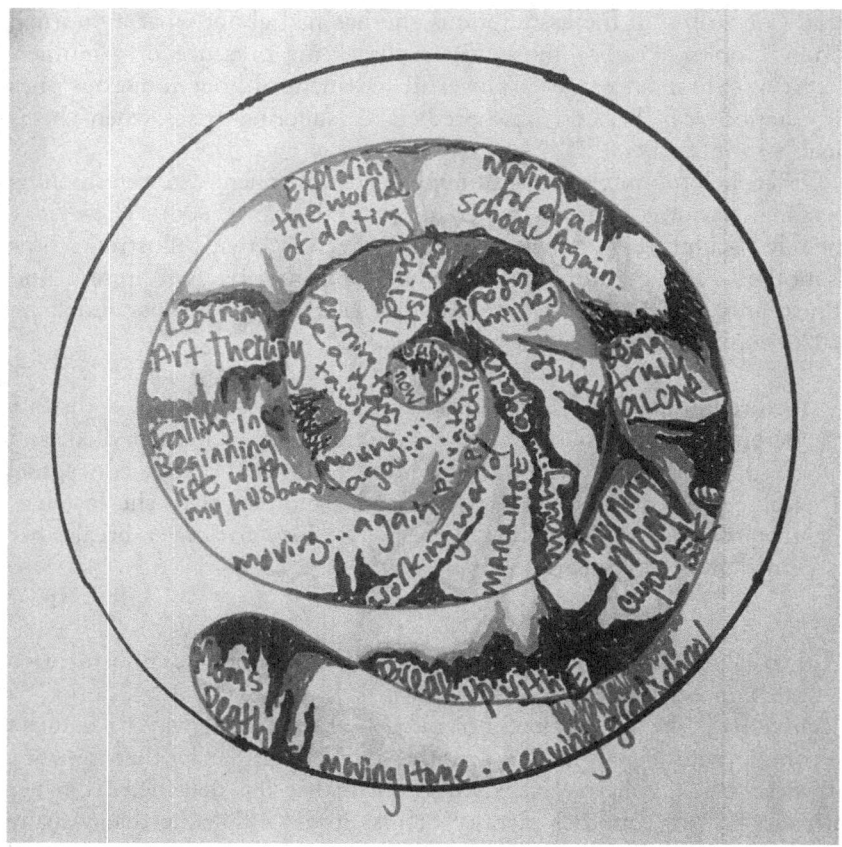

*Figure 10.1* "Mandala Timeline of Loss and Growth" drawing.

has seemed to relate to the persona of strong, wise explorer who has navigated many challenges and is continuing to use her life experience to grow in contentment and wisdom. From an archetypal perspective, Lena appears to embody the initiation archetype in her artwork and verbal narratives about her life journey; she specifically portrays herself as an often-misunderstood heroine who has been transformed by ordeal (Swan-Foster, 2012).

In "The Mountain" (Figure 10.2), Lena portrayed her personal narrative of initiation in an assemblage of a mountain surrounded by a moat with no bridge, made from found materials.

"The Mountain" is a structure representing the mountain of Lena's life, as she describes it. In assembling it, she felt and saw with compassion the difficult journey her life has been and her quest for growth. Lena has used her piece as a visual metaphor for where she has been and

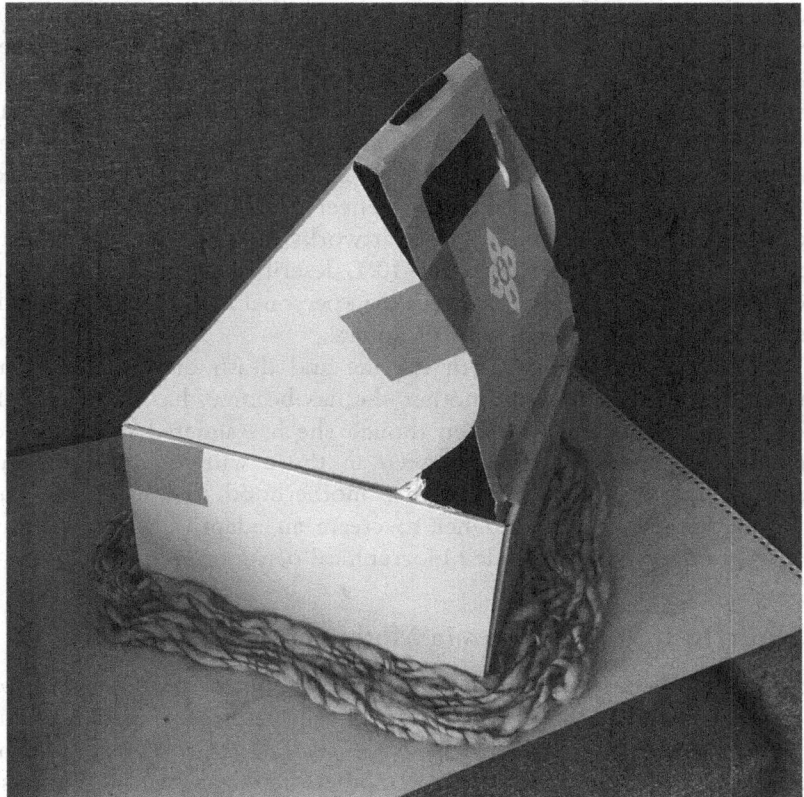

*Figure 10.2* "The Mountain" mixed media.

where she is now, and it affirms her determination to keep growing toward the summit, which she identifies as a life well-lived. The three-dimensional materials Lena used seemed to allow for a broader expressive palate to address the theme of challenge in her narrative than the two-dimensional materials had; seeing and feeling the verticality and hard edges, she appeared to really "get" that her life has been an uphill battle at times and that she has come so far.

While therapists must be careful to not impose their own conceptualizations of meaning in client artwork and narratives, the initiation archetype may help validate the motherless mother's experience of crisis and value in hard-won self-transformation, as it has for Lena in her experiences of loss, pregnancy, birthing, and motherhood. According to Swan-Foster (2012), "by becoming conscious of the archetypal pull through her emotional and creative efforts, [the pregnant woman] uncovers her own mythic story" (p. 210). Lena has achieved this kind of awareness through active engagement with her grief process, pregnancy, birth, and the journey of motherhood. By sharing memories of her pregnancy and birth, Lena appeared to powerfully crystallize her vision of herself as an initiate who has been transfigured by death and birth. Despite living most of her life without her mother and birthing five children over a 20-year period, Lena cried as she described the fear and loneliness of giving birth without her mother. Her births entailed a very real fear of not just labor and delivery, but of dying in childbirth like her mother. Nevertheless, in her artworks, such as "The Mountain" (Figure 10.2) and "The Path" (Figure 10.7, described later), Lena has been able to contextualize her trials in her own personal mythic narrative with herself cast as the wounded warrior-initiate.

Lena's understanding of both the life and death of her mother as integral to the capable, wise mother she has become, has been undeniably critical to her growth. Even though she has suffered physical and mental health issues commonly seen in those with complex trauma histories and these have affected her motherhood, the work she has done in therapy has allowed her to create an adaptive autobiography that has healed and transcended biographical disruption.

## "Can I Do It?": Challenges in Mothering

When a motherless mother enters therapy, she is often longing for someone to validate the lonely, dissonant aspects of her experience, but some women like this also struggle with handling the responsibilities of parenting as upsurges in grief and motherloss-related self-doubt arise (Edelman, 2006; Davidman, 2000).

A motherless mother may be predisposed to feel intense doubt in her ability to be a good mother when she becomes one or even contemplates conceiving. Even if there is another mother figure in her life, the daughter who was left motherless early often misses the intimate modeling of mothering during her own experience of motherhood and when she was actively needing nurturance and guidance as a child (Edelman, 2006). In many, if not most families, it is the mother who explicitly and implicitly teaches relationship building, caretaking, and running a household; if she dies when a daughter is young, there may be little exposure to the rules of the game (Davidman, 2000).

As Edelman (2006) discussed, motherless women tend to worry about the possibility of their own early death. For others, anxiety is more focused on their children and may lead to overprotective parenting as a result of their sensitization to mortality and the vulnerability of the mother–child relationship, as well as the absence of a maternal grandmother for their child. In either case, if the preoccupation with safety and future is extreme, it may ironically interfere with the kind of attuned, mindful parenting that allows children to feel safe and form a secure attachment style. As post-traumatic growth unfolds for mother-less mothers, fear of the possibility of their own early deaths may be tempered with or even replaced by an exceptional ability to be mindfully present and grateful as parents, knowing through loss how precious and brief time with their families may be. When the time is right, such wisdom may be nurtured through art making that is focused on lessons learned from motherloss.

Art processes that allow mothers to practice compassionate awareness of anxiety and engage in somatic self-soothing may be used as a template for responding to anxiety while parenting. These include body outline drawings in which mind–body experience is represented with colors and shapes. Extrapolating from the Acceptance and Commitment Therapy technique of Expansion (Harris, 2019), a common way I help clients build self-compassion and somatic self-regulation skills is to guide them through breathing both breath and compassion into the feelings that are portrayed. This kind of somatically focused art directive can be extremely useful in coping with the intense feelings mothers without mothers—indeed *all* mothers—face.

Awareness of trauma reactions and how to respond in a trauma-informed way is important when exploring the intense feelings of motherless mothers. Having lost a significant person to death, some of these clients may continue to have post-traumatic symptoms long after the loss, especially if the death was sudden, violent, or unexpected.

For Celene, a 36-year-old married woman whose mother committed suicide five years before she started art therapy with me, therapeutic goals have included deepening the grief work she previously began and exploring fears and values around having children. In our sessions, she has wrestled with issues of lifestyle, but also her difficulty imagining herself as a mother. She attributes this to being without her mother's example and support, as well as feelings of abandonment from her mother's suicide and lack of connection to others with children. Celene's doubts also stem from fears that her difficulty understanding and expres-sing her own feelings will negatively impact her ability to parent.

Figure 10.3 is an image of an "inside-outside box" intervention I suggested to Celene.

Hass-Cohen and Findlay (2015) called their version of the inside-outside box directive an "adaptation container," which emphasizes resi-lience and adaptive coping methods. They asserted that "adaptive responses and internal working models of security are evoked when we take thoughtful ownership of our inner space through artistic expres-sion" (p. 242). These art therapist–researchers likened the inner space of the box to the client's inner experience, suggesting that creating a "private sanctuary space" inside the adaptation container with images and other symbolic elements that represent connection, inspiration, and soothing can help in this process (p. 243).

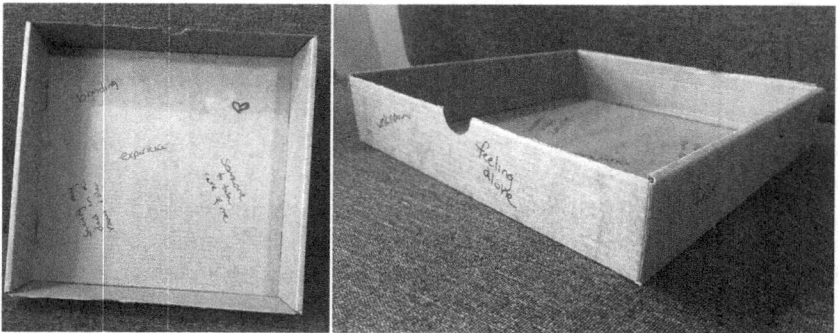

*Figure 10.3* "Hopes and Fears Box" mixed media.

The decision of whether or not to have children or not felt stuck for Celene and her husband; their perceived "cons" seemed to outnumber the "pros," and yet Celene continued to express that she might regret not having children. Given that Celene believed that her fears obscure her reasons for having children, I used elements of the adaptation container directive to help her externalize and normalize her fears on the outside of the box and truly internalize her hopes and values using the "sanctuary space" inside. By supporting a stronger connection to values and a more observant stance toward fears, it is possible to help clients cultivate greater psychological flexibility. This capacity allows for making decisions based on values rather than others' expectations or the avoidance of uncomfortable feelings (Harris, 2019).

In Celene's piece, only one image appears—a small, pink heart. Future therapeutic work may include dialogue with it and listening to what it might say about Celene's decision around conception. Given the depth of her love for her mother, it may also have something to teach her about her mother's place in her process.

In the session that followed, Celene expressed a new calm about her decision-making and shared that she and her husband are planning to start trying to conceive next spring. She attributed her shift to my normalization of her concerns, but it is likely that her artwork also helped her to relate to her fears in a new way, allowing a values-based resolve to emerge.

## "I Don't Feel like a Mother": Barriers to Identity Integration

A more existential estrangement from the Mother identity may be mixed up with feelings around new decisions and responsibilities. This is, of course, not exclusive to women with deceased mothers, but when it is part of the motherless mother story, the reasons are especially complex. Without a close maternal model and active parental support, motherhood is daunting, but there may also be a psychological challenge in identifying as a nurturer when a motherless woman has unconsciously come to define not just her story, but her sense of self, by loss. Reasons for this kind of self-definition are complex, but may include the sense that an ongoing connection to a deceased mother can be maintained only by continuing to identify as bereft. Making loss a central feature of one's identity can be a way to bring meaning to suffering, so it may be difficult for a motherless mother to embody the "nurturing mother" identity if it feels as though the "motherless daughter" inside her will, as a consequence, no longer be seen.

This conflict between identities (self as nurturing mother and self as motherless daughter) may begin with the decision around having children. Art making to visualize oneself as a mother may access intuition about what would be most authentic to one's choice of lifestyle, family structure, and identity. Images can help build confidence, demystify, and soothe the discomfort of uncertainty. To that end, I guided Celene in imagining herself as a mother in a drawing. Figure 10.4 is an image of Celene with her imagined child in the woods, which reflects her hope of continuing to spend much of her leisure time outdoors and sharing her love of nature with her child.

This scene represents some of the personal values Celene imagines she could embody more fully as a mother, despite complicated feelings around identity and responsibility, anxiety and grief, and worries that motherhood will be incompatible with the lifestyle she has enjoyed. While aspirational images do not always gain enough emotional traction to help resolve dilemmas like this, Celene seemed to glimpse a new version of herself that invited hope and curiosity when she created this drawing. Building on what seemed to be accomplished with the inside-outside box, this directive appeared to help Celene find a deeper connection to her values and internalize the idea that a new version of herself is not only possible, but consistent with who she wants to be.

## Identity Challenges of Pregnancy

For all women, pregnancy is a kind of limbo in which we experience the death of who we were and the gradual birth of a new version of ourselves (Swan-Foster, 2012). For mothers without mothers, feelings of loss and insecurity connected to the mother's death may be aroused by this first "powerful psychological feminine initiation" (Swan-Foster, 2012, p. 210) of motherhood.

For me, pregnancy was a journey of fear and faith. Having carried four pregnancies, two of which ended in live births, my relationship to pregnancy is a complicated one. After the loss of my mother when

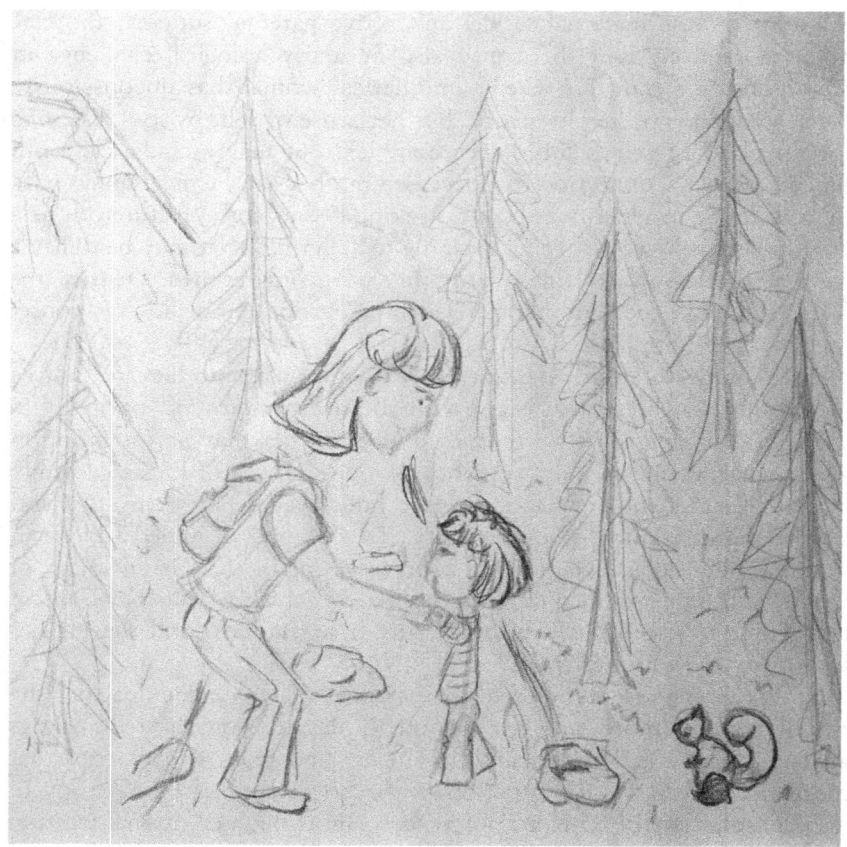

*Figure 10.4* "Imagining Motherhood" drawing.

I was 24, my inclination to one day have children became a spiritual imperative; I knew I would eventually try to recreate what I loved of family before mine was fractured by divorce, illness, and death, and I desperately wanted to create long-lasting, intimate relationships with my own children—as was not possible for me and my mother.

Given my challenges to conceive and maintain a pregnancy, pregnancy meant potential loss but also incredible hope to me. In my ambivalence around identifying with a mother who died, I wanted to relate to her, yet also wanted distance from her. Through a year of trying before conceiving our first child naturally, then a miscarriage, a surgery, and a year and a half of fertility treatment to conceive our second child, the possibility of not being able to have children felt like foreclosure on the life narrative I had already rewritten in my mind and a threat of new grief from which I was not sure I could recover. I processed my experience of this roller coaster in personal art making and art therapy, and even now, at the 20-year anniversary of my mother's death and 11 years into motherhood, I am still gleaning meaning from my experience of loss and motherhood through art.

As my pregnancies proceeded, I struggled to feel connected to my body, my baby, and the Great Mother archetype I wanted to claim as a kind of antidote to loss and the post-traumatic anxiety and detachment I sometimes experienced. To embrace the abundance of my healthy body and growing family sometimes felt like a betrayal of the Motherless Daughter identity I had adopted somewhere along the way. It was almost as though my loss, and therefore my mother, wouldn't matter anymore if I did. I also sometimes felt afraid that I, too, would die relatively young, marking my children's lives in the way that my mother's death had marked mine. But still, I tried for abundance. I worked with a professional body cast artist to create plaster casts of my torso, striving to feel more present with my pregnant body and more deeply connected to the baby growing inside it (Figure 10.5).

The casting process and the outside of the finished casts helped me appreciate the miracles of procreation and this new bond to my mother, but the hollows inside my first cast, with my torn shirt, exposed the ambivalence I sometimes felt about pregnancy. Mostly, though, the casts strengthened trust in my body to live and create life, and they offered me

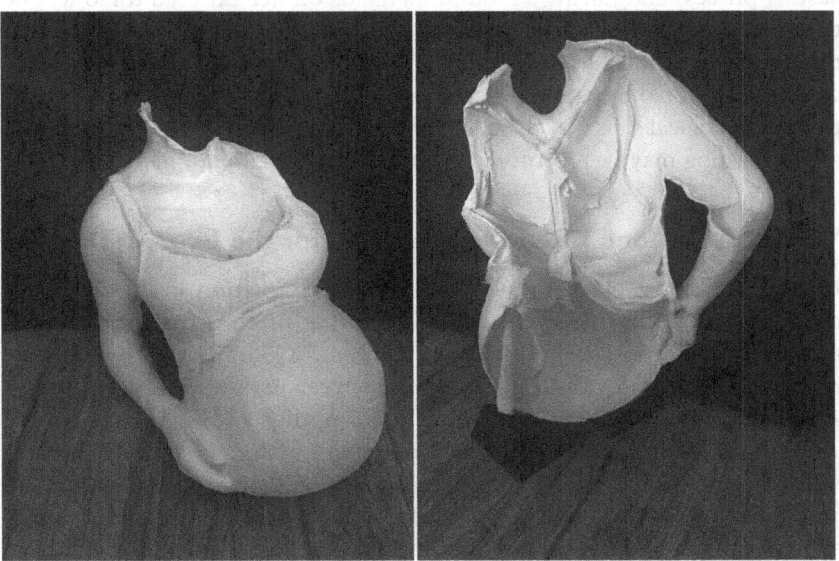

*Figure 10.5* "Pregnant belly cast" mixed media by Juliann Rubijono of Mamacasts (Boston, MA).

evidence of an archetypal connection to my mother. With motherhood, I could have a second chance at the kind of family and mother–child relationship I always wanted, this time from the other side. I also felt closer to my mom than I had since her death; I related to her in living out the feminine potential to gestate and birth a child, and I reveled in beginning to make the same kind of family she did.

Making a plaster belly cast may be helpful in some therapeutic relationships in all the ways it helped me, but it is an intervention to be used with extreme caution. First, it typically requires a longer session than the average individual therapy session, which is to be considered in terms of therapist and client stamina and how the intersubjective dynamic of a casting differs from a typical therapy session. In addition, given the exposure of and contact with a woman's stomach, an often judgment-laden, personal part of the body and something that already receives intrusive scrutiny by others during pregnancy, a belly cast process may feel violating. It may also be experienced as a boundary crossing to have a therapist use touch in session if that has not been part of the dynamic before and a strong trusting relationship has not been built.

Body casts are to be used with caution, also because of their immobilizing qualities. Encasing a woman who may have experienced abuse or other traumas in a hardening substance, which requires her to be still for a long period of time, may trigger a trauma response. For a belly cast to be a successful, trauma-informed art therapy intervention, it must be planned with trauma and body image history in mind, assessing with the client if the casting process and having a therapist's hands on her exposed torso will be triggering, and honestly evaluating the level of safety and intimacy in the therapeutic relationship at the time. When the therapist is skilled in the technicalities of the casting process, however, and takes care to safeguard the psychological safety of the client and sanctuary of the therapy situation, a belly casting may be a profoundly therapeutic intervention.

## "I Miss My Mom": Renewed Grieving for the Lost Mother

In addition to the challenges of identity transformation in motherhood, there is the predictable, renewed grieving that often occurs with transitions, as even positive changes entail loss. Complicated by change-induced activation of old losses, grief may rear its head in a new way as a woman grows to identify with her own mother and contemplates life without a grandmother for her children and a maternal support through motherhood. For some, this new phase of grieving comes with great pain; for others—often those further along in their grief process and those who lost their mothers later in life—the experience may be more bittersweet (Edelman, 2006; Davidman, 2000).

In my personal experience and clinical work with mothers without mothers, it has been confirmed that nurturing an ongoing relationship with a lost mother is a key task of grieving. Doing so tends to lead to a sense of movement in one's grief, a decrease in the frequency and/or intensity of emotional pain and an enhanced sense of existential meaning. Contemporary grief theory affirms this idea (Neimeyer, 2001).

Discussion and art making in art therapy often reveal the ways in which the client's relationship with herself, her children and life itself are enriched by her posthumous connection to her own mother and to loss itself, and literature on grief and motherhood bears this out (Edelman, 2006). This continued connection with a deceased mother, sometimes referred to as "the internalized mother," is the focus of several interventions described below.

Although an initial surge of grief may make the experience of pregnancy or new motherhood more challenging, when we, as motherless mothers validate and tend this grief, it can connect us to the ways our mothers continue to lend meaning and support to our experiences of motherhood and continuity to our lives. Memorial altars, art made as gifts or to represent our mothers' impact on our lives, rituals using handmade objects, masks, and letters may all serve to tend grief and an ongoing relationship with our deceased mothers. They may also promote a connection between our mothers and our children. Cherishing how our mothers' physical and personality traits appear in our children and sharing our memories with our children can be deeply healing and satisfying. The following artwork (Figure 10.6) illustrates how one mother nurtures an inner relationship with her mother.

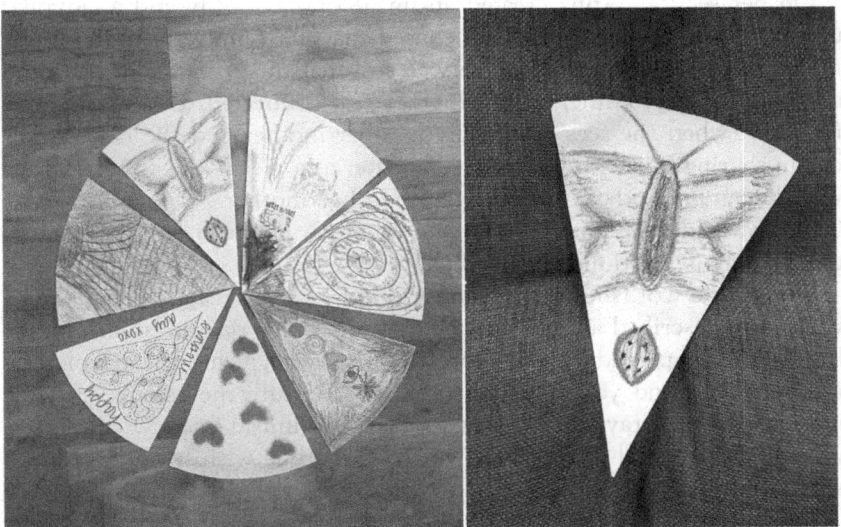

*Figure 10.6* "Mother's Day group mandala" drawings.

On the left is a mandala consisting of sections created by participants in a workshop for motherless daughters that I co-facilitated with a yoga therapist the day before Mother's Day 2019. The section on the right was made by Anna, a 39-year-old mother of a ten-month-old girl whose mother had died almost two years before, due to complications of a blood clot.

On a weekend devoted to cultural celebration of mothers, as therapists, we presumed that nurturance and support for reflection would be beneficial for this population. Awareness of holidays, death anniversaries, and birthdays that trigger grief in the lives of clients and responding with opportunities for self-compassion and creative processing promotes a more meaningful, contextualized therapeutic process for our clients.

My co-facilitator led a yoga sequence as a restorative exploration that would later inform art making. As an art therapist with a holistic approach, trained with an intermodal expressive therapy orientation, I often engage clients in multiple expressive modalities in one session, drawing on the different investigative and expressive capacities of each modality and the potential for crystallization of inner meaning from one expressive medium to the next.

At the end of the yoga program, we invited the women to use sections of a paper circle to respond artistically. The sections were assembled into a mandala as a closing ritual at the end of the workshop as a way to gently engender a sense of solidarity amongst the women, honor their mothers, and normalize the diversity of inner experience related to motherloss.

On her section, Anna created an image of a butterfly and a ladybug, creatures her mother loved. She shared that her family released butterflies at her mother's memorial service and that the butterfly has become a symbol of her mother that helps her feel connected to her; she even feels that when she sees a butterfly it *is* her mother and she has already begun sharing this with her young daughter as a means of connecting her with her grandmother. Through keeping her mother's passions present in her own life and sharing who she was with her own family, Anna is able to stay in relationship with her.

During the workshop, Anna chose oil pastels to create a soft texture, which she described as evocative of the watercolor paintings her mother loved. She employed colors expressively as well, using the purple her mother loved and yellow for the sun, to "capture the essence" of her mother and portray her "brightness and optimism." Anna also used imagery, colors and texture as a way to embody a wish for her: "I hope she feels light and free."

In her piece, "The Path" (Figure 10.7), Lena used imagery to depict her mother's unique spirit as well, but as she drew on themes explored with "The Mountain" (Figure 10.2), Lena put her mother in the context of her

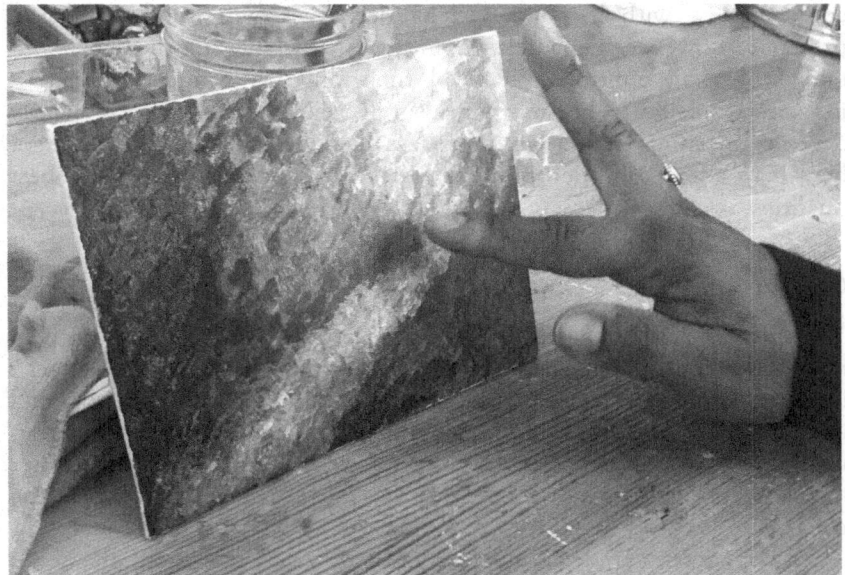

*Figure 10.7* "The Path" painting.

own life story and self-development. In this photograph, Lena pointed out where, on her life path, she feels she is and the direction she is going. Encouraging the use of movement in examining art may help clients to elaborate and more deeply encode their insights in mind-body memory (Hass-Cohen & Findlay, 2015).

More than 3D materials, the capacities of paint to blend and achieve different tones seemed to allow Lena greater access to the shades of transformation she had experienced, capturing the quality of gradual process in her personal evolution. She used the metaphor of light shining through dark clouds to portray her post-traumatic growth as well as her mother's spirit, affirming the value in her trials and her relationship with her mother. Lena calls this kind of light "Heaven's elevators," conduits for "angels like my mother coming up and down, up and down to help us."

Lena described this painting as a symbol of her mother's influence in her life, which began with Lena's conception and early life when her mother was alive, and then transformed into a spirit that continues to serve as a source of support and inspiration. Several sessions after creating this piece, while discussing the birth of her youngest son, Lena shared that she believed her mother was in the birthing room supporting her. She described all five of her births as miraculous, yet profoundly "frightening, isolating experiences," because her mother could not be with her at her deliveries. Even without her physical presence, however, Lena felt an intimacy with her mother that sustained her and continued to feed their ongoing connection. Lena's inner relationship to her mother, even 36 years after her death, clearly deepens meaning in her grief process and strengthens her image of herself as a good mother who embodies her mother's energy and best qualities.

## Conclusion

This chapter has elucidated some of the main ways art therapy can help meet the therapeutic needs of mothers without mothers. Motherloss can impact a woman's experience of motherhood in terms of her identity and integration of her self-narrative, including her grief process and parenting. Yet, when she explores and tends what is unfolding inside her through art, image-making can assuage the struggle and deepen the rewards.

As women who are both mothers and motherless daughters, the needs of our multiple internal identities can sometimes feel insatiable and irreconcilable, but artistic exploration of motherhood can help meet and integrate them. Creative engagement with the tender place where grief and motherhood overlap can help mend a fundamental biographical disruption, reduce the impact of anxiety and grief on parenting and deepen relationships with the lost mother. As a result we invite her into our mothering and the lives of our children.

It is vital to find ways to restore a sense that we are not alone, not entirely cut off from our mothers, when we feel more "vulnerable daughter" than "strong mother." We may also need practical tools for calming the dysregulation of our anxiety and grief reactions so we can be the mindful, authentic mothers we want to be, responsive to our own needs as well as those of our children.

Crafting a meaningful, self-affirming relationship to our lost mother and learning to find abundance where there was once scarcity helps us create strong relationships to ourselves and our children, and furthers the grief process. The healing and meaning-making potential of the creative process and expressive images, along with the reparative safety and nurturance of the therapeutic relationship, enable this inner and outer relationship building. As motherhood rounds out the circle of birth and death in our life narratives, art can connect the dots in its own circle of meaning-making. As we look inward through supported creative expression, we develop confidence in ourselves as good enough mothers (Winnicott, 1971), learning to honor both motherless daughter and mother of origin inside ourselves.

# Note

1 This phrase was borrowed from p. 7 of Edelman, H. (2006) *Motherless mothers*. New York, NY: HarperCollins.

# References

Davidman, L. (2000). *Motherloss*. Berkeley, CA: University of California Press.

Edelman, H. (2006). *Motherless mothers*. New York, NY: HarperCollins.

Epstein, V. (2004). *Ofrendas for the living: The Mexican day of the dead and grief work in expressive therapy*. Unpublished master's thesis, Lesley University, Cambridge, Massachusetts.

Gilbert, A. (2016). *Passed and present: Keeping memories of loved ones alive*. Berkeley, CA: Seal Press.

Harris, R. (2019). *ACT made simple: An easy-to-read primer on acceptance and commitment therapy*. Oakland, CA: New Harbinger Publications, Inc.

Hass-Cohen, N., & Findlay, J. C. (2015). *Art therapy and the neuroscience of relationships, creativity, and resiliency*. New York, NY: W.W. Norton & Company.

Malchiodi, C. (2002). *The soul's palette*. Boston, MA: Shambhala Publications.

Neimeyer, R. A. (2001). Introduction: Meaning reconstruction and loss. In R. A. Neimeyer (Ed.), *Meaning reconstruction & the experience of loss* (pp. 13–31). Washington, DC: American Psychological Association.

Swan-Foster, N. (2012). Pregnancy as a feminine initiation. *Journal of Prenatal and Perinatal Psychology and Health*, 26(4), 207–235.

Winnicott, D. W. (1971). *Playing and reality*. London: Tavistock Publications, Ltd.

# 11 The Use of Japanese Ritual and Art Therapy in Healing from Pregnancy Loss

*Ellen Speert*

Pregnancy loss through miscarriage, stillbirth or abortion is often a highly emotional, indeed traumatic, experience for parents as it blurs the border between birth and death. Yet, American culture lacks rituals that honor and support those who are left behind. Perinatal death often goes unmarked by people outside the immediate family (Davis, 1996). In fact, the unborn child is seldom even mentioned in the US.

This is not true in Japan where *mizuko kuyo*, a ritual commemorating these lost babies, is widely practiced (Smith, 2013; Wilson, 2009). Thousands of statues and carved rocks honoring the Buddhist deity *Jizo*, the protector of these "water babies" as they are known, are seen throughout the forests, along roadsides, and in cemeteries across Japan. Increasingly, this Buddhist observance, along with some simple art making experiences, is being adopted into American communities.

This chapter explores perinatal loss in the United States and the Japanese *mizuko kuyo* ritual. In addition, art making and the adoption of this ritual into multi denominational observances in America will be considered. It is my hope that other therapists will become interested in providing this type of support to grieving parents.

## Part I: Perinatal Loss

It is estimated that more than one million fetal losses occur annually in the United States, most of which are early fetal deaths, also called miscarriages (Hoyert & Gregory, 2014). Only stillbirths—fetal losses at 20 or more weeks' gestation—are generally reported by states in the National Vital Statistics System. In addition, it is estimated that one in four pregnancies end in abortion (Ventura, Curtin, Abma, & Henshaw, 2012).

Even putting aside the politicized American debate of whether abortion should be legal or not, there are often unresolved, emotionally charged responses for women and their families following any of these losses. With no physical remains, no ceremony, no grave site, and little community recognition of the loss, I have found, as well as others (Davis, 1996; DeFrain, 1991; Wilson, 2009) that the emotional effects of these perinatal deaths can linger for years. This may be due in part to the family's inability to talk about the experience and all the consequent feelings surrounding this lonely loss (Wilson, 2009). Due to the dearth of commemorative rituals, there is a vast and troubling silence surrounding pregnancy loss, despite its widespread occurrence. This, in fact, is causing a crisis of spirit (Nathanson, 1989). Without funerals or memorial services, there is a lack of context or language for the fetal death, which further leaves families isolated (Gross & Klaus, 2005; Wilson, 2009).

In the 1980s, following in quick succession the miscarriages of two of my sisters-in-law and the stillbirth of a client's son, I began to research the emotional support (or lack thereof) that the medical system was providing. I questioned my father, who had been a prominent obstetrician/gynecologist at the time, about this phenomenon. He said that in his long career delivering babies, both alive and dead, none of the women he had treated had ever had any emotional issues. As he was part of the old school of American obstetricians, he had never been aware of any emotional issues for the women he treated. As part of the medical model that reflected the patriarchy of male doctors who treated women patients, I wondered, was this the dominant attitude held by the medical community? How could doctors and other birth professionals overlook the pain that appeared so obvious to me? Here is what I found:

Despite the large number of perinatal deaths in the US, the mother's (and father's) need for mourning often goes unmet (DeFrain, 1991). Although parents come together in the joy of birth, they are often left isolated in their grief, a time in which friends and family feel uncomfortable and ill-equipped to discuss this loss (Speert, 1992). Furthermore, mothers told me of feeling left in "medical limbo" as their obstetricians saw their job as finished and the pediatricians had no infant to attend. Medical terminology and sanitized responses along with the medical procedures following a miscarriage, stillbirth, or abortion may inadvertently isolate the parents further. Terms like "product of conception" and comments like "it's nature's way of getting rid of defects" can add salt to the emotional wounds (Speert, 1992).

As therapists, we know that the suppression of grief can exacerbate, prolong, or complicate the mourning process (Seftel, 2006), yet rituals have the potential to help heal human grief, releasing it from the body. Mourning is a grief-infused symbolic action in response to the loss of attachment (Homans, 2000). "In addition to symptoms seen during bereavement (sadness, anger, depression, emptiness and blaming), the mother often experiences guilt, inadequacy, and a sense that the perinatal death reflects her failure as a parent" (Speert, 1992, p. 121). Suicidal thoughts may also appear. The mother may feel responsible for the loss. Many state that they have also lost a part of themselves and their future (Davis, 1996).

Behavioral consequences such as sleep disturbance, isolation, marital turmoil, increased rate of divorce, substance abuse, family violence, and over protection of surviving children are also seen in response to this profound loss (DeFrain, 1991). Additional consequences observed by art therapist Laura Seftel (2006), in her beautiful book *Grief Unseen*, include insomnia, changes in appetite, lethargy, irritability, despair, repetitive thoughts, and guilt, especially if there was ambivalence during the pregnancy.

In *Women's Growth in Connection* (1991), Jordan et al. postulated that female psychological identity and maturation develop through a series of relational stages, with increasingly more complex networks of relationship. Thus, isolation during the period following a perinatal loss denies women their need to be held in a relationship. Carol Gilligan (1982) observed that women's identity is threatened by separation. The loss of a fetus, since it severs the most intimate of human connections, compromises the sense of choice, fluidity, and articulation, all elements beautifully addressed by art making. The mourning that families experience is not just for the lost loved one but also for the lost dreams the family carries, leaving confusion and disorientation in its wake (Smith, 2013).

In addition to these psychological and behavioral symptoms, physical symptoms may appear including deep pain in the chest, aching arms, and hormonal shifts. In the case of a stillbirth, the coming in of breast milk, without a baby to receive it, may trigger additional physical and emotional distress (Speert, 1992).

## Part II: My Work

I have facilitated two women's art therapy groups a week for the past 40 years, and the stories of miscarriage, stillbirth, and abortion occasionally find their way into my art therapy studio. But they are not nearly as common as the statistical occurrence suggests. Is this because there has been an unconscious conspiracy of silence around this issue? The art does open the avenue to safely explore emotions linked with this loss, but the trauma of perinatal death has seldom been the presenting problem which brings a client into my art therapy practice.

In the 1980s, I delved into the study of Buddhism, I learned about *Jizo*, the *bodhisattva* who protects babies who die at birth. *Jizo* presides over *mizuko*, the souls of aborted, stillborn or miscarried babies. According to Japanese belief, babies who have died are not able to cross into the afterlife because they have not performed enough good deeds and have caused suffering to the parents they leave behind. This will be explored in more depth in the next section.

From 1993 to 1995, I began offering a monthly pro-bono art therapy support group for the Empty Cradle, an organization that provides a forum for the open discussion of feelings and concerns over the loss of a pregnancy. Parents were free to share in whatever way was most comfortable for them. I introduced art to these parents, providing materials to safely express and release their myriad and complex emotions. Frequently, the physicality of tearing paper, tissue, fabric and cardboard, which supported the metaphor of destruction, matched their needs, releasing anger, frustration, and tension in the body and psyche. With these shredded materials, new relationship to the loss could be built and explored along with new, solid art structures to navigate the new landscapes of their lives.

During this time period, I was visiting San Francisco where, poking around among a pile of old masonry in an antique store, I came across a stone carved *Jizo*. Delighting in the synchronicity, I commented to the store owner on what I knew of *Jizo*'s significance. The owner then generously donated this carved stone to my retreat center (Figure 11.1).

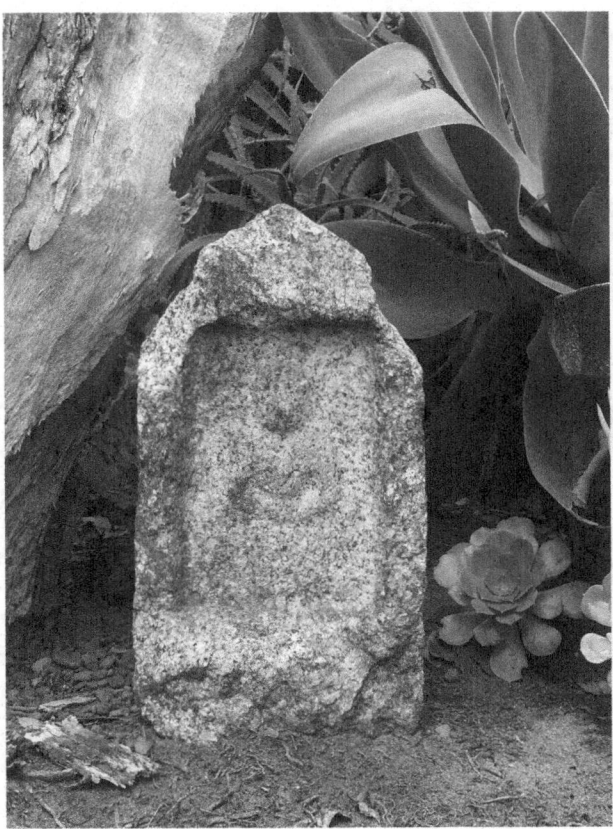

*Figure 11.1 Jizo* stone at the retreat center.

The stone sits among the trees, providing comfort to the grieving who visit the center. The generosity of the gift beautifully parallels the generosity of *Jizo*'s significance.

Another synchronistic event occurred 25 years later, in 2019, when I traveled to Japan to hike the Komano Kodo pilgrimage route. Just as I began preparing for my journey, I was invited to write this chapter, renewing my focus on perinatal concerns, which had settled quietly out of view in my practice for about 20 years. Perhaps I had unconsciously become complicit in overlooking this issue, allowing it to drop away from my awareness.

In Japan, I visited both Shinto shrines and Buddhist temples along the ancient route. My journey began in the village of Koyasan, founded 12 centuries ago as a seat of Buddhist training. The Okunoin cemetery there has over 1000 *Jizo* statues (Figure 11.2).

During the weeks that followed, as I hiked the pilgrimage route, I encountered hundreds more *Jizos* along the forest trails, nestled in

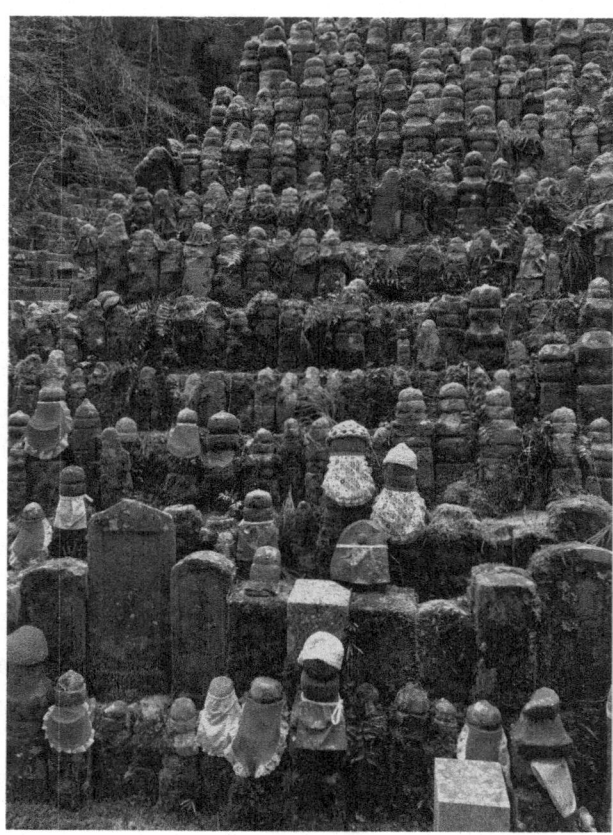

*Figure 11.2 Jizos* in Japanese cemetery.

roadside alcoves, crowded together in cemeteries and lovingly displayed in villages. Most stone carvings or statues were adorned with a bib or cape (almost always red), and had offerings of toys, flowers, or coins. Many were childlike; some looked like miniature Buddhas. I felt called to revisit this work when I returned home to the US. With the recommitment to this therapeutic focus, I carried a shared identification with the pain of perinatal loss as I hiked. As art therapists, we know that creativity is a powerful antidote to distress, so I composed many poems as I walked, lines forming in rhythm with each step. This haiku came to me hiking through the deep cedar forest:

> Moss covered *Jizos*
> A thousand tiny red bibs
> Ancient parents' prayers

This poem formed an invisible bridge—between the suffering of Japanese families and those in the United States—that stretched from my pilgrimage backwards to the families I had previously served and forward to the parents I would be returning to in America.

## Part III: Japanese Practice

> *Jizo* is beloved as the protector of all children—and in the hearts of these grieving parents, *Jizo* brings a special kind of comfort.
>
> (from the The Mizuko-Kuyo Memorial Wall)

### *Jizo*

*Jizo* is one of the most loved of Japanese divinities and is the protector and savior of travelers and children, especially those who die before their parents (Figure 11.3). He helps people at the crossroads of human experience which includes *mizuko*, the souls of aborted, stillborn or miscarried babies. As mentioned previously, such children cannot cross the mythical River Sanzu en route to the spirit world because they have not yet accumulated sufficient good deeds (similar to the concept of purgatory for unchristened babies in Christianity). These deceased babies are doomed to endlessly pile stones on the riverbank as penance, but *Jizo* protects them in his robes, caring for them as a parent would. Statues of *Jizo* sometimes depict him as a shaven-headed monk or with childlike features, resembling those of his protégés (Bays, 2003; Smith, 2013; Wilson, 2009).

### *Mazuko Kuyo*

*Mazuko* means "water baby" and *kuyo* means "to offer" and "to nourish." For centuries the ceremony of *mazuko kuyo* in Japan has been

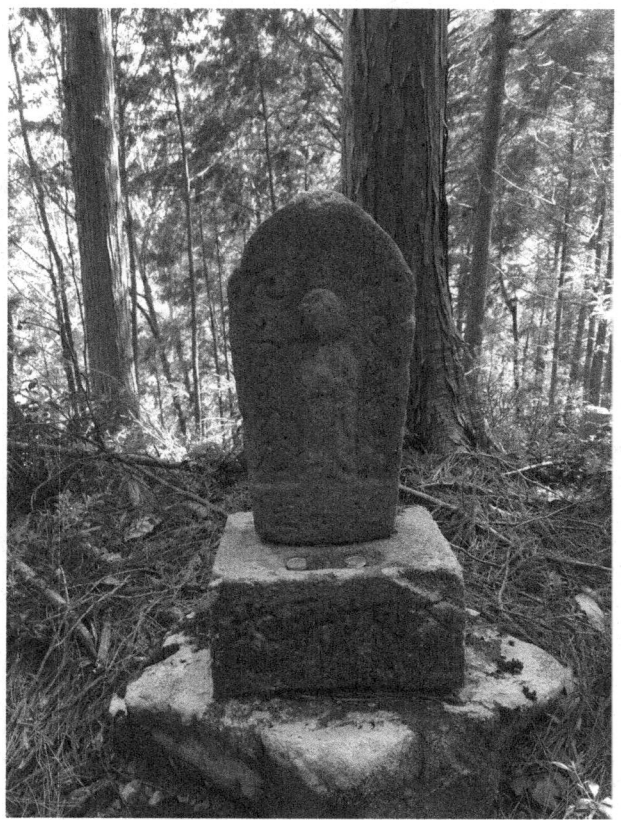

*Figure 11.3 Jizo* in Japanese forest.

observed for babies who have died through stillbirth or miscarriage (Bays, 2003; Smith, 2013; Wilson, 2009). The ceremony became widely practiced at the end of World War II, when abortion became common there (Smith, 2013; Wilson, 2009). Currently, it is practiced thousands of times a day all over Japan in simple rituals in Buddhist temples, at Shinto shrines and at neighborhood and road side altars (Bays, 2003). Water imagery relates to the fact that in Japan cremation is performed after death and the remains return to the earth and from there to the sea (Smith, 2013).

*Mazuko kuyo* "remains a case study of how old and new forms of myth, symbol, doctrines, praxis and organization combine and overlap" (Smith, 2013, p. 6). It began in the 1950s, became a significant movement in the 1960s, and by the 1980s served to memorialize any child who died before its parents (Smith, 2013). Jan Chozen Bays, a Zen Buddhist teacher who is credited with bringing this ceremony to Americans, talks of the concepts of the life cycle that Asian people hold. She explains that for Buddhists, life and death are continuous cycles like waves in the ocean, with no exact beginning or end.

Strong family bonds are held in Japanese Buddhism, especially with the dead who are dependent upon the prayers and ritual activities of their descendants. It is also believed that the dead remain close by, shaping the lives of the living:

> From a certain vantage point, much of the water baby ceremony could be interpreted as a type of psychotherapeutic exercise per-formed in a religious venue. For instance, the sewing of bibs, making of memorials, and drawing of pictures appears as a type of art therapy, while sitting in a supportive circle of fellow sufferers seems rather similar to group therapy.
>
> (Wilson, 2009, p. 103)

Wilson (2009) went on to emphasize the need for others to hear and accept the grief and loss, and found that this ceremony had tremendous appeal to many non-Buddhist Americans in a variety of settings from temples to private homes. *Mazuko kuyo* "provides America with precisely what is believed to be missing: compassionate spirituality, nonjudgmen-tal savior figures and ceremonial practices for an angry, divided, bereaved society lacking in healing ritual" (Wilson, 2009, p. 190). There is a need to keep the memory alive for many parents and this can be supported by creating a physical representation symbolizing the lost one (Smith, 2013; Speert, 1992).

## Part IV: The Ritual and Finding a Voice

Ritual brings us into relationship with the sacred world by removing us for a little while from everyday life (Miller & Ober, 2002). Yet, in discussions of pain around abortion and other pregnancy losses, a major theme that appears again and again is the lack of rituals we have in America. We are culturally and religiously unprepared to help families deal with the pain (Wilson, 2009). In fact, we lack the basic, compassionate terminology for the lost child/fetus/baby. We simply have no words to effectively name, honor or comfort the parents who endured this traumatic event.

In order to emerge from the loss and to heal, we must have the chance to mourn (Smith, 2013). In honoring the "lost presence" in the company of others, we recognize that loss is universal yet each is unique. As one client stated, "I appreciated being heard, held, and seen by the group. Other people expressing their grief allowed me to feel my own." Smith (2013) named three elements needed to experience genuine healing from perinatal loss: (1) a quiet, sacred space; (2) having others there to join in the experience; and (3) the intention to act on behalf of another. As an eco-art therapist, I would add a fourth element: the healing presence of nature.

In adapting this ritual in America two distinct parts have evolved. The setting of the first part is indoors. Sitting in a circle, each parent can express her/his grief and any other emotions that arise. This is followed by creating markers or wooden plaques on which to write wishes or prayers. Bibs to adorn *Jizo*, and other gifts to honor the spirit of the lost being may also be created. Although the bibs are usually red, a color in Japan that represents safety and protection, they can be created of any material associated with the spirit of the lost one. "This giving of form provides the invisible with texture, shape and significance, enabling the formlessness of grief to be woven into a larger body of meaning" (Smith, 2013, p. 247). Or as Wilson (2009) explained, "Pregnancy losses thus are moved from the realm of the imagination into the perceptible world, just as the participant's grief and sadness are moved from the shadows of the heart into the shared circle of the ceremony" (p. 119). At the Zen Center in Chicago, *Jizo* statues are actually wrapped in swaddling clothes and are brought home by the bereaved parents to be kept in a crib for a month before being returned to the temple.

The second part of the ritual is usually conducted outdoors surrounded by nature where the *Jizo* stone or statue is located (Wilson, 2009). This outdoor portion begins with ritual purification through the washing of hands. Ritual cleansing is performed in many religious practices as a preparatory step, separating the sacred act to be performed from the mundane world outside the ritual. Next offerings are made. Here the nourishment is reciprocal—parents offer food, flowers, prayers or incense and in turn are soothed by the sense of connection to their lost child (Bays, 2003).

Both these parts fit with what Wilson (2009) saw as the three primary needs that American women (and I would add men) have following this loss, which include: (1) the opportunity to voice their experience of pregnancy loss in order to counteract the silence they find around them; (2) the chance to do this within a community of listeners—others who are essentially witness to what is unseen by most people; and (3) the structure to perform an action to deal with the loss.

The rituals are congruent with expressive arts therapy in that they utilize all five senses to address the conscious and unconscious needs of the participants: the smell of flowers and incense; the tactile and visual qualities of art making; sound through music, chants, and prayers; the sharing of tea and cookies; and body movement through walking the labyrinth and bowing. These rituals "work through the senses to cultivate wisdom in the bones" (Arai, 2008, p. 194). Ceremonies also include the traditional offerings of the four natural elements: water, earth, air, and fire (Bays, 2003). The inclusion of candlelight and water as symbols of transition, along with the natural setting for the ritual, make the ceremony feel familiar, even to those with a non-Buddhist heritage. As one woman wrote, "The ritual felt sacred and beautiful. It was the first time I felt like I could truly honor their lives. I'm very grateful for the music, chanting, hand washing and incense."

## Part V: Differences between this Observance in Japan and in the US

Let us now look at how this ritual's adaptation into the US differs from its Japanese precursor in order to understand the cultural differences and to be sensitive to cultural appropriation. Here are some of the ways the ritual has been changed:

1. In the US, the emphasis is on the emotional/psychological and spiritual health of the grieving parents. In Japan, the emphasis is on the "trapped" spirit of the baby, which could haunt the parents (Wilson, 2009).
2. In the US, participants are actively involved in the process, expressing their feelings, sharing their loss with others, making objects to clothe the *Jizo* statue and participating in other art making experiences. In Japan, however, they are passive recipients of the ritual, while the priest performs the rites and prayers. There is no art making or discussion among Japanese participants.
3. In the US, both parents are included in the rituals while in Japan, men seldom participate (Smith, 2013).
4. In the US, the dead are departed, removed from daily life, whereas in Japan, though departed, they remain nearby, actively shaping the lives of the living and are somewhat dependent on the prayers and rituals of their descendants (and in this case, parents) (Wilson, 2009).
5. In the US, the service is free and all art supplies are provided, while in Japan, money is charged for the service. In Japan *mazuko kuyo* has, in fact, been seen as corrupt, as priests take advantage of the grieving parents in the sums they charge (Wilson, 2009).

## Part VI: My Approach

I believe in the power of *group* art therapy. Clients find solace and hope in witnessing the images that others create, which frequently mirror their own stories, while, at the same time, the group members can witness and hold in return. My eco-art therapy work has evolved further to include an expanded identification with the natural world. The cycles of the seasons remind us that a fundamental part of all life is change. Rocks and wood can provide strong and stable bases, but most elements in nature, like leaves and flowers, age and die. To observe this ever-present change is a comfort to those who feel that their depression will never lift or their anxiety will never dissipate. I begin most art therapy sessions, whether individual or group, by encouraging clients to let the materials guide them in what is to be explored, rather than starting art making with a concept. I encourage them to notice how the smells, textures and colors of materials, both from art stores and from nature, stimulate associations and heighten our awareness. This focus on media can get us out of our heads and into deeper communion with the creative process.

## Part VII: Adapting the Ritual into an American Art Therapy Retreat

The adaptation of these concepts into a half day retreat has been appreciatively received by the community in which I practice. I will outline what I, along with a Zen Buddhist teacher who is familiar with *Jizo*, have developed. I also invited a friend to play flute music during parts of the retreat to provide a soothing atmosphere.

### The Setting

It is important to have a private outdoor setting available near the art therapy studio for performing the ritual. My art therapy retreat center with healing gardens is illustrated here (see Figure 11.4), but any quiet private garden where ritual can be performed is important.

It is helpful to include an altar with statuary honoring other religious traditions as well as Buddhist beliefs. My altar includes an angel for Jewish participants, a painting of Mary for Christians and Quan Yin as well as several *Jizos* for Buddhists. I also set up a wooden bowl and dipper for the ritual of hand washing and candles and incense for the blessings at the altar. I invite each parent to bring an empty picture frame to symbolize their invisible loss, and honor the missing soul they are commemorating. This is intended to begin their process of preparation for the day. I did not have any participants from other religious traditions, but these should be considered and the ritual modified for attendees of other beliefs.

### In the Studio

We begin by sitting in a circle for a warm up, allowing time for each parent to express his/her intentions and desires for the day. I explain confidentiality and encourage each to share whatever wants to be spoken, asking for no cross talk. As one woman writes, "It was nice to put words to my own loss, to hold the space with others who have shared a similar experience. Being in relationship holds the pain."

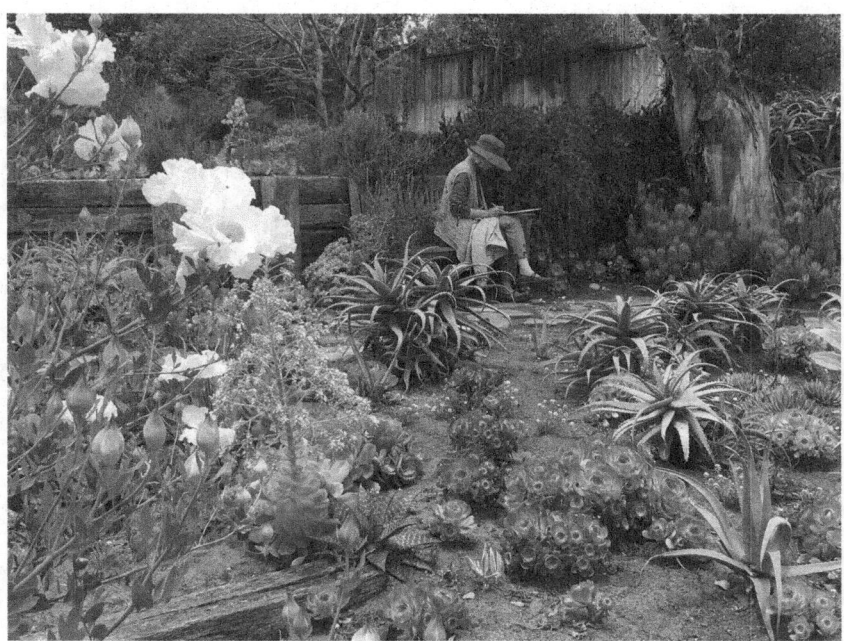

*Figure 11.4* Retreat center.

We then make *"ema,"* commemorative markers, with each baby's name and thoughts for each one. For these totems of remembrance, I offer large colored tongue depressors and permanent markers. These are then positioned in the center of each parent's cardboard circle using a small piece of plasticine. Around the *"ema"* each parent creates a mandala on the cardboard to serve as a peaceful holding place for the pain and the lost baby (Figure 11.5).

Creating mandalas seems fitting as an art directive since it reflects the roundness of the earth, a pregnant belly, and the circle of life and death (Seftel, 2006). Some participants choose to paint their mandalas, and everyone chooses to glue on nature elements for support and protection. I encourage them to choose elements in nature that reflect and express the support they seek. Soon, the mandalas are filled with the textures and colors of seed pods, feathers, shells, and flowers. As one participant writes, "I had a chance to memorialize my babies and express gratitude and grief through my art." The active process of construction has a deeply healing effect as we welcome in the spirit of the lost babies and make the unseen tangible. Then each parent journals whatever feelings and thoughts are emerging from the process. Another participant writes: "I felt like I was able to see my grief for the first time in 3D. It helped me

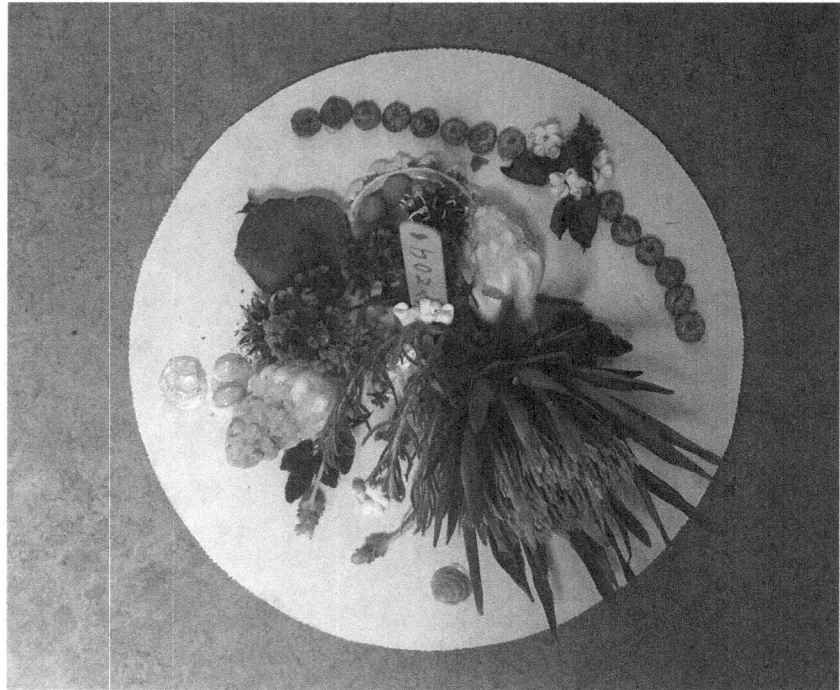

*Figure 11.5* "Mandala" cardboard and nature objects.

to leave behind some of my sadness and know it is being held by the group and by the earth." Another elaborates, "The symbolic nature of creating the art in this way flowed so easily." Those who finish quickly walk the labyrinth in the garden while others linger over the art.

Next *Jizo* and the *mizuko kuyo* ceremony are explained and illustrated by many photos of *Jizo* from different settings in Japan (Figure 11.6).

Red felt pre-cut capes and bibs soon become embellished with the wishes the parents held for their babies. We carry these, with their mandalas and empty picture frames, out into the garden.

### In the Garden

Descending the studio steps, we slowly wind our way toward the altar as flute music softly plays. Each parent mindfully places her/his mandala among the plants surround the altar, accompanying it with their empty picture frame. They each then adorn one of the multi-denominational religious statues with the bib they had lovingly made (Figure 11.7).

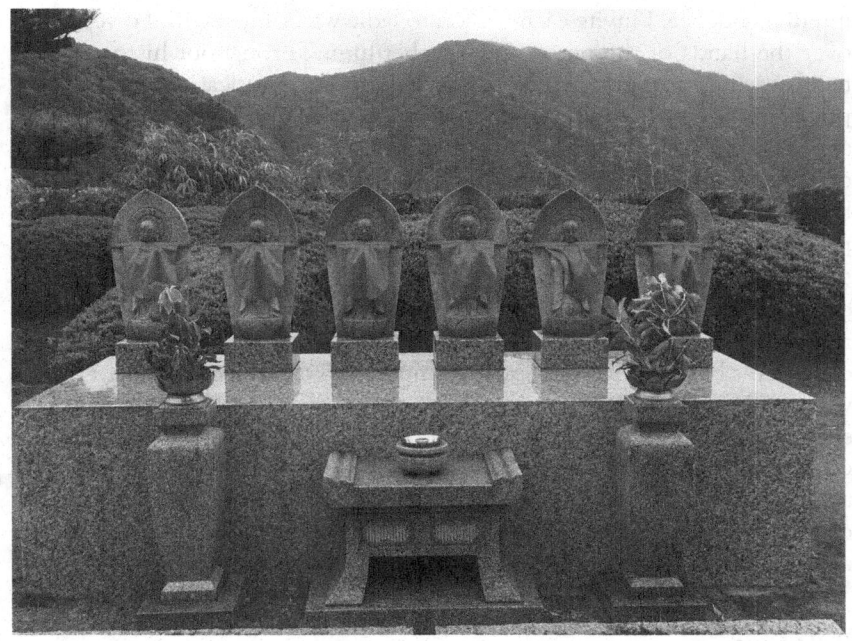

Figure 11.6 *Jizos* with bibs outside Shinto shrine.

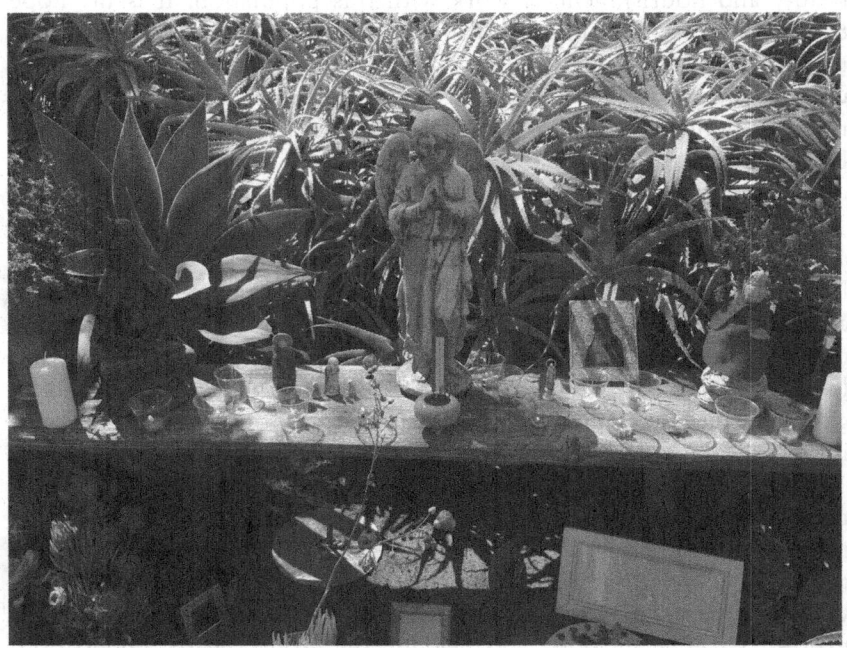

Figure 11.7 Garden altar.

To begin the ritual with purification, and as a way to accentuate our interdependence, I invite each person to ladle water filled with flower petals over the hands of the person next to her/him. Throughout history, ritual hand washing has provided a psychological and physical delineation and preparation for entering the realm of the sacred. We each take our turn approaching the altar, lighting a candle, and, from that flame, lighting a stick of incense. We each then bow to the altar to humbly honor the sacred beings represented there. After a Buddhist chant and lilting flue music, one parent writes, "The ritual gave new insight and awareness. It allows me space to reflect on what the art experience held and gave me courage to consider another way forward." When everyone had taken a turn, we return slowly to the studio. Again forming a circle, each participant pours out her/his heart, expressing much gratitude to be in the company of others who really understand them. Another parent writes, "His little soul was speaking to me so clearly to let go and move on." They then journal and fill out an evaluation and a release form, taking their art with them as a continuing reminder of their experience and to serve as an avenue to open conversations with others about their loss. Another reports, "I had a chance to feel community and not alone in my grief."

## Reflections

Although this format worked well for this group, in this setting, there are many other options that can be designed to support the healing, beauty and nourishment of work with this population. It is my hope that we, as art therapists, will adapt other creative ways to honor perinatal loss and bring it out of the shadows in a way that fits our unique clients. It is advised that any art therapist who utilizes this ritual be familiar with bereavement work and practice regular self-care. Having supervision is also advised, especially if this type of loss is unfamiliar to the therapist.

Some other art therapy directives with this population include creating a personal *Jizo* statue or image. Any medium can be used to create *Jizos* including paint, clay, wood, or papier mâché. Ephemeral earth art such as drawing images in the sand and watching them wash away with the tide is a powerful metaphoric expression of the interplay of creation and loss. The erasure by the waves echoes the impermanence of life. Religious or spiritual traditions other than Buddhism can also be incorporated, utilizing prayers appropriate to the participants.

The parents in this retreat had experienced pregnancy losses ranging from 30 years ago to a couple who had lost their baby just two weeks prior to this gathering. As one woman wrote, "This was lovely, bringing together people at different stages of our grief, and still being able to be with our own experience and share what was needed." Each of them expressed feeling included and held by the group, heard, understood, honored, and supported. For a few, this began a journey of more art therapy, knowing they were no longer alone. All 12 people in the retreat expressed feeling lighter and connected to others who understood their experience. I offered follow-up pro-bono art therapy to anyone who desired it and most expressed interest in doing so. As of this writing, only Anna has continued this art therapy work with me.

## Part VIII: Anna's Story

A year before the retreat described in the previous section, I had begun treating Anna (a pseudonym), a highly educated woman suffering from Dissociative Identity Disorder. In her 30s and after much verbal therapy, Anna was referred to me for art therapy to deal with the trauma of being adopted by a family who had sex trafficked her as a child. During our individual sessions, and later in her group art therapy, she explored many aspects of her identity including the pain and anger of her lost childhood, a time during which she had never been permitted to make art. Our work focused on creating safety, including much time in the gardens. Anna found soothing support in the scents, textures and colors there and frequently gathered lavender and rosemary to use in her sculptures. Themes of protection often appeared in her imagery, including the "Mama Bird Protecting" (Figure 11.8).

Although our art therapy sessions had provided much healing to the complex layers of her past, it wasn't until she participated in the perinatal loss retreat that she was able to access her grief over the three abortions she had been forced to undergo as a result of the daily sex abuse from her past. She sometimes wrote poetry in response to her art pieces:

Gracefully closing out this season
of growth
evolution
and change
Gratitude for this journey
from brokenness
to more freedom
Continually creating boundaries
of safety
to ground
hold
and keep me
No longer alone
and afraid
Nature holds me
as I progress

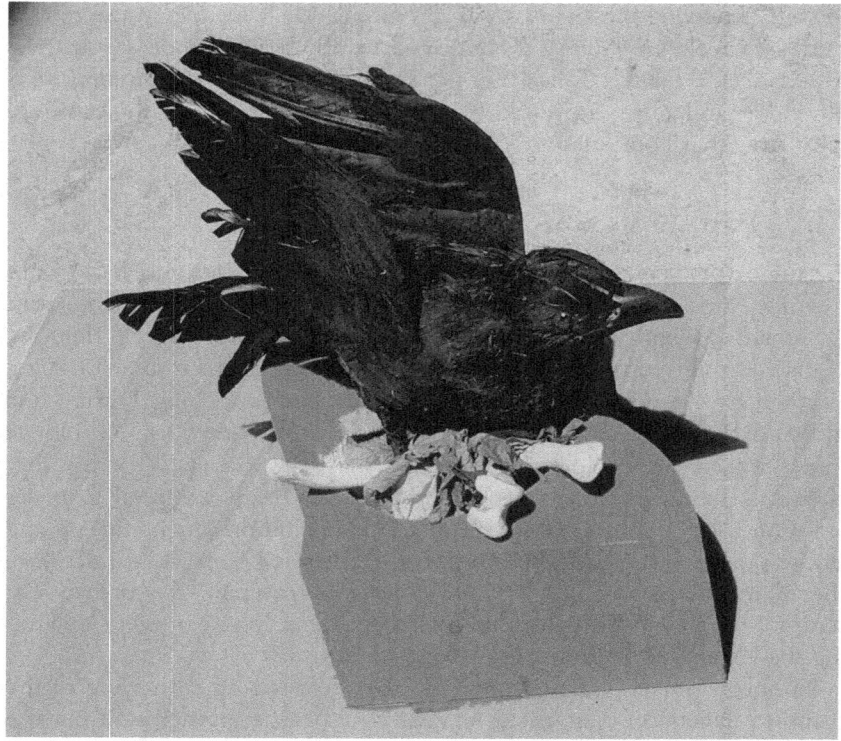

*Figure 11.8* "Mama Bird Protecting" mixed media.

In art therapy sessions following the retreat, Anna chose to sculpt her own *Jizo* in clay. She spent many subsequent sessions embellishing the sculpture and surrounding it with layers of seed pods and flowers. She was not only giving support to her lost babies but to herself, helping consolidate the strength she was discovering (Figure 11.9).

## Conclusion

How can we as art therapists bring light and support to the many parents who suffer from the isolating, traumatic loss of a pregnancy? What can we learn by adapting a Japanese Buddhist tradition into a multi-denominational American therapeutic setting without falling victim to insensitive appropriation? This chapter has presented the underpinnings of the *mazuko kuyo* ritual and how it can be reshaped to serve American parents who are silently suffering the isolation and invisibility of their loss. Although I have outlined the ritual I have developed, it is my hope that other art therapists who work with bereavement and loss will adapt

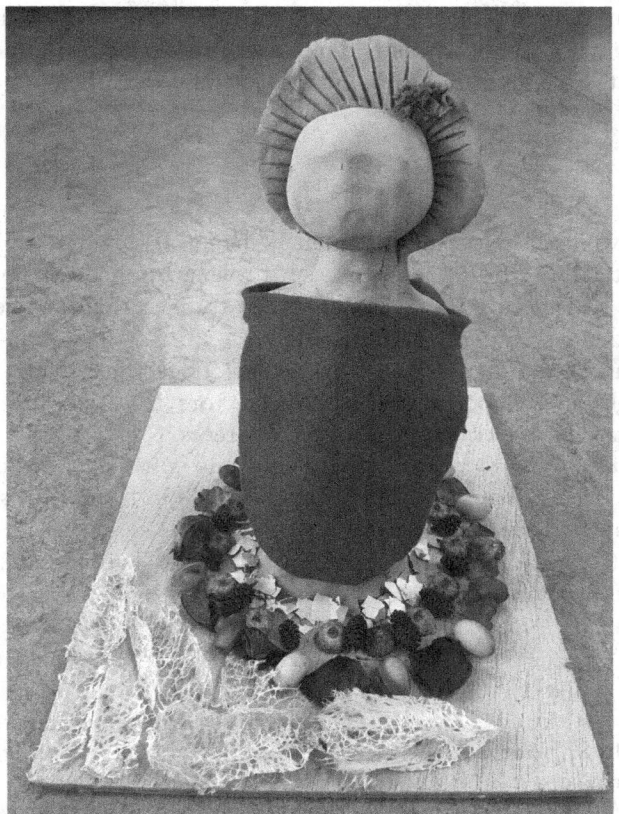

*Figure 11.9* "Anna's *Jizo*" clay and mixed media.

art making and rituals that best serve their specific clients' needs and bring perinatal loss out into the open where the grief can be supported and honored. In the words of Jan Chosen Bays (2003):

> I feel strongly that the *Jizo* ceremony is much needed in the United States. It is needed both to help the individuals who grieve, often for many years after an abortion or a miscarriage or after the loss of a baby, and also to help those with conflicting views regarding abortion find a way to work together in peace with the pain that surrounds this controversial and difficult issue.
>
> (p. 14)

I am deeply grateful to Nicolee McMann, the Buddhist teacher and friend of over 40 years who helped lead the ritual and chanting, and to my friend Karen Sorriano Wolfe, a gifted musician who played her flute during our retreat. This ritual was a salve to them, to me and to the brave parents, many of whom had never met or worked with me prior to this retreat. I feel honored to be on this journey with them.

## Terms

**Bodhisattva** (Sanskrit) an enlightened being (similar to a saint in Christianity) who is able to reach nirvana upon death, but delays doing so out of compassion in order to save suffering beings and help them attain enlightenment.

**Ema**  Japanese commemorative markers for one who has died.

**Jizo**  the Japanese bodhisattva who protectors travelers and children, especially those who die before their parents.

**Mazuko kuyo**  *mazuko* means "water baby" and *kuyo* means "to offer" and "to nourish". The ceremony of *mazuko kuyo* in Japan is observed for babies who have died at birth.

**Nirvana** (Sanskrit) a place of perfect peace and happiness (similar to heaven in Judeo/Christian or Islamic belief).

## References

Arai, P. K. R. (2008). Women and Dogen: Rituals actualizing empowerment and healing. In S. Heine & D. Wright (Eds.), *Zen ritual* (p. 194). Oxford: Oxford University Press.

Bays, J. C. (2003). *Jizo Bodhisattva: Guardian of children, travelers & other voyagers*. Boston: Shambala Publications, Inc.

Davis, D. L. (1996). *Empty cradle, broken heart: Surviving the death of your baby*. Golden Colorado: Fulcrum Publishing.

DeFrain, J. (1991). Learning about grief from normal families: SIDS, stillbirth and miscarriage. *Journal of Marital and Family Therapy, 17*(3), 215–232.

Gilligan, C. (1982). *In a different voice*. Cambridge, MA: Harvard University Press.

Gross, R. E., & Klaus, D. (2005). *Dead but not lost: Grief narratives in religious traditions*. Walnut Creek, CA: Alto Mira Press.

Homans, P. (Ed.). (2000). *Symbolic loss: The ambiguity mourning and memory at century's end*. Charlottesville: University Press of Virginia.

Hoyert, D. L., & Gregory, E. C. W. (2014). *Cause of fetal death: Data from the fetal death report*. National vital statistics reports; vol 65 no 7 Hyattsville, MD: National Center for Health Statistics.

Jordan, R. K., Kaplan, A. G., Miller, J. B., Stiver, I. P., & Surrey, J. L. (1991). *Women's growth in connection*. New York, NY: The Guilford Press.

Miller, S., & Ober, D. (2002). *Finding hope when a child dies: What other cultures can teach us*. New York, NY: Fireside Publisher.

Nathanson, S. (1989). *Soul crisis: One women's journey through abortion to renewal*. New York, NY: New American Library.

Seftel, L. (2006). *Grief unseen*. London: Jessica Kingsley Publishers.

Smith, B. (2013). *Narratives of sorrow and dignity: Japanese women, pregnancy loss, and modern rituals of grieving*. New York, NY: Oxford University Press.

Speert, E. (1992). The use of art therapy following perinatal death. *Art Therapy: Journal of the American Art Therapy Association, 9*(3), 121–128.

Ventura, S. J., Curtin, S. C., Abma, J. C., & Henshaw, S. K. (2012). *Estimated pregnancy rates and rates of pregnancy outcomes for the United States, 1990–2008*. National vital statistics reports; vol 60 no 7. Hyattsville, MD: National Center for Health Statistics.

Wilson, J. (2009). *Mourning the unborn dead: A Buddhist ritual comes to America*. New York, NY: Oxford University Press.

# Part IV

# Art Therapy

Special Topics of Childbearing
Women

# 12 Where It All Begins

## Anthropology as a Method for Engaging with Menstruation and Uncovering Art Therapy Explorations

*Fiona Swan Foster*

Menstruation is the beginning—a threshold to cross—that determines a body is now capable of bearing offspring. Human females are biologically unique in the way they menstruate. For the majority, irrespective of culture or location, menstruation is a given at some point in a woman's life. It is illuminating to see, therefore, the variety of ways in which cultures interpret and deal both socially and psychologically with this physiological process that so autonomously takes over a woman's physical body each month. Cultural anthropology is a way to engage with these different expressions of menstruation.

Anthropologists are never comfortable with universalities, and so while the discipline has identified some overall patterns, perspectives on menstruation are "strikingly variable, both cross-culturally and within single cultures" (Buckley & Gottlieb, 1988, p. 3). The questioning nature of anthropology is a valuable foundation for asking probing questions that appear simplistic and yet produce complicate answers such as what is menstruation? How is it perceived? What is its function? (Delaney, Lupton, & Toth, 1988). These questions can produce fruitful responses, images, and narratives from menstruating women.

The lens of anthropology reveals cultural structures and patterns, while art therapy brings a deeper understanding through visual documentation of the personal psychobiological experience, both of which are potential catalysts for transformation within the individual. Transformative processes like menstruation lead a woman to "experience her own creativity" (Neumann, 1955/1974, p. 31). And a transformative process like art therapy is a nonverbal expression of both the power of the image and the psyche—one's own inner creative force.

This chapter will begin with an overview of cultural attitudes towards menstruation—both the empowering and the taboo—to highlight the multiplicity of ways in which cultures celebrate and scorn monthly blood. It will then look at cultural interpretations of menstruation in the US, especially where it comes into contact with institutions: jails, schools, and poverty. These examples illuminate where art therapy might be incorporated as group or individual mental health services or programs focused on reproductive literacy or psychosocial education that visually addresses the emotional relationship to menstruation.

## Menstruation as a Backdrop for Pregnancy and Internal Temporality

The physical transition from girlhood to womanhood is one where a young person comes to realize her biological potential for pregnancy and motherhood. There are many cultures across the world that link menstruation to fertility, pregnancy, and birth (Buckley & Gottlieb, 1988). Menstruation therefore is integral to childbearing issues; a woman becomes attuned to an internal cycle. Tangentially, it can also be associated with dual feelings of loss and relief, especially if pregnancy is desired or feared. Each month, a woman undergoes a range of emotional reactions and physical sensations unique to her (Bernstein, 1995; Vick & Sexton-Radek, 2005).

Women sometimes correlate menstrual cycles with the cyclical nature of the moon. The English etymology of menstruation contains *menses* from Latin, *menses* meaning month. This lunar connection appears in some cultures' social rituals or mythology (Buckley, 1988; Buckley & Gottlieb, 1988). One mythological example of this connection with the moon is from the Amazonian Barasana, who believed that the moon would have sex with menstruating women and then during a lunar eclipse, the moon itself would become a ball of menstrual blood and come down to Earth to fill the house (Barnard & Spencer, 2002). The myth is an expression of the physical experience when a woman comes to "determine time" (Freeman, 1987, p. 267), in that she has her own understanding of time that is nonlinear and separate from the chronological concept. Thus, the "body is regarded as a sort of symbolic template for the communication of gnosis, mystical knowledge about the nature of things and how they came to be what they are" (Turner, 1987, p. 16). It is the disconnection from this internal knowing that many feminist psychologists suspect causes splits within the psyche and mental health issues associated with being unseen, devalued, and unimportant. Art therapy offers a way to bridge this disconnect and explore the underlying feelings in a tangible way.

## Menstruation as Initiation into Women's Temporality

Cultural attitudes towards menstruation are not always restraints foisted upon women, they can express a larger concept of world order. This section will provide two examples of how initiation and menstruation can connect a girl with her fertility and her culture in a positive way. Menstruation marks the physical transition from girlhood to womanhood and this shift may be recognized or facilitated with a ceremony, or *rites of passage*, that acknowledges the cultural importance of this shift (Neumann, 1955/1974; Turner, 1987). The liminality of initiation culminates in a deeper understanding of cultural norms and a new role within the society (Turner, 1987). Recurring monthly blood can be a powerful time for a woman, one where she is connected both to her internal self and wider cosmological purpose (Buckley, 1988; Buckley & Gottlieb, 1988).

One example of a menstruation initiation ritual that connects a woman to her fertility and creativity is the Navajo kinaaldá. This ritual takes place after a girl's first menstrual cycle that recreates the mythology of Changing Woman, who became the first woman to bear children. During the four-day ceremony, the girl is physically pressed in order to symbolize "molding" her into a woman that is "beautiful" in the eyes of Navajo culture: "strong, ambitious, and capable of enduring much ... friendly, unselfish, and cheerful" (Lincoln, 1981, p. 95). Once the ritual is complete the woman is connected to her fertility and also "more creative, more alive, more ontologically real" (Lincoln, 1981, p. 104) within the Navajo culture.

Monthly blood also represents a continued connection to cosmology. The Beng people of the Ivory Coast have traditionally worshiped "the Earth," although many have now converted to either Islam or Catholicism. In the Beng belief system, restrictions that surround menstruating are "part of a wider system of symbolic classification of space and fertility" (Gottlieb, 1988, p. 73). One custom, among others, is that menstruating Beng women who have been initiated or married must not enter the forest and fields. From the outside, these beliefs might be seen as a way to restrict women; however, for the Beng it has to do with a cosmological perspective on fertility. Fields and forests symbolize the Earth's fertility, while menstrual blood is a symbol of human fertility. As one Beng man, and a Master of Earth said:

> Menstrual blood is special because it carries in it a living being. It works like a tree. Before bearing fruit, a tree must first bear flowers. Menstrual blood is like the flower: it must emerge before the fruit—the baby—can be born.
>
> (Gottlieb, 1988, p. 58)

Therefore, women and fields/forests are parallel in that they both undergo a harvest cycle; they both bear fruit. To protect the fertility of each, it is believed that they must be kept separate. The Beng are an example of a respect and acknowledgement of a woman's fertility. Little, if any, research was found regarding menstruation and art therapy, suggesting this is an area that could be explored in greater depth through psychosocial groups that support individuation.

## Menstruation as Restriction and Taboo

For some cultures, menstruation can also be deemed "risk laden." It is a time when women can be negatively affected, or be a negative effect to the world around them. Taboos associated with menstruation are varied and complex. They can center on the food, hunting or body-related taboos such as not allowing menstruating women to view the sunlight (Barnard & Spencer, 2002, p. 363). Given the wide range of restrictions on women, it is difficult to make a generalization and say that cultures with restrictions view menstruation as "bad" (Buckley & Gottlieb, 1988, p. 3). Often, it is necessary to dig far deeper into the culture itself to understand the origins of a particular belief. The aim is not to suggest a return of these traditions or claim they are not harsh; some have even resulted in death, such as a 21-year-old Nepal woman who suffocated in her menstrual hut during an outlawed Chhaupadi practice, which "consider women impure during their periods and after childbirth" (BBC News, 2019). Cultural traditions like these act upon specific beliefs (in this case, maintaining community purity) in a physical manner (Tan & Hara, 2019).

Art therapy can provide a way to deal with the physical and psychological impact of a belief system that may be damaging. In the case of Chhaupadi, "Art to Healing" (Tan & Hara, 2019) is a creative arts resource program in Nepal that provides therapeutic support to women and girls who have been gravely impacted by this menstruation practice and other forms of abuse. It is important to hold in mind how cultural beliefs influence the creative process and also to respect individual defenses and privacy. To remain concise, I will provide three further examples of menstrual taboos related to food, physical separation, and religion. We can relate these cultural practices to art therapy in the US by considering how such beliefs could be acted upon symbolically through art.

There are many cultural taboos associated with food, such as the Kharwar of India who ban menstruating women from the kitchen. Other taboos are connected to animals or hunting, such as the Bukka who do not go into the sea for fear of killing the fish or Habbe men in western Sudan who do not go hunting if their wives are menstruating (Delaney et al., 1988). In European history, too, there are superstitious associations with menstruating women spoiling food. Around AD 77–79, Pliny the Elder thought that menstrual blood "turns new wine sour, crops touched by it become barren, grafts die, seed in gardens are dried up, [and] the fruit of trees falls off" (Weiss-Wolf, 2017, p. 5).

Taboos surrounding menstruation can also involve a physical separation, prohibiting men from coming into contact with menstrual blood or menstruating women. For example, the Mae Enga of Papua New Guinea believe that contact with menstruating women or menstrual blood would cause a man's slow decline and eventual death (Delaney et al., 1988). However, when considered in a cultural context, the Mae Enga perspective can be seen as taboo and also as a metaphor for the cultural distrust of outsiders (Buckley & Gottlieb, 1988).

Religion is a place where rules about menstruation are delineated; however, these rules also are complex and layered in their meaning. In Islam, a menstruating woman is not allowed to fast, pray, or have sex. While this could have a negative or restrictive interpretation, as in women are unable to be pure during this time, some also see menstruation as way of paying spiritual dues, exempting women from other ritual tasks. Gnostics, Kabbalists, and some Christians believe that menstruation is part of the "Curse of Eve" that came with enjoying the fruit, and also correlates with uncleanliness because of a passage in Leviticus 15:19–30 that specifies a menstruating woman is "unclean" and "impure" (Nagy, 1987; Weiss-Wolf, 2017).

While it does not apply to all examples of menstruation, Mary Douglas's (1966) famous theory of symbolic pollution as a pollutant being "matter out of place" aligns well with the Christian and also American idea of menstruation as a pollutant. In their theoretical appraisal of menstrual symbolism, Buckley and Gottlieb (1988) argue that the application of "pollution" to all theories of menstruation is overly simplistic and reductionist. The authors state that the "the elegance of pollution theory itself can thus manufacture the illusion of overwhelming negativity" (p. 32). I agree with this assessment and feel that much of the menstruation literature takes examples out of their cultural context. While I have also cherry-picked my examples, it is in an attempt to demonstrate the wide ranging types of taboos and also some of the cultural-specific thinking that creates these taboos. For art therapists, these amplifications might encourage symbolic thinking that could inspire conversations and visual interventions, while also encouraging compassion for diverse beliefs.

It is also my hope that the various examples of menstruation I have provided will be helpful when considering the cultural context in the United States and how particular views settle into individual beliefs and influence emotional reactions. The experience of US women is no less complex—particularly as it is a country made up of diverse cultures and religious beliefs—and is still infused with themes of fertility, creativity, temporality, as well as "negative" associations such as uncleanliness, restrictions, and hassles within a woman's everyday life.

## Menstruation in the United States

While America is not solely a Christian nation, negative associations derived from Christianity have indeed taken hold in the culture, dominating the viewpoint of menstruation (Buckley & Gottlieb, 1988). Many women and men alike associate menstruation with uncleanliness and shame. In 2019 a study found that 80% of teenage girls who were polled felt that menstruation is repugnant or unsanitary and 64% felt that it was "society" that taught them to be ashamed of their period (Thinx & PERIOD, 2019, p. 1).

Since the 1920s, menstrual product advertising in the United States has focused on hiding and controlling menstruation with the right products. This way of thinking represents an "ideal" American lifestyle of "simplicity, self-sufficiency, and self-control" (Weiss-Wolf, 2017, p. 15) that does not take into account women's true individual experiences. With regards to art therapy, it is noteworthy to consider the parallels between the creative process and the biological process. Menstruation denotes the destruction or loss of fertility, but reveals the inside of a woman, in particular remnants of her uterine lining. In a similar way, the image reflects an isomorphic expression of a woman's subjective and emotional world. The person and the temperature of the culture come together through images. The question then becomes, are the images drawn from within her or they foisted upon her? The expressive arts could be utilized as an important way for women to break free of this dichotomy and work with their bodies, menstruation, and pain (Cohen, 1983).

In the 1960s and 1970s, second-wave feminism and publications of books like *Our Bodies, Ourselves* introduced menstruation as a possible (even if not acceptable) topic for public discourse. Women became interested in their bodies and self-education took place in a way that had not happened before, especially within such a public format. This coincided with the 1972 passage of the ERA (Equal Rights Amendment) that resulted in women taking to the streets without bras or going to work in male dominated environments whether they were menstruating or not. Birth control that would eventually regulate, and even halt menstruation, became vogue.

Vaulting ahead, current public discourse has shifted to activism. A *Newsweek* article published in 2016 noted that "[f]or the first time, Americans are talking about gender equality, feminism and social change through women's periods" (Jones, 2016). National organizations like "PERIOD" and "Free the Period" are fighting for menstrual equity through legislative equality. In addition, a pending House bill (Menstrual Equity for All Act, 2019–2020) is seeking to eliminate some of this financial burden by having menstruation products covered by Medicaid in schools, jails, and homeless shelters.

While activism is making huge strides, it does not address the "significant, cultural and structural obstacles" (Thinx & PERIOD, 2019, p. 1) that create the shame surrounding menstruation. This is where art therapy can make a difference in the United States.

Art therapy offers a way to reflect and confront these complex feelings. Even though little psychological and social research has been recorded in the area of art therapy and menstruation, it could easily be implemented into larger research projects or community assessment programs. Holding in mind the diverse cultural views on menstruation, art therapy research could touch on other topics such as race, income, inequality and transgender rights. Three areas in which we might see the psychological effects of menstruation when it comes into contact with American institutions are schools, jails and extreme poverty. I will use Colorado as a regional example of the discourse that is happening in these particular areas and the way women are affected. Throughout this section, I will use the word "menstruator" to represent the larger group and the word "woman" to reflect the language of the research literature or discourse in the space.

## Colorado: A Case Study in Menstruation

Colorado, as a purple state with both farming and tech economies, is a thermometer for the United States in this new decade. As such, the examples presented here in some ways also represent the middle ground of the conversation. Menstrual products are taxed as a luxury item and any attempts to repeal this statewide tax have been unsuccessful. However, in March 2019, the city of Denver voted to eliminate the 4.3% city sales tax on all menstrual products (Garrison, 2019).

### Homeless, Unsafely Housed, Low-income Women

Studies have shown that tax on menstrual products disproportionately affect low-income women (Weiss-Wolf, 2017). Homeless women and transgender people face unsanitary, uncomfortable and unsafe challenges while menstruating. First-person accounts contain stories of people using anything they can find as a sanitary product: socks, newspapers, rags, toilet paper or bleeding into their clothes. Unreliable restroom access can make changing a tampon or washing underclothes difficult or, for transgender people, life-threatening (Weiss-Wolf, 2017).

Across the state, several organizations provide homeless, unsafely housed, and low-income menstruators with the sanitary products they need. "Period Kits" is a Denver-based organization that builds a three-month supply package with everything from products to underwear. Twenty percent of what they build goes directly to people who live on the streets and the other resources are split between low-income families. Menstrual products are not covered by Supplemental Nutrition Assistance Program (SNAP is pending elimination) and shelters often do not stock menstrual products; the CEO of "Period Kits" explained that this is because "men are running the programs and this stuff is not on their radar" (G. Davis, personal communication, December 6, 2019).

Davis also noted that a homeless menstruator experiences untold burdens, issues and trauma that are made even more invisible by the image we have of a homeless person as "an alcoholic man" (G. Davis, personal communication, December 6, 2019). What if these women had art therapy groups where their untold burdens could become known, visible to each other and more visible to the world? This is a complicated demographic often with comorbidity of addiction, abuse, and mental health issues. While activism is stepping in to solve the logistical problem, nobody is addressing the underlying psychological effects of menstruating while homeless. This could be a rewarding opportunity for art therapy research. Davis also mentioned how important menstrual education is for boys because it is a way to alleviate stigma and improve knowledge (G. Davis, personal communication, December 6, 2019). This topic is largely unexplored yet has great potential for art therapy.

### Menstrual Products in Schools

One might not associate menstruating girls skipping school with a rich developed nation such as the United States. However, this is a significant a problem in the US. Nearly one in five teens struggle to afford or are not able to purchase period products and nearly 25% of students in both public and private schools have missed class or know someone who has missed school because of a lack of access to period products (Thinx and PERIOD, 2019, p. 1).[1]

In Denver, student activists are working to pass a bill sponsored by Representative Brianna Titone that would provide free period products to students in a Denver school district (Hindi, 2019). This bill would not only assist the students who are missing class due to unaffordable menstrual products, but could go some way to normalizing the stigma— after all, toilet paper is provided free of cost. Currently, students have to manage not only class attendance, but also when to leave class and risk missing content to change products, or ignore their condition while suffering underlying worry about leaks and stains that cause embarrassment and even bullying. Negative associations such as these that surround menstruation have contributed to self-objectification and body shame (Stubbs, 2008). In fact, 57% of teenage girls feel "personally affected by the negative association surrounding periods" (Thinx & PERIOD, 2019, p. 2). Psychologically, this level of stress and anxiety becomes an imbedded message of restrictions and double binds: a damned if you do and damned if you don't scenario.

Through increased psychosocial support, we must confront these negative cultural associations and the way they manifest in schools in order to normalize menstruation. Until then, there is no choice but to conform to the message that monthly blood is a devalued bodily function, a shameful and inconvenient event. It is indeed "out of place"

(Douglas, 1966) in schools. Art therapy gives menstruation a place visually, and provides the opportunity to change the emotional and psychological consciousness that impacts our schools. Additionally, it could help to raise student's self-esteem an issue that is concurrent with menstruation and puberty (Franklin, 1992; Hartz & Thick, 2005).

## Menstrual Products in Prison

Like many structures in our society, prisons were designed with male bodies in mind. There are a large number of women in prison and in many states there is a lack of access to menstrual products, which is degrading, inadequate, and immoral. Across many states, women are not being guaranteed access to sufficient or absorbent enough pads for their flow. In one New York prison, women had to present blood-soaked pads when requesting new ones because the medical director needed evidence that the sanitary napkins had been used (Weiss-Wolf, 2017). And yet, toilet paper does not fall under the same restrictions, illustrating how the patriarchal system continues to denigrate and shame women for their bodily functions. Many female inmates are forced to purchase tampons from the commissary, which for women who usually come from poverty, is a luxury they cannot afford.

Similar to other states across the country, Colorado has historically given women access to sanitary napkins. But recently, the State has addressed the issue of women's access to tampons as well. Representative Leslie Herod introduced a 2017 bill for Federal prisons because she discovered women were bargaining and trading for tampons. "I was shocked and appalled. It's dehumanizing" (Herod as cited in Paul, 2017).

Trading and bargaining for tampons created a dehumanizing and unsafe condition in the jails that could have led to violence and assaults. Denver Sheriff Department Chief Elias Diggins commented,

> by forcing women to pay for an item that is a basic need, we created a system where an individual may feel pressured to barter or borrow the item and be placed in the uncomfortable and vulnerable position of owing another inmate.
>
> (Paul, 2019)

Arguably, the access to tampons will not improve the underlying shame of menstruating while incarcerated. In a 2012 letter published by the Committee Against Political Repression, one inmate reported that menstruating in prison is "an experience that ... intentionally works out to degrade inmates ... Prison makes us hate part of ourselves; it turns us against our own bodies" (Weiss-Wolf, 2017, pp. 80–81).

Art therapy groups that focus on menstruation and the burdens of menstruating in prison could supplement the statistical research, but also bring awareness to these personal challenges and the general situation by creating more visibility. A nonverbal process of art therapy matches how the prison industrial complex silences these women. Instead, women are forced to fit into the patriarchal system and opportunities for art therapy would offer them a safe space to explore their psychobiological experience and build self-esteem (Hartz & Thick, 2005).

## Conclusion

Menstruators in prisons, schools, and the homeless are three examples of populations that are vulnerable and in need of art therapy groups or individual art therapy. There is a shame and stigma in the American culture surrounding the taboo of menstruation that all women carry into the world, which ultimately influences their personal narrative, identity, and confidence. These experiences are compounded in situations where menstruators' bodies are simply "matter out of place" (Douglas, 1966), particularly in institutions where men's bodies are the primary consideration. Until we give consideration, through such avenues as art therapy, to the emotions surrounding menstruation, we will not find a way to shift our treatment.

As a concrete matter that often goes unnoticed, menstruation is also metaphorical and the pragmatic experiences can be worked with creatively and nonverbally through art therapy services. Anthropology offers us a wider and richer understanding of how previous and current cultures grappled with similar challenges. Menstruators are engaged in a monthly rhythm that is either devalued and hidden or celebrated and respected. At times, menstruation means yet another loss for a woman interested in having a child, in experiencing gestation, childbirth, and motherhood, while for others, the sight of blood is a sign of health, aliveness, and relief.

Integrating art therapy into the research data and creating supportive programs could have beneficial long-term effects, improving women's mental health by decreasing stress and anxiety, and building community. While it was not the focus of this chapter, bringing men into the education and dialogue about menstruation offers the opportunity to grow community beyond the bounds of gender. If we improve the psychological, social and economic services in prisons, schools, and homeless communities, then American women can grow with confidence into their bodies and feel more encouraged to live a full and unrestricted life.

## Note

1 It is important to note that this study identified their survey participants as "girls" and did not specify if they spoke to transgender boys who were still menstruating.

# References

Barnard, A., & Spencer, J. (Eds.). (2002). *Encyclopedia of social and cultural anthropology* (3rd ed.). New York, NY: Routledge.

BBC News. (2019). Nepal man arrested over death of woman in 'menstruation hut'. Retrieved from www.bbc.com/news/world-asia-50691387

Bernstein, J. (1995). Art and endometriosis. *Art Therapy: Journal of the American Art Therapy Association, 12*(1), 56–61.

Buckley, T. (1988). Menstruation and the power of Yurok women. In T. Buckley & A. Gottlieb (Eds.), *Blood magic: The anthropology of menstruation* (pp. 187–209). Berkeley: University of California Press.

Buckley, T., & Gottlieb, A. (1988). A critical appraisal of theories of menstrual symbolism. In T. Buckley & A. Gottlieb (Eds.), *Blood magic: The anthropology of menstruation* (pp. 1–50). Berkeley: University of California Press.

Cohen, B. M. (1983). Combined art and movement therapy group: Isomorphic responses. *The Arts in Psychotherapy, 10*(4), 229–232. doi:10.1016/0197-4556(83)90023-0

Delaney, J., Lupton, M. J., & Toth, E. (Eds.). (1988). *The curse: A cultural history of menstruation* (2nd ed.). Urbana and Chicago, IL: University of Illinois Press.

Douglas, M. (1966). *Purity and danger: An analysis of concepts of pollution and taboo.* New York, NY: Praeger.

Franklin, M. (1992). Art therapy and self-esteem. *Art Therapy, 9*(2), 78–84. doi:10.1080/07421656.1992.10758941

Freeman, J. M. (1987). Turnings in the life of a Vietnamese Buddhist nun. In L. C. Mahadi, S. Foster, & M. Little (Eds.), *Betwixt & between: Patterns of masculine and feminine initiation* (pp. 264–278). La Salle, IL: Open Court Publishing.

Garrison, R. (2019, March 27). Denver city council votes to eliminate 'tampon tax' on feminine hygiene products. *Local News, The Denver Channel.* Retrieved from www.thedenverchannel.com/news/local-news/denver-city-council-votes-to-eliminate-tampon-tax-on-feminine-hygiene-products

Gottlieb, A. (1988). Menstrual cosmology among the Beng of Ivory Coast. In T. Buckley & A. Gottlieb (Eds.), *Blood magic: The anthropology of menstruation* (pp. 55–74). Berkeley: University of California Press.

Hartz, L., & Thick, L. (2005). Art therapy strategies to raise self-esteem in female juvenile offenders: A comparison of art psychotherapy and art as therapy approaches. *Art Therapy, 22*(8), 70–80. doi:10.1080/07421656.2005.10129440

Hindi, S. (2019, November 27). Student-advocated bill would help Colorado public schools provide free tampons and other feminine hygiene products. *The Denver Post.* Retrieved from www.denverpost.com/2019/11/27/colorado-schools-tampons-feminine-hygiene-products/

Jones, A. (2016, April 20). The fight to end period shaming is going mainstream. *Newsweek.* Retrieved from www.newsweek.com/2016/04/29/womens-periods-menstruation-tampons-pads-449833.html

Lincoln, B. (1981). *Emerging from the chrysalis: Studies in rituals of women's initiation.* Cambridge, MA: Harvard University Press.

Nagy, M. (1987). Menstruation and shamanism. In L. C. Mahadi, S. Foster, & M. Little (Eds.), *Betwixt & between: Patterns of masculine and feminine initiation* (pp. 223–238). La Salle, IL: Open Court Publishing.

Neumann, E. (1955/1974). *The great mother: An analysis of the archetype*. Princeton, NJ: Princeton University Press.

Paul, J. (2017, May 3). Women in Colorado prisons will get free tampons under amendment that offers 'a small piece of dignity'. *The Denver Post*. Retrieved from www.denverpost.com/2017/05/03/colorado-prisons-free-tampon-amendment/

Paul, J. (2019, March 19). Colorado's prisons offer free tampons to female inmates. *The Colorado Sun*. Retrieved from https://coloradosun.com/2019/03/19/color ado-jails-tampons-house-bill-1224/

Stubbs, M. (2008). Cultural perceptions and practices around menarche and adolescent menstruation in the United States. *The Menstrual Cycle and Adolescent Health*, 1, 58–66.

Tan, A., & Hara, A. (2019). Menstruation is not a curse: Menstrual discrimination, gender based violence, and sex trafficking in Nepal. Unpublished manuscript.

Thinx & PERIOD. (2019). State of the period: The widespread impact of period poverty on US students. [Report]. Retrieved from https://cdn.shopify.com/s/files/1/0795/1599/files/State-of-the-Period-white-paper_Thinx_PERIOD.pdf?455788

Turner, V. (1987). Betwixt and between: The liminal period in rites of passage. In L. C. Mahadi, S. Foster, & M. Little (Eds.), *Betwixt & between: Patterns of masculine and feminine initiation* (pp. 223–238). La Salle, IL: Open Court Publishing.

Vick, R., & Sexton-Radek, K. (2005). Art and migraine: Researching the relationship between artmaking and pain experience. *Art Therapy*, 22(4), 193–204. doi:10.1080/07421656.2005.10129518

Weiss-Wolf, J. (2017). *Periods gone public: Taking a stand for menstrual equity*. New York, NY: Arcade Publishing.

# 13 Penalizing More Than One
## Art Therapy with Prison Inmates Struggling with Pregnancy, Birth, and Motherhood

*Casey Barlow, Shannon Schmitz, and Dave Gussak*

Prisons in the United States were originally constructed to house men deemed to be reprobates and criminals; the notion of housing women who committed infractions against societal norms became an after-thought, resulting in female inmates housed in environments constructed for—and by—men. Even when separate institutions were developed for women, they continued to follow the male-dominated construct—never mind the very different needs for women, and the manner in which they respond to incarceration. As a result, the system does not always account for their needs, resulting in compounded marginalization, loss of iden-tity, and degenerating self-worth. This is made even more complicated in an environment that is just not equipped to address the needs of the female inmates who are either pregnant, giving birth, or dealing with being a new mother. Thus, their struggles are amplified by loss, grief, remorse, isolation, and pain.

As supported in the literature, art therapy has been found effective in addressing the various issues that women face inside. Two of the authors of this chapter have relied on art therapy to address and mitigate the complications of pregnancy, birth, and loss of a newborn for several imprisoned women. To provide a context in which to understand such a population, this chapter will begin by highlighting additional concerns about this environment, and, in particular, how it pertains to the challenges and benefits of using art therapy with this population. This will be illustrated through several case vignettes.

### Women in Prison

Early in the history of the American penal system, women were impri-soned far less than men—more likely for "moral turpitude" (Pishko, 2015) than for a violent offense. As a result, women were held in the same institutions as men; as there were so few female offenders, most states simply didn't have separate facilities. In one of the earliest prisons, men had access to the entire institution while women were constrained in the facility's attic. It was not until the late 1800s when women were finally placed in separate institutions. However, separation did not improve conditions. Early women's prisons were overcrowded, and the inmates received inhumane treatment. Some were even gagged and kept in straitjackets.

Given that such institutions were created and primarily staffed by men, stereotypical perspectives shaped the limited reformation that occurred; women were not held to the same standards as men, as it was believed that they were not able to make free choices (Gartner & Kruttschnitt, 2004). Women were—and remain—doubly marginalized in the correctional milieu.

The number of incarcerated women has continued to increase over the ensuing years (Sawyer, 2018). Over a 40-year period the amount of women in prison has increased 834%; in the 11 years between 1993 and 2004, the women's prison population has increased from 7% to 12%; during the same time period, the number of women in jail increased by 468% (Elias, 2007). Yet, given the historically male-oriented institutions, the specific needs of women are simply not addressed. This includes protection against sexual assaults, gender-specific mental health issues, family care and, in particular, reproductive concerns, including pregnancy and birth (Braithwaite, Treadwell, & Arriola, 2005).

### The Pregnant Inmate

Clearly, women in prison are increasingly more marginalized than their male counterparts. To compound matters, many women who enter prison are pregnant and oftentimes give birth during their sentence. Between 5 and 10% of women enter a penal institution pregnant. As a result, 2,000 babies are born a year inside the fence (Clarke & Adashi, 2011; Clarke & Simon, 2013). Despite this propensity for housing pregnant women, little is understood or done to address this specific population. If they are unfortunate enough to give birth while still incarcerated, women are treated heartlessly. Many are forced to wear shackles during labor, which increases medical risks, psychological trauma, and continues to dehumanize the new mothers (Sichel, 2008).

To aggravate this painful ordeal, while some states are attempting to develop "prison-based nursery programs that house mothers and their newborns in special units" with various degrees of success (Clarke & Simon, 2013, p. 782), the majority of new mothers are separated from their infants at birth (Tracy, 2010). In addition, the chances of them having their children returned to them upon release is extremely slim according to Clarke and Simon (2013):

> Because the average sentence for women in prison is 18 months, by the time parents are released it is likely they will no longer have

custody of their children. Thus, a sentence as short as 15 months can result in the lifelong separation of a mother and her children.

(p. 782)

Therefore, challenging issues are compounded exponentially as these experiences further attack mental health and well-being within the prison.

## Creativity and the Female Inmate

Similar to their male counterparts, art making is a natural by-product of being imprisoned. Women in prison already have a tendency to create art for display, providing an opportunity for their own self-expression (Lazzari, Amundson, & Jackson, 2005). Therefore, art therapy has provided a viable intervention for those inside.

Art and other creative activities were found to support and enhance empowerment (Leberman, 2007). When older female inmates took part in organized art workshops, they became demonstrably more connected with one another, eventually exhibiting empathy for others (Hongo, Katz, & Valenti, 2015). Gibbons (1997) discovered that when imprisoned women were offered opportunities to create through welding, carpentry, poetry, gardening, and mural painting, it was "therapeutic and cathartic, (facilitating) women prisoners' quest to maintain and define self, despite legal and social structures designed to discredit and stigmatize" (p. 79). Merriam (1998) recognized that art therapy with incarcerated women:

> (offered) autonomy, (strengthened) self-esteem and (provided) a safe and acceptable way of releasing feelings such as anger and aggression. Art therapy can be important for this population of highly traumatized women whose unspeakable feelings often lead to emotional withdrawal and isolation, or the practice of destructive, tension-releasing activities.
>
> (p. 169)

In a study on the effectiveness of art therapy with male and female prison inmates, women demonstrated a significantly greater improvement in mood and internal locus of control than the men (Gussak, 2009). Their mood and their internal LOC increased significantly more than the men's. Yet, as the numbers revealed, it wasn't that the women were a lot less depressed and had better internal control than the men at the end of the intervention; rather, the men and the women displayed similar post scores, indicating the women had more of a deficit to overcome than the men. These conclusions supported the literature that incarcerated women may be more susceptible to depression (Butterfield, 2003; Harris, 1993) and have a greater external locus of control (LOC)

(DeWolfe, Jackson, & Winterberger, 1988) as revealed by the crimes they committed.

Regardless, the data further supported that the women prefer alternative therapies including art, and also benefited from the group interactions that the art therapy sessions provided (Day & Onorato, 1997; Zingraff, 1980). Although men generally responded well to the art therapy groups, they had more of a tendency to be concerned about the final product; "their natural competitive tendencies compelled them to produce good art" (Gussak, 2009). Yet...

> (i)n the sessions observed, the women seemed content with creating the art piece, but did not concentrate on the final result as much as the men. That is not to say that the women did not care that they produced good art. While they complimented each other's work, the women did not focus on whether their art was better or worse than someone else's in the group ... the women were able to use the art making process as a catalyst to facilitate discussion and empathic interaction. In other words, the women seemed content simply with the interactions, drawing energy from the group cohesiveness and socialization, with the final piece of secondary importance.
>
> (p. 205)

Simply put, the women seemed to enjoy more empathic support from the others in their group when making art. The women also seemed to respond to, and be affected by, the overall mood of the group.

As indicated, depression, helplessness, and feelings of marginalization and dehumanization are further exacerbated when contending with pregnancy, giving birth, and losing their families, while incarcerated. The following several vignettes reveal complications and subsequent interventions for those inmates addressing such challenges, loss and fear.

### Megan

In one rural women's prison nestled halfway between two larger historical cities in the South, one inmate, a 26-year-old White woman, Megan (not her real name), was experiencing an even higher level of hardship than normal for the institution. She was six months pregnant, and requested a mental health therapy appointment as she was greatly frustrated with others in her wing. She appeared calm when recounting the agitation she felt about her living situation.

This facility is not only a maximum security prison holding the most violent and behaviorally deviant offenders, this prison is also home to those inmates that have been designated acutely physically and/or mentally ill, requiring the highest medical needs available. The population includes death row inmates, civilly committed patients, those suffering terminal diseases, the intellectually disabled, and inmates that have been placed in behavioral modification programs. It also includes pregnant women.

Typically, pregnant women are designated a bottom bunk on the bottom tier of the wing. Such a bed is more highly valued within most of the pods in this prison for a variety of reasons; it is a valuable and limited commodity. Megan explained that some of the interpersonal conflict she was experiencing arose due to her bed assignment and roommate situation. There was one individual on the wing who she felt was giving her a particularly hard time.

Additionally, Megan was dealing with some of the many challenges of being pregnant while incarcerated. One such adversity is that the pregnant inmate is not informed of her scheduled doctor's appointments until the day appointments are held, as they are transported outside of the prison. While such a policy has been established for security concerns, it leaves the pregnant woman guessing and unsure of the potential outcomes. Clearly, being incarcerated during a pregnancy limits a woman's choice in her child-bearing options. When asked about this, Megan shrugged, indicating that she had accepted it as "the way it is." She further explained that her grandmother, who had raised her, planned to care for her child after she gave birth until she was released from prison in a few years.

Given Megan's openness to the art therapy, and her interest in exploring her frustration, anxiety, and helplessness through art, she was offered the opportunity to complete an open directive that focused simply on how she was feeling on that day. Provided with several different materials to choose from, she chose oil pastels to apply color to a cut out medium-sized mandala. She had never used oil pastels before and liked the strong colors they produced. She scribbled frenetically, pressing down on the paper with the oil pastels so firmly that hardly any white could be seen on the paper through her lines. She used almost all of the available colors within the pack, and layered them around the circle. While she indicated that she chose the colors merely because they were pretty, her sense of energy and implied force clearly suggested that she was transferring her anger and frustrations onto the paper. When she finished filling the entire circle up with layered colors, she released a deep breath, seemingly more at ease and relaxed than when she came to the session. Unfortunately, while she was eager to attend another session, she was unable to schedule one prior to the birth of her child.

### Allison

In the same prison as Megan, Allison (not her real name), a White woman, was recently returned after giving birth at a local hospital. She had only been back at the prison for a day or two, so a session was arranged while she was still in the infirmary wing. Often in the chaos and commotion of a prison schedule, mental health staff are sent to certain individuals "on the fly" and may not have access to their chart prior to meeting with the inmates. In this case, the clinical supervisor simply indicated that a woman had recently returned from giving birth and needed to be checked on, which is typical protocol for this situation. Not much information was available about her, and standard of such check-ins, the session was fairly short. She was 32 years old.

In speaking with her, she expressed that she was "fine," but admitted to feeling sad about leaving her child so abruptly. While she was initially reserved when offered blank paper and markers to express some of her feelings through art, she slowly began to open up.

She half-laughed nervously as she indicated she was not artistic. Yet, with reassurance, she began to draw a circle in the center of the paper that eventually became her baby's head. Despite initial attempts to draw the baby realistically, she became frustrated at the outcome, and resorted to a stick figure baby, albeit with slightly more characterized facial features.

As Allison drew, she talked about her baby and tried to process and reconcile her feelings that she was abandoning her child. She admitted to mourning not being able to hold her baby and physically touch her soft skin. She was invited to reflect this longing on her page. She added bright colored hearts and flowers in the empty spaces surrounding the image of the baby. As she drew, she talked of the soft petals, the sweet smell of the flowers and the warmth of the radiating hearts.

While seemingly superficial in content and imagery, it was clear she was genuinely trying to articulate her loss and her sensory desires. She kept repeating that most of all she wanted her daughter to feel loved. Before finishing the piece, she added a semi-circle in the top right corner, similar to the way a child may draw a schematic sun. Adding two eyes, a nose, and a small line for a mouth, she indicated that this image represented herself, and that while she might not be physically present, she wanted her baby to "feel" loved.

Before the session ended, we discussed additional coping skills and available options during her brief, remaining time in the infirmary were discussed. Although Allison was encouraged to request further sessions, this was the last time she was seen in art therapy; she simply did not follow up. However, even this singular experience seemed to provide her at least a brief opportunity to reconnect with her lost infant.

## Rachel

Motherhood is difficult when a woman is separated from her child, but can be even more painful when trying to reconcile that she was the cause. At 22 years old, a Black woman Rachel (not her real name), was left feeling overwhelmed, exhausted and alone after a medically complicated labor. Returning home to an empty house as her husband was serving in the military overseas, and unable to count on her family for support, she became overwhelmed and began to experience serious postpartum depression. She sought help from community resources, but was only offered to be placed on a wait list for a group that was starting several months later. Her child was one month old when a moment of intense grief resulted in unintentional infanticide. She was charged and subsequently incarcerated in the same prison as Megan and Allison for second-degree murder, child abuse, and neglect. Divorce followed, which added an additional layer to her grief.

Rachel held a job in the prison helping other inmates who had challenges living in the general population because of severe intellectual disabilities and/or mental illness. Outwardly, she exhibited selflessness and compassion as she engaged with the other women; however, inwardly, she struggled with low self-esteem, perfectionism, and the inability to forgive herself for her crime. Highly intelligent, she was in the process of earning an advanced degree, but would often become stuck "in her own head." Consumed with unbearable guilt, she was terrified of what it would be like when she was eventually released. She could not fathom others forgiving her when she was unable to forgive herself. While she entertained hopes of one day having another family, she was afraid that it just was not possible; and if by chance she could begin another family, she was paralyzed with the fear her postpartum depression would return.

During art therapy, Rachel focused on confidence, self-acceptance, and forgiveness. In an earlier session, she created a collage of images identifying her perfectionistic drives, unattainable high standards for herself and the factors that contributed to her lack of self-worth. Once these issues were identified, Rachel was able to focus on recognizing and reinforcing her personal strengths; she did so by providing personal challenges and raising her confidence by exploring materials she was unfamiliar with. Once a rapport was established and confidence improved, she was willing to explore self-forgiveness.

She chose watercolors to represent different emotional layers she hoped to examine throughout the process. She started with a rich shade of blue, and added more water to let the color run thin in certain areas and saturate others with the richness of the color. She moved the paper around to watch the watercolor run across the circle and seep into different parts of the paper. She continued to add the same rich blue, but began to alternate it with a lighter grey-blue tone. She watched as the colors tentatively began to mix. She then chose light purple and began to let the colors bleed together. Gradually, as she became more comfortable with the natural blending of colors occurring on the paper, she added watered down layers of black watercolor, which changed the blues and purples that had already seeped into the paper into hazy, obscured versions of their earlier brightness. Before finishing, she added two small spots of yellow that appeared to be peeking out from within the muddled blur of darker cool tones (Figure 13.1).[1]

Reflecting on her piece, she explained that while it was not intentional at first, she began to enjoy and respond to the "messiness" of the piece. She felt it more accurately reflected the unresolved, disorganized grief she was carrying within. Once this grief was recognized, she began to focus more on finding her way through the haze.

### Karen

In some cases, when the inmate's identity is focused on her role as a mother, removing her from her children becomes extremely detrimental

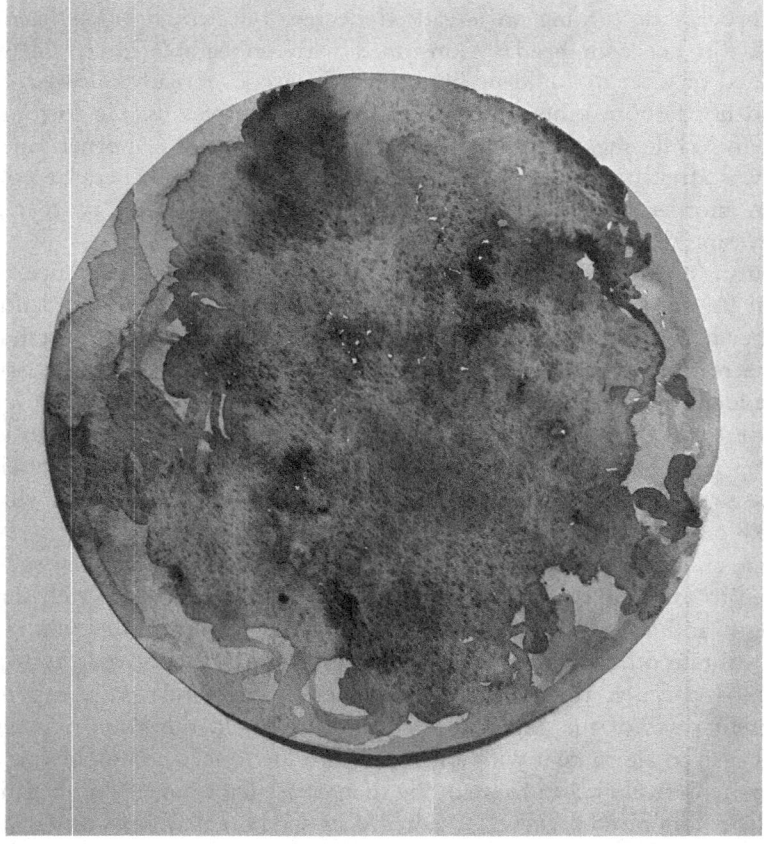

*Figure 13.1* Rachel's watercolor (recreated by author).

to her health and well-being. When working in the mental health department of a women's prison located in a major city in the Midwest, one of the authors worked with Karen (not her real name) a White woman whose depression worsened the longer she was away from her infant daughter.

Karen was in her mid-20s when she was arrested and imprisoned in the facility after driving under the influence multiple times. Her daughter was eight months old when she was imprisoned.

Prior to her arrest, Karen struggled with addiction, primarily alcohol and pain medication, which contributed to her crime. Diagnosed with Major Depressive Disorder, she struggled with symptoms that would naturally increase in intensity when she heard of her child meeting many milestones throughout her first year of life.

Karen participated in an open studio art therapy group with five to seven other women. She would often cry as she worked on her art therapy pieces. Much of the time she focused on creating different art and craft projects to send home to her daughter, "so that her daughter knew her mother was thinking of her all the time while she was away." This was common with many of the women; drawings and paintings, coloring pages, and various craft projects would often be sent home to their children to maintain the mother–child connection while separated through incarceration.

Karen would sometimes work on coloring sheets of cartoon characters that she believed her daughter would like. She meticulously colored and shaded these pictures for hours and would often seek reassurance that she chose the correct colors for each character. Other times she would create whimsical paintings of fairy tales and princesses, frequently sprinkling glitter somewhere on them. On one occasion, Karen used red, black, and yellow geometric shapes on white paper to create a sort of paper quilt as she had heard that these colors were the first ones that babies could discern and wanted to make something that was age appropriate for her daughter.

Karen often struggled with recognizing an identity outside of being a mother to an infant. While incarcerated, she began engaging in detrimental behaviors, such as trading and selling her commissary goods for substances, fighting with other inmates, and stealing. It soon became clear that after these incidents she would feel guilty and shameful for compromising her values; as a result, her depression deepened. In the sessions, she slowly came to realize how her environment affected her and the difficulties she faced in managing the time away from her daughter. She began to recognize that such dangerous behaviors "were an attempt to numb the pain of not being able to hold her daughter." She was ashamed of behaving like an "inmate" rather than a mother. After many of these scenarios, Karen focused her attention on making even more artwork that she could send home to her daughter in order to make amends and remain connected with her. Regardless of the impetus for the increased productivity, this allowed Karen to channel her feelings of loss and grief into a much more acceptable form of expression while providing a natural bridge to who she was outside. Eventually, her dangerous behaviors decreased, and her intense guilt and shame dissipated as she focused on being reunited with her daughter.

### Danielle

Within the same Midwestern institution, Danielle (not her real name), a White woman in her early 30s, was serving a sentence for a sex offense. While married at the time of her incarceration, she had been estranged from her husband since she was imprisoned. She was a mother of two children—a five-year-old boy and a three-year-old girl. As a result of her crime, she had minimal contact with her children while in prison, but would receive vague updates about them through family members who still maintained contact.

Danielle was soon diagnosed with Major Depression Disorder and Borderline Personality Disorder; it also became clear that she herself had been sexually molested as a child. She struggled with emotional instability, self-harm, and suicidality throughout her incarceration. These symptoms increasingly heightened due to her separation from her children.

It became clear that Danielle's identity was strongly based in her role as a mother. She would often reference this identity in the artwork she created in the group and individual art therapy sessions she was referred to. In one collage representing her strengths, she included that she "was good at cooking, keeping traditions, planning her children's birthday parties, growing her own food and playing games with her children" (Figure 13.2).

Much like Karen, when her work was not about her identity as a mother, she would create pieces to be mailed to her children as an attempt to maintain her albeit precarious connection, mostly in the open-arts studio sessions. Even when the art therapy directives were more specific, Danielle would often find ways to create imagery that was appropriate to send to her children while still addressing the directive.

As Danielle continued to struggle with the separation from her children, their developmental milestones and birthdays would become overly difficult, prompting extreme emotional dysregulation and maladaptive coping, exacerbating her tendencies towards self-harm and suicidality. An inability to be with her children during these important times was "too much (for her) to bear." She admitted that the acts of self-harm gave her a different type of pain—physical rather than emotional—to focus on. Such pain was easier to experience and allowed her to punish herself for not being the mother that she desperately wanted to be. Frequently during these incidences, she would be placed on a crisis level to ensure her physical safety. Counterintuitively, during these

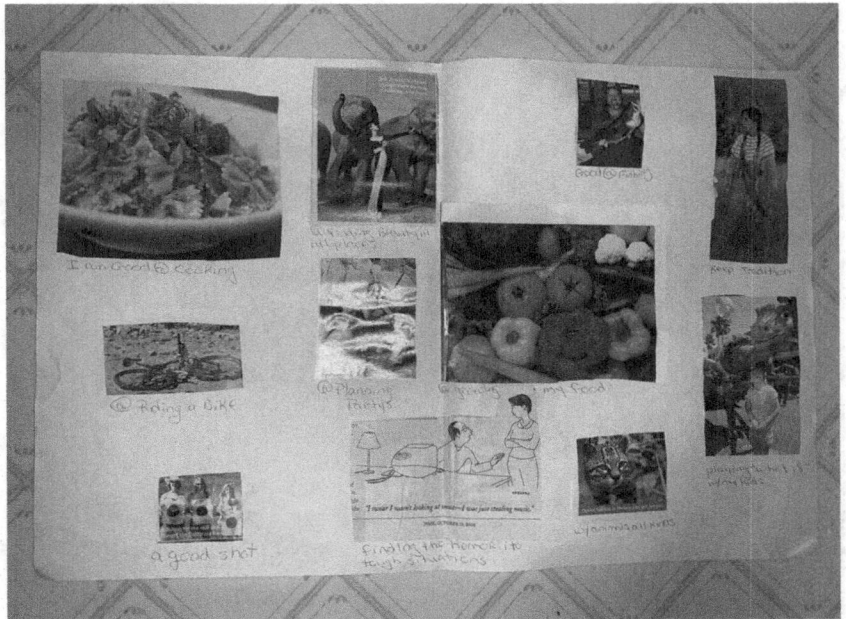

*Figure 13.2* Danielle's collage.

times, the art directives would focus less on family and would be designed to express and contain her intense emotions, identify healthy ways to cope with her distress, and provide productive ways to change her reactions and behavior.

Danielle had been placed on a crisis level following an incident of self-harm and suicidal ideation around Christmas. Upon the therapist returning after the New Year, Danielle created Figure 13.3 to symbolize her experience. The sparse composition is made up of several simple forms drawn with markers.

She explained the Christmas tree represented how she missed seeing her children open presents. The small table and empty chairs represented her desire to make decorations with her children as they had done in the past. The black rectangle with lines represented the one year anniversary of her incarceration. She admitted that these missed traditions and the anniversary propagated her intense emotional dysregulation. The HELP sign with a circle and a slash depicted her failure to ask for help from the mental health staff and failure to engage the coping skills she had developed. The dry erase board with an animal drawn on it, the two small green dominoes, and the brown dog in the corner depicted moments of happiness; however, after drawing them, she admitted, she felt guilty for any feelings of happiness while separated from her

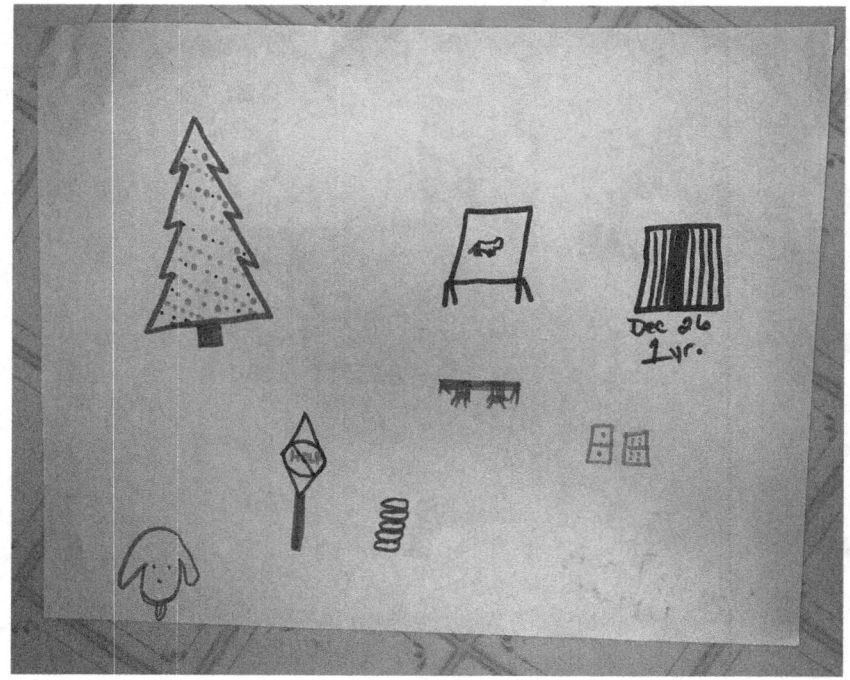

*Figure 13.3* Danielle's Christmas drawing.

children. Finally, the blue and pink ovals represented the medication change she experienced while on a crisis level.

As Danielle lost her identity as "mother" during her incarceration, she struggled immensely with identifying who she was, which resulted in trauma and emotional pain.

### Providing Security and Nurturance: The Baby Blanket Group

There are unique ways in which these women may address their own loss. In the same facility where Danielle and Karen were housed, a group of incarcerated mothers, comprising White, African American and Latina women, developed a community service project. They crocheted baby blankets for newborns and mothers identified by a local hospital as experiencing financial hardship or in need of extra support. This popular group continuously had a lengthy waiting list of incarcerated women who wanted to provide nurturance and security.

This crocheting group, ranging from five to eight women, operated very much the same as a sewing circle and provided a safe and nonjudgmental space for incarcerated mothers to discuss their families and children, while reflecting on their challenges and feelings about mother-hood with others who understood.

The rate at which these group members completed blankets was impress-ive. Large trash bags filled with dozens of blankets were frequently dropped off at the local hospital by staff members. Donations of skeins of yarn were provided as quickly as the bags of blankets were completed. Group members talked about how they felt more relaxed, the uplifting brightness of the colored yarns against the stark prison environment, and their positive feelings around contributing to children and mothers.

While not necessarily a "therapy group," it often resembled one as the women would talk about their struggles. Many times, the conversation developed into storytelling about their children and their achievements; anecdotes about the joys and tribulations of raising their children circulated the room. Some would provide different strategies for rearing children, some recounted experiences with their own mothers, and some would lament about missing their children's first days of school, first dance, or other activities. They provided witness to each other. Towards the end of each meeting, the conversation slowly dwindled until a pregnant silence would come over the small room. This silence seemed to contain the sadness each woman was experiencing so distant from their own children.

## Final Reflections

The experience of prison for women is extremely difficult, particularly for those that may simultaneously be experiencing pregnancy, birth or motherhood. It is only recently that some facilities are considering the needs of this sub-population, and are developing childcare units and longer visitation with their families. Even still, such progress is slow and inconsistent. As a result, many women, who already suffer from depression and anxiety, develop debilitating grief and loss as the system continues to minimize their needs. When available, art therapy has provided a voice for these women who are otherwise silenced by dehumanizing and objectifying institutions, giving them an opportunity to implement and maintain connections with those they lost, and poten-tially offer prospects to develop new identities that will herald a chance for reconnection and personal triumph.

Still, of all of the sub-populations that need attention within the prison milieu, this one is by far the most challenging, and—in all honesty—heart-rending. The art therapists who provided the services in these cases not only drew upon the art but also their own identities in order to elicit empathy and compassion so desperately needed to meet the needs of these women while still maintaining their own integrity and boundaries. One of the authors admitted that although her own experi-ences as a young mother working inside a women's prison resulted, at times, in self-examined "countertransference and judgment," her own identity allowed her to

> validate my clients' feelings and experiences as mothers and the difficulties experienced with maintaining an identity while raising children. Being a mother is clearly a part of my identity but, unlike so many of my clients, is not the crux of my identity. I soon accepted that this was okay; it did not make me a bad mother. I learned to accept all styles of parenting, and was able to find the identity that best served me and my children without sitting in judgment of myself or others. This allowed me to provide the best services for these women.

Since another author had not had children one author indicated that she couldn't completely relate to the pregnancy-related issues faced by some of the women she worked with. However, she clearly "recognized the special bond between a mother and child." As a result, working with these women "kept me grounded as an art therapist and allowed me to meet them wherever they may be in their individual journeys."

Still, the third author, a father, understood how important it was to not ascribe his preconceived biases and privileges onto these women, recognizing that the patriarchal penal system simply does not account for such struggles. Over the years Gussak (1997, 2009, 2019) has often cited that one of the many benefits of art therapy in prison is that it provides a bridge between the inside and outside cultures. All three authors would argue that the art, in these cases, provided a connection between the incarcerated woman and her lost family, and quite frankly, between herself and her own identity.

## Note

1  Please note, given the rules of the particular institution, this author was unable to photograph Rachel's art. As a result, Figure 13.1 was recreated by the author to represent the work completed by the artist.

## References

Braithwaite, R., Treadwell, H., & Arriola, K. (2005). Health disparities and incarcerated women: A population ignored. *American Journal of Public Health*, 95(10), 1679–1681.

Butterfield, F. (2003, October 22). Study finds hundreds of thousands of inmates mentally ill. *The New York Times*. Retrieved from http://query.nytimes.com.

Clarke, J. G., & Adashi, E. Y. (2011). Perinatal care for incarcerated patients: A 25 year old woman pregnant in jail. *Journal of the American Medical Association*, 305(9), 923–929.

Clarke, J. G., & Simon, R. E. (2013). Shackling and separation: Motherhood in prison. *JAMA: The Journal of Ethics, 15*(9), 779–785.

Day, E. S., & Onorato, G. T. (1997). Surviving one's sentence: Art therapy with incarcerated trauma survivors. In D. Author & E. Virshup (Eds.), *Drawing time: Art therapy in prisons and other correctional settings* (pp. 127–152). Chicago, IL: Magnolia Street Publishers.

DeWolfe, T. E., Jackson, L. E., & Winterberger, P. (1988). A comparison of moral reasoning and moral character in male and female incarcerated felons. *Sex Roles, 18*(9/10), 583–593.

Elias, G. (2007). Facility planning to meet the needs of female inmates. In *New jail planning: Bulletin from the jails division of the national institute of corrections* (pp. 1–11). Washington, DC: National Institute of Corrections, Retrieved from: https://info.nicic.gov/nicrp/system/files/022247.pdf

Gartner & Kruttschnitt. (2004). A brief history of doing time: The California Institution for Women in the 1960s and the 1990s. *Law & Society Review, 38*(2), 267–304.

Gibbons, J. A. (1997). Struggle and catharsis: Art in women's prisons. *The Journal of Arts Management, Law, and Society, 27*(1), 72–80.

Gussak, D. (2019). *Art and art therapy with the imprisoned: Re-creating identity.* New York, NY: Routledge.

Gussak, D. E. (1997). Breaking through barriers: Art therapy in prisons. In D. Gussak & E. Virshup (Eds.), *Drawing time: Art therapy in prisons and other correctional settings* (pp. 1–11). Chicago, IL: Magnolia Street Publishers.

Gussak, D. E. (2009). Comparing the effectiveness of art therapy on depression and locus of control of male and female inmates. *The Arts in Psychotherapy, 36*(4), 202–207.

Harris, J. W. (1993). Comparison of stressors among female vs. male inmates. *Journal of Offender Rehabilitation, 19*(1/2), 43–56.

Hongo, A., Katz, A., & Valenti, K. (2015). Art: Trauma to therapy for aging female prisoners. *Traumatology, 21*(3), 201–207.

Lazzari, M. M., Amundson, K. A., & Jackson, R. L. (2005). "We are more than jailbirds": An arts program for incarcerated young women. *Affilia, 20*(2), 169–185.

Leberman, S. (2007). Voices behind the walls: Female offenders and experiential learning. *Journal of Adventure Education and Outdoor Learning, 7*(2), 113–130.

Merriam, B. (1998). To find a voice. *Women & Therapy, 21*(1), 157–171.

Pishko, J. (2015). A history of women's prisons. *JStor Daily. (Jstor.org).* Retrieved from https://daily.jstor.org/history-of-womens-prisons/

Sawyer, W. (2018) The gender divide: Tracking women's state prison growth. *Prison Policy Initiative.* Retrieved from www.prisonpolicy.org/reports/women_o vertime.html

Sichel, D. L. (2008). Giving birth in shackles: A constitutional and human rights violation. *Journal of Gender and Social Policy Law, 16*(2), 223–255.

Tracy, C. E. (2010). Pregnant inmates—the most forgotten of the forgotten. *Legal Intelligencer.* Retrieved from www.law.com/jsp/pa/PubArticlePA.

Zingraff, M. T. (1980). Inmate assimilation: A comparison of male and female delinquents. *Criminal Justice and Behavior, 7*, 275–292.

# 14 Working with the *Huecos*

## The Art Therapy Space for Undocumented Latina Mothers

*Paula De Oliveira Santos*

There are social structures inside which we are constantly—and often blindly—sitting inside of and/or unconsciously desperately trying to get out of. Some of these social structures may feel like oppressions where our power of choice is stripped. Worst of all are the oppressions we are creating unconsciously in our positions of power, such as our role as an art therapist. As Freire (1970) points out, "Leaders who do not act dialogically, but insist on imposing their decisions, do not organize the people—they manipulate them. They do not liberate, nor are they liberated: they oppress" (p. 178). Framing the chapter, Freire's concept of oppression is emphasized as decisions made for others instead of mutually engaging with dialogue; he wrote extensively about oppression and how it shows up within larger systems in which we play out our roles. Throughout this chapter, his words are incorporated to frame the work, and to remind us of the self-reflective nature required to become social justice art therapists.

I wrote this over and over and each time I rewrote this chapter, I insisted that it fit within the constructs of scholarly writing; however, in each version, I found that the open dialogue mattered more than describing this work in a scholarly, singular, concrete representation of what art therapy with undocumented Latina mothers looked like. Instead, this writing emerged from discussions with colleagues and friends, and I felt it was important to bring the dialogue into written form. Using the lived standpoint of a Latin American immigrant—now legalized American citizen—as the basis for this discussion, I began to tell the story of the art therapy space with undocumented Latina mothers. I questioned whether to include such countertransference experienced through writing on this topic, and wondered if it had any value for the reader. Does my countertransference as the author engaging with the topic of oppression shine a light on the parallel experience of navigating the *huecos* (holes) of art therapy with undocumented Latina mothers? I find my experience of countertransference within the therapeutic relationship just as informative, if not more than, any methodological lens I apply in treatment. I believe that most art therapists agree that transference and countertransference exist within art therapy, and presume that it also shows up while condensing such experiences into words. So why not consider the process of writing on this topic as equally informative to the work I do in the office?

I experienced resistance in writing this chapter first and foremost because I felt that what I had to say about my experience within the therapeutic space with these women didn't look like textbook art therapy. This matters because we often forget the Eurocentric lens from which most art therapy literature stems from. I felt that not having the therapy space reflect my education, made it invalid to be written about. But like the metaphor that was birthed in sessions with these women, *huecos* was where the work began in the room and on this page—and I had to consider the different ways art therapy shows up for diverse populations. In the art therapy process, the experience of missing parts was reflected in a client's beautiful sentiment of *"Tengo huecos"* (I have holes) and the narrative that described the missing parts of life left back in her home country. Another client also described a similar feeling of *huecos "cuando vengo aquí, les digo a mis hijos que voy a ver alla doctora del alma porque hablar con alguien que se preocupa por mí me permite no sentir mis huecos y mis cicatrices"* (when I come here, I tell my kids I'm going to see the soul doctor because talking to someone who cares allows me to not feel my *holes* and my scars).

Since I have been working in the field, I feel that art, for the art therapist, is often viewed as a "heal all" universal language. Although all cultures have forms of creative expression, the value of art depends on a cultural organization and categorization. Artistic expression itself is not value free, even though art therapy is a more indirect form of expression from traditional talk therapy and we can often mistake art as a universal form of communication. However, as a field, art therapy is bound with specific cultural assumptions and structures of a Eurocentric society. We often then, in multicultural art therapy, categorize and make decisions of what form the space takes while still comparing it to this Western/Eurocentric lens. We add academic coursework to include "multicultural" art therapy, and assume that learning about diversity in itself qualifies as enough training to work with different populations without doing harm. Even though we love to include words of inclusivity when speaking to multiculturalism in our curriculum, we do not consider enough the importance of true social justice, intersectionality, privilege and oppression, and how these show up within the constructs of our field. Gipson (2017) explained this as Neoliberalism, which

> communicates otherwise contradictory values, granting society permission to access (and consume) diversity while denying an intersectional analysis that could contest ideology and collectively build intercommunity resources. Neoliberal diversity politics offer a multicultural color

blindness that attempts to heal traditional colorblind racism with a love of diversity.

(p. 114)

I believe there is a naiveté within our field that loves to look at a third world culture, pick up all the art supplies and go rushing into the middle of chaos to make things well, to save. Until we can as a field address the prevalent "white savior" mentality, we cannot even begin to talk about art therapy with oppressed populations. In the color blindness of the field, we can forget to see that certain clients and populations require additional fundamental resources and steps to develop trust in art therapy. Gipson (2017) spoke to color blindness as the component that empowers white professionals within the field "to name racial difference without questioning their participation in the hyper invisibility and homogeneity of *whiteness*" (p. 114). I have questioned my participation in oppression and reflected upon my personal discomfort in not making art with clients in my sessions. As a result, instead of art making, I have spent a foundational amount of time in talk therapy, learning about the ideological, institutional, interpersonal and internalized oppression my clients endured—and most importantly becoming an ally. Sound multi-cultural art therapy requires being comfortable with a space that looks non-traditional rather than forcing the target population to fit within the limited Eurocentric constructs of the field; it also requires evaluating its appropriateness to each client's experience and personal meaning (Bermudez & Ter Maat, 2006).

In writing a chapter about art therapy with undocumented Latina mothers or mothers to be, I feared it might become yet another script categorizing a certain population based off beliefs and over-generalizations. The therapeutic work with undocumented Latina mothers requires creative adaptability much more than concrete theories. To categorize the work as a finite truth is yet another form of oppression for an already vulnerable population. To assume a singular approach to a pluralistic population objectifies the population, and in turn strips the population of its diversity and attempts to make it fit the constraints of Eurocentric therapeutic practices. Thus, the informal structure from which this chapter took shape is intended to emphasize that this information is not prescriptive to working with undocumented immigrant Latina mothers, but rather emphasizes the personal reflection necessary to do social justice work well.

There is a great importance in doing the personal work and identifying the *huecos* within ourselves and the system, so that we don't blindly create more pot holes for our clients to climb out of. It is the work of dialogue to organize all that is presented by our clients versus imposing decisions of what we consider is best for them. In our eagerness to help, in our naivety that we hold the power to liberate another, we are but contributing to oppression. As Lilla Watson, an Indigenous Australian,

Murri visual artist, activist, and educator said in a speech at the United Nations, "If you have come here to help me, then you are wasting your time. But if you have come because your liberation is bound up with mine, then let us work together" (Watson, n.d.).

## Filling the *Hueco* of Accessibility

The Hispanic community is currently the largest minority in the United States. According to the US Census Bureau (2018), "Hispanic" is the term commonly used to refer to people of Spanish origin and those from Latin America. There is a linguistic question of how to refer to people of Latin America, and because this chapter includes undocumented immigrants from Brazil, we will be using the term "Latina" instead of Hispanic.

> [T]he more radical the person is, the more fully he or she enters into reality so that, knowing it better, he or she can transform it. This individual is not afraid to confront, to listen, to see the world unveiled. This person is not afraid to meet the people or to enter into a dialogue with them. This person does not consider himself or herself the proprietor of history or of all people, or the liberator of the oppressed; but he or she does commit himself or herself, within history, to fight at their side.
>
> (Freire, 1970, p. 39)

Freire's quote serves to frame that idea. Although we will be talking about undocumented Latina women, this chapter does not intend to become the proprietor of this work, but rather to unveil, confront, question and open dialogue about the important nature of this work within this population.

Undocumented immigration is a focal topic in our current political climate even though the United States is widely known as a nation of immigrants. Over the course of history, immigration policies have fluctuated between restrictive and inclusive. With President Trump as America's current president, immigration has been widely discussed and should equally be deliberated in clinical research. In a time that this population is increasing rapidly and becoming more vulnerable due to restrictive policies and systemic barriers, the mental health of undocumented immigrants requires special consideration. Very little has been written about art therapy and the undocumented population living in the United States, and I wonder if the limited research on such a topic relates to the accessibility of services. Despite the lack of research, we cannot ignore that oppression has an impact on mental health, not to mention access to mental health services. This chapter does not present political discourse on the topic of immigration, but I found that I cannot separate the way current policies impact the undocumented Latin American population in an art therapy setting. The conversation about art therapy with undocumented Latina mothers or mothers to be must begin outside of the office space.

Undocumented Latina women who give birth to American citizens struggle to receive adequate perinatal medical and mental healthcare. Research suggests that about 7% of American births are to undocumented parents each year in the United States (Fabi, 2019). Although contrary to some public beliefs that immigrants come to the United States and go on welfare, undocumented immigrants are not allowed to obtain most welfare services such as Medicaid or Medicare coverage, nor are they allowed to purchase plans that are available from the Affordable Care Act (Kelly & Tipirneni, 2018). Due to the Welfare reform of 1996 and continuing through the Affordable Care Act of 2010, undocumented immigrant populations have no access to federally funded programs with an exception to emergency conditions and active labor thanks to the Emergency Medical Treatment and Active Labor Act of 1986 (Fabi, 2019). The birth and medical procedures the baby may need will be billed to the child who is born an American citizen, but any medical services unrelated to the baby cannot be obtained unless considered an emergency. This means limited or no access to perinatal care. Such systemic barriers have an impact on undocumented Latina mothers' mental health as stressors increase due to lack of adequate resources, not to mention the well-being of the fetus during postpartum.

Cultural beliefs, language barriers, culture shock, acculturation, social isolation, and fear of deportation also contribute to reluctance and difficulty in accessing services. Particularly significant with undocumented Latina women regarding access to mental healthcare is the lack of funding. The lack of mental health insurance coverage and providers is a significant contributor to being able to access treatment for mental health needs. Access to clinicians or organizations who offer sliding-fee scales or free mental healthcare is limited in America. Depending on geographic location, there are centers and nonprofits that serve oppressed populations and offer mental health services free of charge, but often these agencies are restricted by grants that have target populations such as domestic violence victims, sexual assault victims or other populations. Affordable mental health services for undocumented immigrants are rare, especially for childbearing related treatment. Further, there are very few mental health clinicians and art therapists who are willing to work with affordable sliding scales or medicaid, and even fewer who offer bilingual services. I see many profiles on psychology marketing websites of bilingual therapists who offer services in Spanish, but often profile descriptors and logistics are not translated into Spanish. It becomes critical to promote services in a way so that those seeking help will be able to have understanding and access. Sharing information in Spanish opens a door for access to services for those with language barriers.

Another contribution to reluctance in seeking treatment is the cultural values within the Latin American culture. In my lyrical conversations with clients, I found repeated metaphors early in treatment used to describe the shame they felt in seeking help such as, "*La ropa sucia se lava en casa*"—similar to "Don't air your dirty laundry in public" (NAMI, n.d.). This fear was described in regards to documentation status and also as a cultural belief to not publicly share personal matters because of privacy concerns. We, as therapists, often assume the course of mental health treatment is information readily understood by all, and we forget that knowledge regarding confidentiality and disclosure agreements are not widely known factors in certain populations. An undocumented Latina woman may have a misunderstanding that seeking professional help will lead to the reporting of her illegal status. These barriers result from a lack of information. Without proper information, the stigma associated with mental health issues increases. Many undocumented Latina women additionally do not seek treatment for fear of being labeled as "*locas*" (crazy), feeling that they should be able to handle their emotions on their own. The stigma that mental health treatment is for serious mental illness only (*locos*) is widely known in Latin American culture. Furthermore, within Latina gender roles, mothers are expected to bear all family demands without support or assistance. Along with these gender roles, Latina mothers often place their children's needs above their own, thus seeing their own needs as less significant.

Within the Latin American collectivist culture, family and community support is emphasized. Many immigrants from such cultures can often feel displaced in entering an individualistic culture, such as the United States, where values differ. Often immigrants leave their families and communities behind and experience social isolation. An understanding of such differences in cultural values and social roles allows us to support a healthy environment and context for undocumented pregnant mothers to enter into a dialogue about their experience. Understanding and respecting prevalent cultural themes such as *marianismo* (selfless and prioritized devotion to the maternal identity) and recognizing the need for strong cultural support throughout maternity are essential in treatment of undocumented Latina women. Common stereotypes may also appear related to spiritual themes and, if not careful, there can be an overgeneralized belief that Catholic themes have high importance for Latina clients. It is important to respect the diversity also present within cultures that may have a dominant set of guiding principles. Although Catholicism and concepts like *marianismo* or *machismo* and general collectivist cultural values are dominant in Latin American cultures, we cannot assume cultural or religious orientation and values. Working from what is presented allows a lower risk of therapists bringing pre-existing, perhaps well-intentioned, beliefs or assumptions about our clients.

By being inquisitive with what is present for our clients allows us to consider other external factors in their course of treatment. If pregnant mothers already have children, there are other barriers to consider, such as childcare. The lack of childcare contributes significantly to the accessibility of therapy. Many mental health clinicians practice on weekdays during business hours, which overlaps this target population's work hours. Depending on social supports and the presence of a partner, more flexible treatment hours would contribute to accessibility. Another consideration is the location of such practices. Many clinicians forget to take public transportation into account and how it impacts accessibility. When working with undocumented populations, it can be assumed that many do not possess a driver's license and thus are limited to locations and hours that are reachable by public transportation.

Understanding the system that undocumented mothers are navigating allows us to understand our first role towards social justice for this population: that of filling the *hueco* of accessibility. To fill the gap of accessibility for undocumented Latina mothers becomes a creative way of navigating in order to provide attainable care and accessible information for our communities in which we serve. These are the only walls worth talking about regarding the undocumented immigrant population, and to fight on their side means to be open to changing the scopes of our practice to make mental health and art therapy, first and foremost, accessible to these women.

## Art Therapy without Art?

Art therapy with undocumented Latina mothers, or mothers to be, begins by first understanding the external systems present in the oppression of these women and then understanding how these show up within the therapeutic relationship and space. In social justice art therapy, we then abandon the notion of artistic universality and other Eurocentric judgments about art, and allow our clients to make decisions about how to process their own subjective experience of the world. As Freire points out,

> Any situation in which some individuals prevent others from engaging in the process of inquiry is one of violence. The means used are not important; to alienate human beings from their own decision making is to change them into objects.
>
> (Freire, 1970, p. 85)

In other words, if we prevent our clients from questioning and deciding what is best for themselves, we too become part of the violence and contribute to the oppression.

I found the ego "white savior" within me who wanted my clients to create art in sessions, so I could translate the lyrical conversations into symbols through art making. Even though my roots are deep in Latin American culture, I was educated through a Eurocentric lens, and my race is white. In having such certain privileges, I had to do some hard looking at myself as to how dominant culture oppressive themes still showed up in my work. Sullivan (2006) suggested that white people avoid examining their *whiteness*, especially because certain discoveries could disrupt their sense of feeling morally good. Ownership is hard work, especially owning where, in our eagerness and well-intentioned desire to help, we may be causing harm.

The *whiteness* in me wanted art to be made that neatly and visually represented my clients' inner childbearing related experiences—I wanted that textbook sublimation, the Eurocentric ideal art therapy session to unfold. Alas, that was not what happened. After many sessions, as I continued to communicate with my clients with words alone, I began to feel I was failing as an art therapist. The way art therapy unfolded in these sessions forced me to wonder, "is it art therapy if there is no art made?" I found that yes, in fact this is art therapy—it is *social justice* art therapy. Instead of manipulating my clients to make art for my own comfort in the process, I wanted to understand the abusive cycle of oppression, and how wanting to save someone is a sure way to dehumanize and strip one of their power.

Since my clients didn't make art, I turned to response art to explore their experience (Figure 14.1) and my own countertransference. Response art is art made by art therapists to contain, explore, and express clinical work (Fish, 2006, 2019). Still, I wondered if bearing witness to my clients was enough (Figure 14.2). I remember one pregnant client that I had invited to join me at the art therapy table, where I had a buffet of supplies set out. With a polite rejection, she sat on the couch stating her desire to not "do" anything but rather her need to *desahogar* (vent). At the time, I wondered how art or art therapy can be seen as an act of doing, when some clients may require an act that fulfills a different need.

During childbearing, women need time and space to grow, heal, rest, and prepare, time to reflect; however, often undocumented Latina mothers are not able to fulfill such needs due to working multiple jobs, caretaking other children, and the lack of resources that prevent pregnancy and postpartum from being a space of rest. It could be that some clients spend so much time working and doing, that simply having the choice to say no to doing is an act of power. Art therapy then needs to adaptively become a space to make room for such unmet needs and expressions. Talking was a way for these women to hear themselves away from their busy life and demands of childrearing. Rather than making art, talking with someone who could understand and easily communicate with them, offered an opportunity for us to build a sense of trust, safety

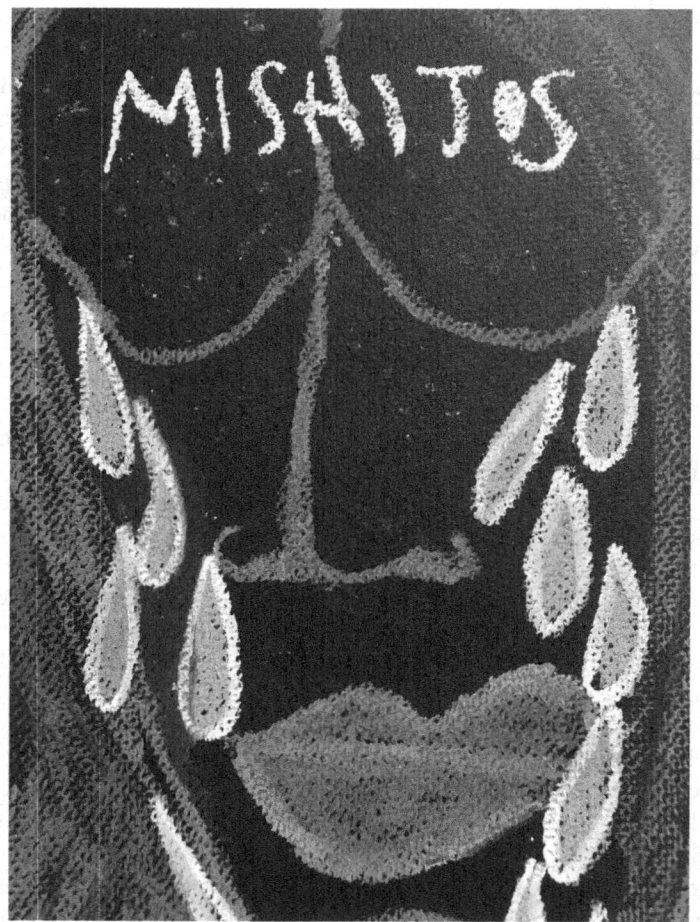

*Figure 14.1* "Mis Hijos" pastels on black paper.

and comfort. The art therapy space became the place where some of the undocumented Latina mothers were able to talk about themselves and prepare for the changes that come with adding another baby to their families.

For me, art often serves as a chaotic discharge and documentation of an emotional state. Some women do not have such a relationship with art making, and so it can be overwhelming and feel like another new thing to learn when they are already stressed. Essentially, it becomes more of a work task than a time for creative self-reflection. It seemed likely that my feeling of inadequacy about not having art made in art therapy sessions was a reflection of the parallel experience my clients

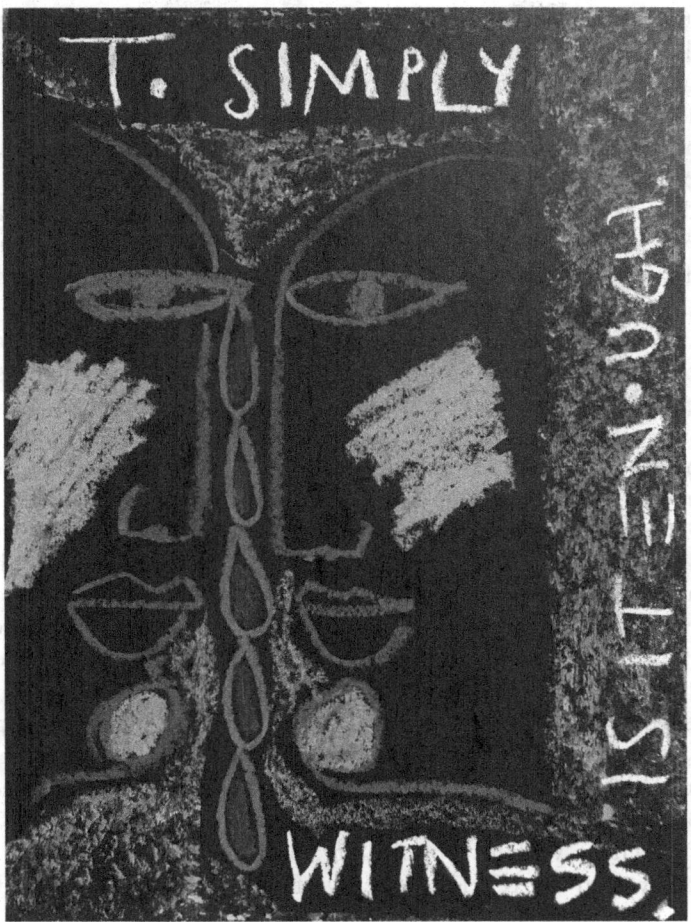

*Figure 14.2* "Discomfort of Witnessing" pastels on black paper.

faced regarding acculturation. As an immigrant, there is a deep desire to hold true to cultural roots and yet a certain need to assimilate for survival, which has a learning curve. Perhaps I experienced a similar desire for my role as an art therapist and the unfolding of a session to reflect the dominant culture of art therapy.

Had I forced my clients to make art, and not allowed for trust building with the women, the experience of art therapy would have been akin to the culture shock experienced by many Latin American immigrants. Then I, too, may be contributing to their oppression, to the unspoken expectation that they embrace without question as a foreign practice. In the field of art therapy, I feel it is imperative that we be open to the fact that art therapy can be too ambiguous or abstract within certain cultural contexts. Some clients prefer and want a more direct, verbal style and with childbearing issues, talking and being listened to in their native language is initially more important as they prepare for the major transitions and inherent vulnerabilities that come with pregnancy, child-birth, and postpartum. So as not to contribute to the oppression, women need to feel supported in how they make use of art therapy.

If I had prematurely forced or directed art making for the sake of filling my *hueco*, the place in me that feels that if art is not made I am not providing adequate enough care, then I too am part of the problem. While I learned to accept my client's resistance to art making, it was useful for me to make art as I considered my feelings around working with these women. In so doing, I chose to reflect in my art the stories and experiences they shared with me of living undocumented, pregnant, in a foreign land. Talwar, Iyer, and Doby-Copeland (2004) said it best: "Ethnocentric monocultural approach is a tool for oppression in a pluralistic society like the United States" (p. 44). Thus, the result is a need for an open dialogue about our role as art therapists within sessions, particularly when working with some Latina women who are confronted not just with the oppression of being undocumented, but also with becoming objectified as a medical problem or burden on a developed society that struggles to have a responsible and ethical healthcare system. I now trust that art therapy needs to look many ways, even as a space without art. The images that come through the words can be incredibly useful and emotionally expressive as in the word *huecos* used by two of the women. If we meet our clients with respect and collaboration, which means "being honest about the impact of discrimination on client welfare, opportunity, and choices" (Potash, 2019, p, 207), it is within the relational creative flexibility that a sense of liberation occurs.

## Considerations for the Art Therapist

As much as the art therapy field loves to emphasize a social justice lens and the careful treading into different cultures, we need to underscore the manner in which this process cannot be done without careful consideration. "To simply think about the people, as the dominators do, without any self-giving in that thought, to fail to think with the people, is a sure way to cease being revolutionary leaders" (Freire, 1970, p. 85). In fact, there is no singular, prescriptive approach that could encompass such personal obstacles and oppressions of others from diverse cultures. As Freire suggests, if we do not consider our role in the work with vulnerable populations, and we simply decide what is best for the people, we cease to create a space for liberation to occur. Creating art requires a certain level of comfort, and when there are too many barriers beyond what our clients are already facing in their external world, our job is to build that safety in the therapeutic space first and foremost. While the talking is art in its own way, and is creating the initial relationship where clients know that what they share will be heard and not be judged, eventually the art will become the next step in treatment. While talking remains ethereal, when trust is established and moves into art making, then the eventual tangible products of creativity will document their journey and deepen the therapeutic relationship. In fact, the art from art therapy would eventually become the living document to these undocumented Latina mothers. As trust is built through talking, it is still important to incorporate art therapy directives regarding safety and containment. To create and explore safety through art is recommended when traumatic histories, lack of social supports, and lack of resources are present. Art becomes a third relationship in the room, and though trust is established with me as therapist, it becomes another task to cultivate trust between art making and the client.

The art therapy space, once art making begins, may re-address the topics presented through talking. Art making would tangibly fill the *huecos* interwoven in the experiencing of self-esteem, cultural identity, perinatal stressors, oppression, isolation, acculturation, shame, social roles and loneliness. I imagine the transition into art making happening organically, incorporating already birthed metaphors and turning them into visual form. I could beautifully foresee creating art around the metaphor of *huecos*, a clothing line of shame and celebration, with images or tangible art products that focus on hopes and fears, protections, walls or social barriers, and other topics that had already been discussed while we were establishing a trusting relationship through talking about their role as a mother.

Additionally, there may be anticipation of the unborn child's needs, and some mothers may have an interest in creating things for the child, such as a mobile. One mother I worked with hinted at a desire to create her dream home and nursery though she didn't want to engage with the process of using collage materials. Many of the women I worked with lacked resources, worked multiple jobs throughout the entire pregnancy, and felt isolated and alone. Once we enter the art making phase, I would address these feelings, while paying close attention to the needs of the client, trusting her desire in what to create. I would gently educate and normalize the possibility of postpartum adjustment and depression and encourage her to define her support system, however limited. Given the lack of choices and resources that these women often face systemically, art therapy could become a buffet of choices—art then, could become a space to create visual anchors of safety and nourishment as much as to imagine solutions and possibilities. These women may also have some fears or uncertainty as they anticipate childbirth, navigate the hospital system or consider postpartum. If a woman is undocumented and does not speak English, she is incredibly vulnerable to medical decisions being made without her knowledge, consideration or consent, especially if no one speaks Spanish when she arrives at the hospital. Some hospitals have a service that connects the pregnant woman with an advocate who speaks her language and can relay medical information. Nevertheless, her body is at risk to become an object of yet another system and any trauma history will be activated, particularly if she is ill-treated or an emergency arises during her antenatal journey. During this antenatal journey, the undocumented woman becomes dependent on the goodwill and compassion of those around her; any childbearing related concerns, fears, and social barriers benefit from her having the therapy space to explore and for her voice to be heard—in art or in words—through discharge and sublimation or simply to *"desahogar"* (to vent).

I think that given the current political climate, the Latin American undocumented immigrant population is already under a significant amount of stress and art therapists need to take all of these factors into consideration. The work of liberation is then founded not on pre-existing values, but rather rooted in cultural humility and honest self-reflection.

Ultimately, when we can recognize our place as art therapists within the dynamics of these interchanges, then we can start doing the real work. This way we can rethink who we are and what we do and start to perceive our roles in how we partner up in the art therapy space with our clients. So many of us lump ideas of treatment into finite truths, and I invite our field to re-consider our Eurocentric approach to art therapy through open dialogue lest we become another invisible hand stripping power from the already oppressed.

## Description of Response Art

### Figure 14.1 *"Mis Hijos" Pastels on Black Paper 11×17*

I created Figure 14.1 after a session where I felt helpless in hearing the amount of barriers my client was facing due to her undocumented status. She was pregnant with a child whose father wasn't present, had other children, and with the Immigration and Customs Enforcement (ICE) raids, detaining undocumented immigrants, sweeping across the nation, there was a powerful sensation of hopelessness. The image says Mis hijos (my children), reflecting my client's endless concern for her children, prioritizing them always, even in the decision to relocate to a place where there was social isolation and no community support for their future— just as my parents once did for us.

### Figure 14.2 *"Discomfort of Witnessing" Pastels on Black Paper 11×17*

In Figure 14.2, I explored the "fix it" attitude that arises in me when the pain I witness is so great. This reflects my "white savior" wanting to heal, save, and do something. In creating this image, I experienced a sense of shame in my inability to sometimes sit with discomfort. To witness sometimes feels harder than to engage with art making, or even talk or implement solution-focused therapies. To simply witness oppressions in another human being felt like a whole new experience—one that became so important for my work with these undocumented women.

### Figure 14.3 "Invisible Hands" Pastels on Black Paper 11×17

Figure 14.3 is of a pregnant woman with no arms; her heart is glowing in a red circle and a small red glow is also representing the baby's heart. Blue hands are reaching for her, with red between the hands and her,

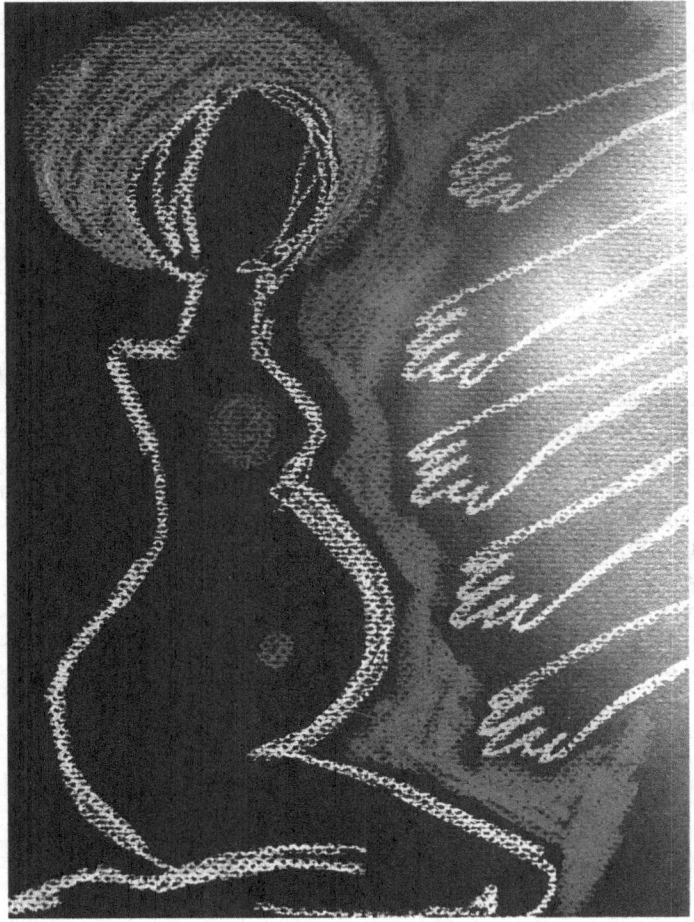

*Figure 14.3* "Invisible Hands" pastels on black paper.

describing the experience of a million prescriptive suggestions from others—medical professionals, family members—targeted towards my clients who sit there feeling helpless (armless) and powerless without being given much choice due to their oppressions.

# References

Bermudez, D., & Ter Maat, M. (2006). Art therapy with Hispanic clients: Results of a survey study. *Journal of the American Art Therapy Association, 23*(4), 165–171.

Fabi, R. (2019). Why physicians should advocate for undocumented immigrants' unimpeded access to prenatal care. *AMA Journal of Ethics, 21*(1), 93–99.

Fish, B. J. (2006). Image-based narrative inquiry of response art in art therapy (Doctoral Dissertation). Retrieved from ProQuest Dissertations and Theses database. (UMI No. AAT 3228081).

Fish, B. J. (2019). Response art in art therapy: Historical and contemporary overview. *Art Therapy: Journal of the American Art Therapy Association, 36*(3), 122–132.

Freire, P. (1970). *Pedagogy of the oppressed.* (M.B. Ramos, Trans.). New York, NY: Seabury Press.

Gipson, L. (2017). Challenging neoliberalism and multicultural love in art therapy. *Art Therapy, 34*(3), 112–117. doi:10.1080/07421656.2017.1353326

Kelly, A. T., & Tipirneni, R. (2018). Care for undocumented immigrants— rethinking state flexibility in Medicaid waivers. *The New England Journal of Medicine, 378*, 1661–1663.

NAMI. (n.d.). Retrieved from www.nami.org/find-support/diverse-communities/ latino-mental-health.

Potash, J. (2019). Relational social justice ethics for art therapists. *Art Therapy: Journal of the American Art Therapy Association, 35*(4), 202–210.

Sullivan, S. (2006). *Revealing whiteness: The unconscious habits of racial privilege.* Bloomington, Indiana: IU Press.

Talwar, S., Iyer, J., & Doby-Copeland, C. (2004). The invisible veil: Changing paradigms in the art therapy profession. *Art Therapy, 21*(1), 44–48. doi:10.1080/ 07421656.2004.10129325

U.S. Census Bureau. (2018, March 7). About. Retrieved from www.census.gov/ topics/population/hispanic-origin/about.html.

Watson, L. (n.d.). About. *Lilla: International Women's Network.* Retrieved from https://lillanetwork.wordpress.com/about/.

# 15 Infertility to Motherhood

## Collective Voices in Art Therapy Challenge Social Constructs

*Mary Andrus*

Social norms convey the message that, for women, motherhood is expected, yet public perception of motherhood often contradicts the realities and truths that women experience. How do we deconstruct the existing narratives that continue to marginalize or conceal the humanity of women's experiences? Art therapists who work with women have an opportunity to give voice to those who are silenced, and create space for an emergent collective story that challenges the dominant discourse.

## My Journey

I am a white, able bodied, cisgendered, middle-class woman, with privilege and freedom to move in the world with few barriers. When I was pregnant with my first child, I was slightly oblivious to the complexities and challenges women experience when pregnant. After having my daughter, I was attuned to the importance of connecting with the baby in utero and awakened by the inequities many other pregnant women in my community face.

As I moved through the balance of working and parenting, I longed for another baby. I tried to conceive and unfortunately experienced three miscarriages spaced two years apart over the next six years. Through these losses, I became acutely aware of the injustice that women endure in their hidden grief. This led me to my doctoral research, which examined the experiences of women related to infertility, pregnancy loss, and stillbirth. This chapter will explore the many voices of women in art therapy, honoring their experiences, art expressions, and validation of their collective stories.

## Background and Theory

My work is informed by a narrative feminist approach. Existing power structures and public policies have defined and shaped how women are viewed in society. Through the lens of social construction, when we examine our relationship to power and how that power has been asserted in society, it informs an understanding of our experiences as women. As art therapists, we must challenge the unjust socially constructed narrative, using art to shed light on and challenge these inequities.

## Childbearing Issues in Art Therapy

There is a need for more art therapy literature aimed to deconstruct social norms related to pregnancy and childbearing issues. Early contributions to the art therapy literature (Speert, 1992; Swan-Foster, 1989) held some feminist principles that challenged the medical model, explored images created by pregnant women, and acknowledged grief associated with perinatal loss. Hogan's (2003) book emerged with a feminist orientation that deconstructed gender constructs and challenged stereotypes in pregnancy and childbirth. Seftel (2006) offered a personal reflection of pregnancy loss, but lacked an acknowledgement of the impact of her social location or a deconstruction of the socio-political constructs related to childbearing and pregnancy loss. This chapter aims to contribute to this gap.

## Power and Feminism

Women are socialized to accommodate and submit to the power imbalance in relationships. The feminist theorists that emerged in the 1960s began asserting themselves against this power imbalance and many were viewed negatively for their outspoken behaviors. This was followed by feminists positioning the personal as political with the emergence of the term, *body politics* (Allegranti, 2013).

In the United States, women still experience sexist oppression within systems. These systems illuminate the power imbalance within the intersections of race, sex, and class oppression (hooks, 2015; Inhorn, 2006). hooks posited that feminism is a struggle to end sexist oppression, where anti-racist work is in tandem with sexist oppression. Feminism pushes against exploitation and domination to move systems into structures that benefit women and men equally.

Reproductive justice aims to organize activists around basic human rights. Reproductive oppression exists within public policies that favor elites and oppress communities of color (Ross, Roberts, Derkas, Peoples, & Bridgewater Toure, 2017; Schneider & Ingram, 2005). These policies benefit people who hold power and those who need services are viewed as burdensome. For example, viewing non-white women as "pathological or deviant" (Ross et al., 2017, p. 24) or creating caps for those who are eligible for welfare, thus punishing women who are on public assistance when having more children (Miller, 2017; Romero & Agènor, 2017). Through the social construction of motherhood, public policies define expectations, categorize women, and define the value of women based on their contributions to meet these goals. Patriarchal ideas in society perpetuate this dynamic.

Women in socially powerless groups experience structural discriminations or hermeneutical injustice (Fricker, 2007). Some examples are "sexual harassment as flirting, rape in marriage as non-rape, post-natal depression as hysteria, [and] reluctance to work family-unfriendly hours as unprofessionalism" (p. 10). Previously, women's experiences of sexual harassment were not taken seriously or seen as valid or socially acceptable to share. Recently, the landscape has shifted, bringing more attention to the importance of raising awareness to inequity, challenging patriarchy, and speaking out about the misogyny. In 2017, millions of women rallied across the world to assemble for a women's march to collectively stand up against sexist oppression. The awareness of corruption and abuse of power by president Donald Trump, and the awareness of sexually inappropriate behaviors by Harvey Weinstein, Jeffery Epstein, and R. Kelly have contributed to this shift. In the #MeToo movement (Burke, 2017), women who had held in secret stories of sexual assault found solace in their collective voices, and realized that moving their stories out of the private into the public gave them strength, acknowledgement, and helped them claim their collective power toward liberation.

However, some women experience negative consequences for taking the risk of speaking publicly. In the 2018 controversy surrounding conservative Justice Brett Kavanaugh, Dr. Christine Blasey Ford publicly testified at the cost of not being believed, and despite her efforts to tell her story of being sexually assaulted by him, he was appointed to the Supreme Court. She faced criticism and public humiliation in her attempts to express her concerns. In the instance of Larry Nassar, the gymnastics coach who was found guilty of sexually abusing over 265 individuals, 150 of the women collectively spoke out about the abuse in his public sentencing hearing. When Jon Lapook (2017) interviewed many of these women on *60 Minutes*, the women found strength in their collective voice of knowing that they were not alone in their suffering and felt motivated to speak up for the first time after hearing others share.

As women, it is isolating to navigate through life without a collective affirmation reflected back to us that we are not alone and our experiences have value when shared with one another. White and Epston (1990) drew from Foucault's theory of knowledge and truth when they wrote "we are subject to power through normalizing truths that shape our lives and relationships" (p. 19). In the construction of these truths, norms are formed that constitute people's lives, and through shared reflections of people's truths, an objective reality emerges.

According to Foucault, examining the act of objectifying people creates a discourse with an emphasis on their control over social norms (Foucault as cited in Madigan, 1992). This act brings our attention to an externalized gaze to the culture around us which holds power, and in doing so we create a fictitious idea of what is considered "normative" or desirable. This practice creates a dynamic of "power over" and distances people from one another. This results in an internalized negative societal message of how we are inadequate and unable to identify with the culturally constructed normative ideals. Fricker (2007) stated:

> when you find yourself in a situation in which you seem to be the only one to feel the dissonance between received understanding and your own intimated sense of a given experience, it tends to knock your faith in your own ability to make sense of the world, or at least the relevant region of the world ... that it may prevent one from gaining new knowledge and more generally, that it is likely to stop one gaining certain important epistemic virtues, such as intellectual courage.
>
> (p. 17)

We tend to police ourselves over each other and shape the acceptable behavior, which creates norms for some things and oppresses others. This results in a socially constructed meaning of being female that is not neutral. Foucault (1982) critiqued the social objectification and categorization of people, which provided social control by determining what was considered normative. This results in situations where people who do not fit into these categories are judged or condemned (Foucault, 1980, in Madigan 1992). White and Epston (1990) posited that in therapy we move through the spheres of knowledge and power; we need to make explicit facets that lead to social control and contest the practices that suppress persons into a dominant ideology (p. 29).

## Unequal Policies

From the 1973 Supreme Court ruling of Roe v. Wade, which supported women's rights to choose, we have slid backwards into a misogynistic culture shaped by conservative state legislation where women are expected to fulfill their role to reproduce, and are left to hold the responsibility of primary caretaker with limited support from employers for maternity leave or affordable childcare (Hogan, 2003). An emphasis on a capitalist driven agenda has shaped this point in our society where women are viewed as serving their assigned role to reproduce. According to Ross et al. (2017), the role of ultraconservative religion is equally problematic in

> denying the responsibilities of the state or religious institutions to provide economic, educational or social opportunities to women. Fundamentalists deploy masculinist rhetoric against social justice movements, while inciting religious, ethnic, gender, anti-immigrant,

and racial hatred. Religions that oppose women's rights offer little sustenance to those seeking self-determination over their lives and bodies.

(Ross et al., 2017, p. 21)

Today, new abortion laws throughout the country are reasserting this narrative and shaping the landscape; currently, 43 states prohibit abortions (Guttmacher Institute, 2020). In May of 2019, several states passed bills banning abortion around six weeks, such as Georgia and Kentucky. Alabama passed the most prohibitive law, banning it altogether with very few exceptions (The Hill, 2019). These laws, coupled with a conservative majority Supreme Court, create a difficult landscape for women to attempt to navigate body politics.

In order to understand the dominant discourse of motherhood in society, Schneider and Ingram (2005) examined the social construction of reproductive policies that organize women into categories. Table 15.1

*Table 15.1* Created from text found in Schneider and Ingram (2005) and Stabile (2016)

| The Advantaged: (Positively portrayed and powerful) | The Contenders: (Negatively portrayed but powerful) |
|---|---|
| • Married heterosexual women embracing motherhood | • Postpone childbearing for career<br>• Have the privilege and financial means for infertility treatments |
| **The Dependents:** (Positively portrayed and powerless) | **The Deviants:** (Negatively portrayed and powerless) |
| • Able bodied white mothers who miscarry<br>• Surrogate mothers | • Seeking abortions<br>• Forgoing motherhood<br>• Poor women who became pregnant<br>• Those who engage in sexual activity without the intent to reproduce<br>• Women seeking to form non-traditional families via non-traditional methods<br>• Women using government benefits |

provides a digestible framework to examine these constructs, exploring the contrast of social location and structural (dis)advantages. Women are categorized based on their choices and are ranked in society as to how they ascribe to this discourse. Public policies are written to support the advantaged and look negatively upon those who make choices that are not in line with these constructed norms. Stabile (2016) concluded that "U.S. public policies affecting reproductive choices have conformed to attitudinal distinctions about motherhood itself" (p. 18).

### Access to Care

Women are at a disadvantage as it relates to healthcare treatment and access. In the medical model, normal bodily processes such as "'pre-menstrual syndrome,' 'fibrocystic breast disease,' 'estrogen deficiency disorder' or the moral 'disease' known in the United States as 'teen pregnancy'" are framed as pathological and convey the message that women are abnormal (Inhorn, 2006, p. 355). Dominant discourses convey eugenic messages (O'Connell, 2017; Ross et al., 2017) to pregnant women, which instill fear of an abnormal child or a potential problem delivery. This results in attitudes toward labor and delivery shifting away from natural methods that use relationally attuned midwives to a medicalized approach using epidurals, episiotomies and limited time with the doctor to meet capitalist agendas (Inhorn, 2006; Ross et al., 2017).

### Racial Disparities

Statistics show that African American women are three to four times more likely to die in childbirth than European American women because of barriers in access to care, especially women of lower socio-economic status and those who faced racial discrimination (Roeder, 2019). The Centers for Disease Control and Prevention (CDC, 2019) report significant disparities related to death in pregnancy among racial/ethnic groups. Between 2011 and 2015, per 100,000 live births, 42.8 deaths were reported for what they termed as "black non-Hispanic women", whereas 13.0 were reported for what they termed as "white non-Hispanic women". Reagan (2003) reflected that United States society is more apt to sympathize with a white woman who mourns for her loss than a black or brown woman who is struggling with her living children (p. 371).

### Infertility

For some women, the idea of being able to conceive is viewed as a gendered entitlement (Whitehead, 2016). Many women from this group express an entitlement toward motherhood as they expect it is a role they can claim with little to no problems. Whitehead found that many of these women were unable to conceive and sought refuge in posting to social media forums where they found a community of people who had similar struggles. They reported that they chose to work or go to school, attempted to get pregnant in their mid-thirties and struggled with conception due to their age (Stabile, 2016; Whitehead, 2016).

Layne (2003) expressed that ethnography is at its best when it "gives voice" to peoples' lived experience by including narrative and stories as essential components of the ethnographic text. Often women are unaware of the universality of their experiences because there are no existing spaces where they can openly talk about and look at these inequities.

## My Experience with Miscarriage

I experienced an inferred message within the power differential of care that conveyed to me that if I follow the doctor's orders then I will be able to carry the baby to term. During these first critical weeks, my body was going through tremendous changes; my hormones were shifting and I was gaining weight and was expected to hide it. One of the miscarriages required me to have a dilation and curettage (D&C) procedure. I was emotionally devastated and received a medicalized detached response from the practitioner with an expectation that sending me home with a pamphlet was sufficient, and I could return to work after a few days.

With each experience of discovering I was pregnant, I was told to withhold this information for three months, which was unfair. I comprehend this as a hermeneutical injustice (Fricker, 2007). This "secret" serves as an unjust burden on the mother to keep this information from others, and for some women it could lead to discrimination at work and/or different treatment by others. It also puts the expecting mother in a position of protecting society from the potential of her loss. I attuned to the growing fetus and envisioned a future with my babies, and then found no space to grieve. There was no public language to honor my experiences, only public misunderstanding. I learned that if I lost the baby I should not burden others with my pain. The invisibility of my loss was devastating.

### Power and Liberation through Art

As a therapist, it is important for me to examine power from critical, social constructivist, and systemic constructs. Paulo Freire (2000) provided a pedagogical framework to examine and empower the collective experiences of the oppressed. He posited, in order for liberation to occur within oppressed groups of people, they need to transition through phases of understanding toward transformation into liberation. Through the struggle, together they experience praxis, or reflection and action upon the world in order to transform it (p. 51). They examine the consciousness of themselves as the oppressed group and the consciousness of the oppressor. They may acknowledge that they have been emotionally dependent on the oppressor (p. 65). Then, they consider the lens in which both groups view the world, their behavior and ethics. It becomes praxis when, in solidarity, they uncover awareness and undergo profound rebirth once they become engaged in the fight for freedom, seeing the oppressor objectively, and then take action with serious reflection (p. 65).

Art therapy groups are spaces where, through the process of praxis, women can validate their isolated experiences, examine their relationship to the dominant narrative, and their oppressor, and take effective action through creating artwork that represents their story. Watkins and Shulman (2008) wrote about the need for liminal spaces—a space for exploration of individual awareness where cultural assumptions are challenged and transformed—as a shared space where people can come together and find *communitas* (p. 156).

The act of being listened to and validated by others as a collective is when people are able to see outside of the individual isolated experience. When witnessing artwork that represents an individual's experience, Buk (2009) wrote that "what is required from the viewer is keen aesthetic sensitivity and a strong affinity and empathy for visual images to perceive and experience the aesthetic dynamics inherent in each image" (p. 62). Connection occurs through embodied simulation (Freedberg & Gallese, 2007) or the human ability to "make sense of the actions, emotions, and sensations of others" as if we were engaged in a similar action or experiencing the same emotion or action (p. 198). This process of meaning making through witnessing creates an empathic resonance between the artist, the artwork and the witness, which builds attunement and community.

Art therapists who work with women, particularly around the issues of reproductive rights and choices, are uniquely positioned to examine, reveal, and give voice to collective private experiences, challenging public expectations of womanhood. Hogan (1997) wrote about the process of engaging women in creating artwork that provides them a process to explore the social and cultural intersections and reflect upon where the meaning shifts from feeling incarcerated to liberated (p. 38). This sentiment was echoed by Sajnani (2013) who urged an intersectional framework by looking at the collective experiences in order to allow emergent evocative responses to social and political issues, shifting the focus from the individual to the collective experience so as to acknowledge societal oppression. Further, as is explored later in this chapter, reflecting on the artwork in public spaces helps give value to the stories and reveals hidden or unspoken aspects of women's experiences externally to the world. The act of moving the private story into the public to raise critical consciousness around issues related to oppressive socio-political systems can be done in group art exhibitions, panel discussions, and disseminating or screening video or films that represent the collective voices of the oppressed groups.

Video can be a uniquely effective method or tool in therapy for providing a format in which clients can gain perspective and distance from artwork or emotionally charged material (Cohen & Orr, 2015). This reflective distance within the intersubjective space is important for developmental growth from the trauma story. Through watching a video of themselves, clients can see through a different lens, and step outside of themselves and into the role of the witness. I believe a similar process takes place when the artwork is shared in a public exhibition. The public offers that reflective distance, allowing a woman to be someone who has overcome a painful experience, rather than a victim of a traumatic event. They can see themselves as a part of a community of people who have experienced similar things. They can identify what was expressed in others' art that is like themselves and see themselves objectively.

## Pregnancy Group

### Context

When I was pregnant with my daughter, I was employed by a small urban nonprofit hospital in the community I lived in that primarily served uninsured, underinsured, and marginalized immigrant, African American, and Latinx populations. The hospital was located in a part of the city with a high crime rate, frequent gang activity, and lacked access to a train line or accessible grocery stores. Many of the employees at the hospital were first generation immigrants to the United States. I worked in the inpatient psychiatric unit where people were often held against their will and longed to connect with people who wanted support out of their own volition.

I saw an opportunity of interest convergence (Bell, 1980) as the women's health center had been recently renovated with a visible campaign marketed to the community. Being the only art therapist in the hospital, I leveraged my social location to propose an outpatient art therapy support group for pregnant women. I was connected with the director of the women's health center who introduced me to the medical director, a doctor who had research interest in prevention and perinatal depression. He helped me craft a pre-investigative research study examining the impact of art therapy on perinatal depression.

### Process

I designed the group to be free to any women who was between 20 and 24 weeks pregnant and could commit to the six sessions, meeting twice weekly for three hours over three weeks. The group ran approximately three to four times a year over three years. It was attended by patients, employees, and community members. To measure the impact of the group, I designed both qualitative and quantitative data collection. Each participant completed the State Trait Anxiety Intervention (STAI) and the Patient Health Questionnaire (PHQ-9) as a pre and post-test and at the end, a short narrative survey was provided for written feedback.

The women who participated ranged in ages from 15 to 34. Many of the referrals to the group came from the women's health center, and I recruited art therapy interns who were bi-cultural and Spanish speaking to help co-facilitate the groups. I was able to build a connection with a neighboring high school and coordinated transportation from school to the hospital with the school counselor and with a taxi voucher home from the hospital.

### Outcome

The disparity was alarming. The pregnant teens who participated were managing a much wider range of challenges. There were some who were navigating the foster care system, did not have a relationship with the father of the baby, and were attempting to manage an unstable living situation without a working cell phone. As they left the sessions, there were days where they were unsure where they were going to sleep that night.

The group evolved into a space where the women could find support and understanding within the common experiences of womanhood and pregnancy. Each week we would start by coloring a mandala as a check-in, and then move into the project for that day. They learned how to assemble a handmade book, which became a place to set intentions for the baby, paste ultrasound images, or create space for letters to the baby from both parents. They shared their experiences of dealing with hormonal changes, body image, coping with gestational diabetes, and other health issues. They each made a belly cast (Figure 15.1) and carefully painted it with intent and presence of the life inside of them.

The women found refuge and comfort in being able to connect and offer support to one another through their shared experiences. They described that the group offered them a quiet, reflective space for them to relax, connect with their unborn babies and find support from the other women.

One woman in the group, a 21-year-old African American, cisgender female from a low SES, was about 20 weeks pregnant with her first baby. She had recently emancipated from the foster care system and reunited with her birth mom who was working on her own sobriety with a long history of drug use. She was sleeping on the couch in the home of her mother and had a tenuous relationship with the father of the baby. One week we taught her how to crochet and set up a pink hospital plastic tub

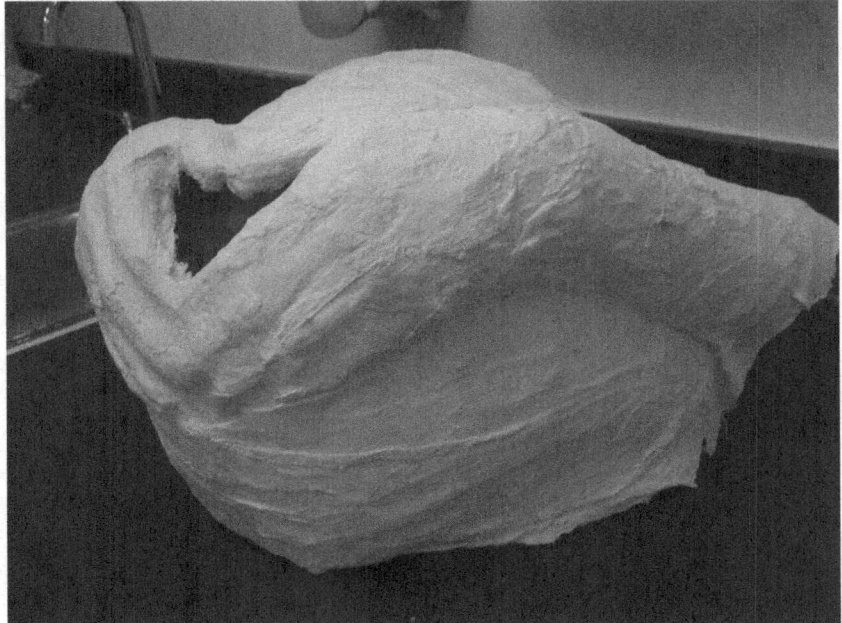

*Figure 15.1* Belly cast from pregnancy group.

for her to soak her feet in. She expressed her intention to be the mom to her baby in ways that her mother was unable to be for her. At the end of the session, we offered to give her the pink plastic tub. Tears formed in her eyes and she said it was the first thing she had been given for her baby and she was excited to use it for the baby's first bath. She reflected on stepping into the role of being a new mother, embellishing a mask and setting an intention for the mother she wanted to be (Figure 15.2).

When working on her mask she shared the following:

> Yellow is for the little bit of sun I will see in the first three months of being a Mom. Red is for love. Blue is for being tough and giving tough love to my little girl. Speckled red on the mouth for accepting that there will be some hard times for me and my daughter. She's got the power. Soon 2-B Mami. Pampers signature moments. I plan to raise my daughter to be a well-mannered girl.

Another group participant was a 30-year-old cisgender female from mid-SES. She was in a recent arranged marriage, had immigrated from India and was now attempting to navigate living in a one-bedroom apartment with her new husband and in-laws. She found the women's group to be

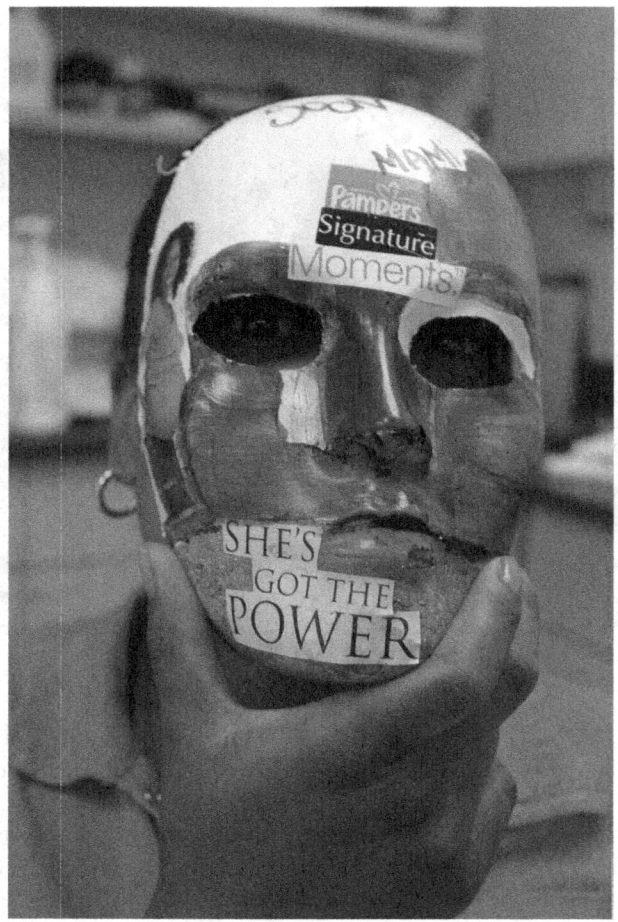

*Figure 15.2* Mask created in pregnancy group.

a quiet refuge where she could set some intentions for her future role as a mother. She found that the group offered her support and affirmed her need for space to connect with her baby, and have reflective distance from her home life. Almost every week she would work until the very end of the group. Many participants shared that they did not want to leave, voicing that they wished they could stay and make more art.

In one session, the opening conversation centered around experiences of morning sickness, needing significant diet changes, nausea from taking prenatal vitamins, swelling in their feet, and the isolation they felt in their excitement. A group member who was struggling with gestational diabetes connected with another participant who was 24 weeks pregnant with a baby that had been diagnosed with possible spina bifida. The group was able to offer support by processing the implications for these women and their families. Later in the session, while painting their belly casts, the women openly discussed the shared phenomena when people are compelled to comment on the size of their bodies and attempt to touch their bellies without permission. This discomfort was affirmed throughout the group and many realized that they were not alone in attempting to navigate in society where being pregnant triggered unwanted comments and encroachment of personal space from strangers. One member shared:

> Before I came to this program I felt alone, like a person going through a new experience [of] my first pregnancy. When I came into this program, I really felt, [sic] accompanied and I felt this was a beautiful experience. We were permitted to be able to express ourselves, to be able to express through art and I felt … well we don't want it to end. It has helped me a lot; it has helped me make decisions, to decide what is good for me and my child without fear.

### Bearing Witness Film: Private Stories into the Public Context

As I adjusted to motherhood, I longed to have another baby. I was the youngest of three, and I wanted my daughter to have a sibling. My husband and I experienced a new pregnancy three times, but each one ended in a devastating loss. As I was grappling with my own grief, I was working on my Doctorate in Art Therapy with an interest in trauma. I was connected with a colleague who had put together two art exhibits four years earlier entitled "Bearing Witness," by women who experienced pregnancy loss from miscarriage, repeated infertility, and death of a child from stillbirth (Andrus, 2017). It was an opportunity for me to better understand and explore the complexity of these losses. With IRB approval from Mount Mary University, I designed a research study to explore the impact of these women's experiences.

Dealing with infertility, miscarriage, and stillbirth is devastating, isolating, and painful. The women in the study had people in their lives who were well-intentioned but made comments that were unsupportive and harmful. It was the lack of understanding from family, friends, and society that further isolated them in their pain.

### Process

The study examined the impact of moving the story out of the private into the public and how or if this was helpful for the women. I interviewed a select group of women and made a film deconstructing their stories and impact of the exhibitions. I blindly paired three of the

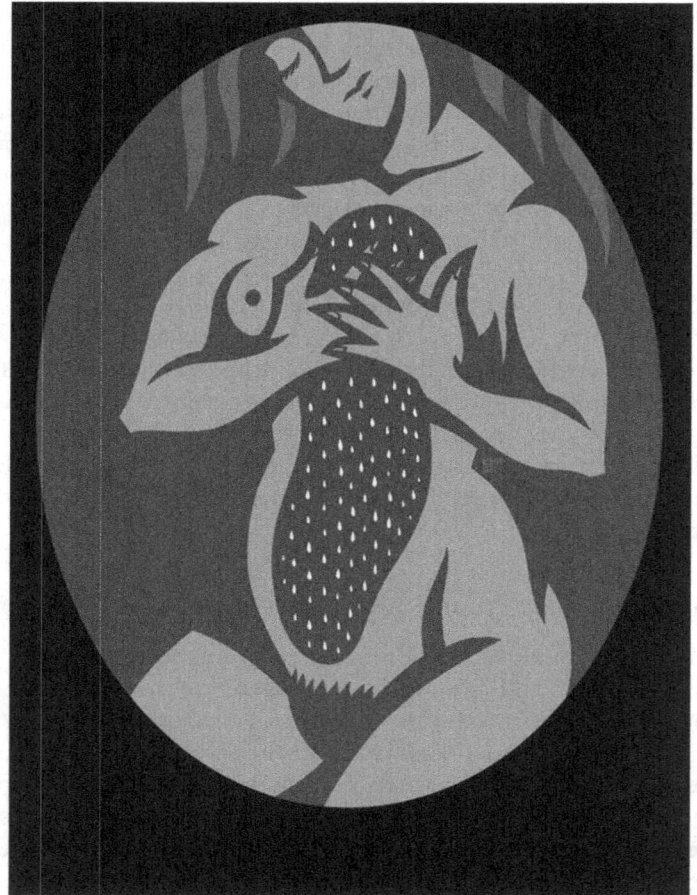

*Figure 15.3* "Internal Weather" by Molly Hayden from Bearing Witness film (Andrus, 2017).

women with three different art therapists for a one-time mock art therapy session. Prior to them meeting, I shared the original artwork (Figures 15.3 and 15.4) from the show, and had the art therapist make response art (Figure 15.5), while I captured the discussion on film.

This is further contextualized in my article that examined how response art can be useful to explore social constructs to help aid in a meta view for the client to explore in therapy (Andrus, 2020b). The recorded session provided a space to further explore the meaning of the original artwork and examined if the response art would help provide a contextual societal understanding for the women that would affirm their experiences and thus provide more healing for them.

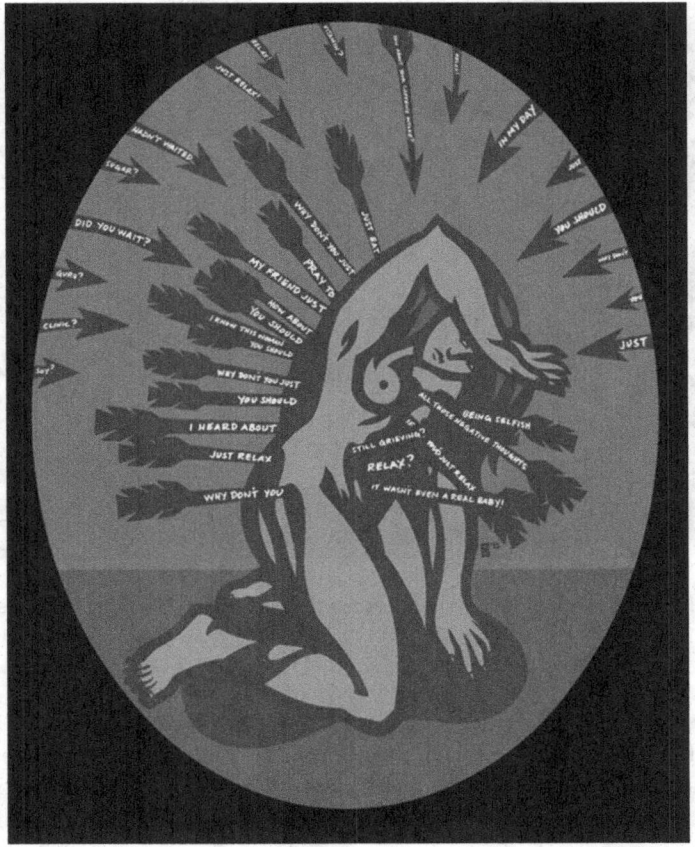

*Figure 15.4* "A Second to a Thousand Arrows" by Molly Hayden, from Bearing Witness film (Andrus, 2017).

### Outcome

The artwork in the film expressed a deep isolation and hidden grief for the pain they were experiencing. One of the artists, Christy, had multiple losses. She shared:

> I had this thing that I would be pregnant when we'd get together for Christmas, I had that secret, it was early enough I had not told anyone, I was so hopeful … and then I would lose the pregnancy and then my sister would have her baby and it was too late for me to share, it was all that more invisible.
>
> (Andrus, 2017)

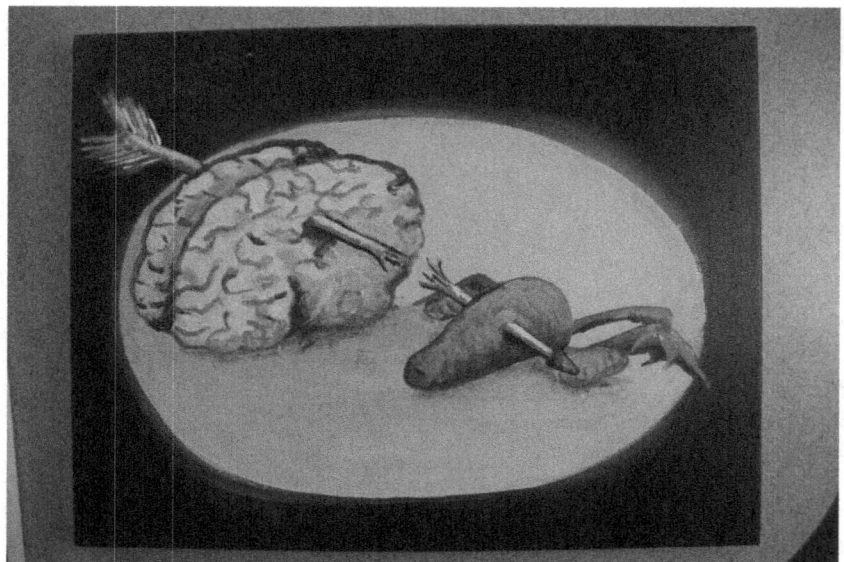

*Figure 15.5* "Response Art" By Heather Jeffries, from Bearing Witness film (Andrus, 2017).

Another artist, Molly titled her piece, "Internal Weather" (Figure 15.3).

She felt isolated in her grief, was unable to openly talk or express her losses and had to process her feelings without the support of a group of people who understood the intensity of her pain. She shared she did not know anyone who had a miscarriage and people questioned if she was ever pregnant. In the film she acknowledged,

> It ain't nobody's fault, and you know what, nobody knows why it happens . . . that's one of those things, and all the culture thinks they have all these answers to it.

> (Andrus, 2017)

The artwork in the exhibit acknowledged the painful comments that were made by family and friends that were intended to be helpful but caused harm. Another participant in the film, Liska, reflected on the comments by people in her life. Often these were hurtful and not supportive. She said, "They would say, why are you trying again? Why don't you just adopt?" (Andrus, 2017). Another participant, Kristen, reflected that she felt guilty that she would tell her friends that she was pregnant and then have to tell them that she wasn't pregnant anymore. There were friends who did not want to hear that she wasn't pregnant anymore. She concluded, "Well I am going to tell this story whether or not it makes you uncomfortable because it is my story to share" (Andrus, 2017).

When Molly reflected on her second picture entitled "A Second to a Thousand Arrows" (Figure 15.4), she described it as being angry at everyone who "felt like they could weigh in with their opinions" (Andrus, 2017). Many people talked to her saying that they really connected with her image because it expressed "being attacked by everybody else's expectations," but Molly noted that she was reacting to everyone's reactions (Andrus, 2017).

Another participant, Jennifer, reflected on Molly's artwork commenting, anyone who "would respond with 'why don't you just'" made her angry (Andrus, 2017). She resonated with the image created by Molly because it really spoke to how she felt.

In the film, art therapist Heather discussed Molly's artwork, noting the socially constructed pressures placed on women surrounding fertility and procreation. Heather described how Molly's art reflected that she was alone in her "secret" and how there are these experiences that define womanhood, which validated Molly's vulnerability. Heather stated, "By caring for that suffering and pain inside, you can integrate that and bring it into something strong . . . the beginnings for new growth" (Andrus, 2017).

Heather created response art to Molly's original artwork (Figure 15.5). She acknowledged that society tells us that "you are on your own" and reflected that we do not have language to be able to openly talk about pregnancy losses.

When looking at Molly's piece, Heather stated, "There was no support, and in fact, all those comments felt like they were pushing away the emotions and the body in a way that was not supporting, but hurting" (Andrus, 2017). Molly responded:

> I found that when I started to get pregnant I knew very little about my body, so in a strange way when trying to get pregnant all the sudden I was paying so much attention . . . and the Doctors talk to you like *you are your uterus* . . . At first I was joined with my body, then the stress of dealing with all of this broke it off, my brain was distancing itself from my body . . . I did not want to be angry with my body but having all this pressure created a division between these two parts of myself . . . [your artwork] brought me back emotionally to where I was when I created these, . . . it was like having it emotionally honored and transformed into something that you had never imagined.
>
> (Andrus, 2017)

Through her response art, Heather was able to deconstruct (with Molly) the societal messages of how women are expected to manage these losses in silence and move on with their lives with little space to acknowledge the gravity of their experiences. Through examining the original artwork and the response art in the film's mock session, they were able to honor Molly's experience, connect through the art image, and give voice to the experiences of many women.

The film served as a means for the women to reflect the value of their voices, reinforce their shared experiences, and continue to make meaning of their pain. What the research revealed is that there is therapeutic value in moving the trauma story and artwork out of the private space into a shared public space. Doing so helps people to connect with hidden aspects of their own private experiences that are expressed in one another's artwork. The women were able to make meaning and see that their story is valuable, they are not alone, and that other people feel the same way that they do. They were able to acknowledge that their loss was real through the externalizing of their experience in the artwork. By pushing back on the dominant discourse, people who have had the experience of pregnancy loss or infertility can make their voices known. Art therapists create space to share images and words to externalize the internal experience, and extract the counter narrative that emerges through collective sharing and dialogue.

The film served as a living document, one that honored these women's experiences and was able to affirm hidden pain. It became an externalized piece of art that they could reflect on, allowing them to see value in educating the public and sharing their stories with others who have been impacted by similar circumstances. Their art with their story and thus the resulting film made the invisible visible. They were able to externalize their pain and re-author their story with a new narrative.

## Summary

From my work at the hospital with pregnant women to the interviews with the women in the Bearing Witness film, I deduce that the dominant discourse from society kept them feeling isolated and unaware of the inequities of their experiences. Their artwork was healing and integrative, which provided a tangible reflection of their isolated experiences, so they could be shared with others for further meaning making.

Shifting out of the private into the public to examine taboo topics of miscarriage, infertility and pregnancy loss validates and normalizes the experiences of women. As art therapists, we are uniquely equipped to remap the territory, challenge the dominant discourse, and amplify the voices of our clients by providing spaces where they can share their experiences, retell their stories and bring the far experiences near for understanding and connection.

# References

Allegranti, B. (2013). The politics of becoming bodies: Sex, gender and intersubjectivity in motion. *The Arts in Psychotherapy, 40*, 394–403.

Andrus, M. (Producer & Director) (2017). *Bearing witness film*. [Doctoral research film]. United States: Mount Mary University.

Andrus, M. (2020a). Exhibition and film about infertility, miscarriage and stillbirth: Art therapy implications. *Art Therapy Journal, 37*, 1. doi:10.1080/07421656.2019.1697577

Andrus, M. (2020b). Response art, intersubjectivity with social construction in art therapy; co-constructing meaning. *The Arts in Psychotherapy*. (In press).

Bell, D. A. (1980). *Brown v. Board of Education* and the interest convergence dilemma. *Harvard Law Review, 93*(3), 518–533.

Buk, A. (2009). The mirror neuron system and embodied simulation: Clinical implications for art therapists working with trauma survivors. *Arts in Psychotherapy, 36*(2), 61–74. doi:10.1016/j.aip.2009.01.008

Burke, T. (2017). In *Wikepedia*. Retrieved January 29, 2018, from https://en.wikipedia.org/wiki/Me_Too_movement

Centers for Disease Control and Prevention. (2019). Pregnancy mortality surveillance system. Retrieved on January 26, 2020 from www.cdc.gov/reproductive health/maternal-mortality/pregnancy-mortality-surveillance-system.htm

Cohen, J. L., & Orr, P. P. (2015). Film/video-based therapy and editing as process from a depth psychological perspective. In J. L. Cohen, J. L. Johnson, & P. P. Orr (Eds.), *Video and filmmaking as psychotherapy: Research and practice* (pp. 29–42). New York, NY: Routledge.

Foucault, M. (1982). The subject and power. *Critical Inquiry, 8*(4), 777–795. The University of Chicago Press.

Freedberg, D., & Gallese, V. (2007). Motion, emotion and empathy in esthetic experience. *Trends in Cognitive Sciences, 11*(5), 197–203. doi:10.1016/j.tics.2007.02.003

Freire, P. (2000). *Pedagogy of the oppressed*. New York, NY: Bloomsbury.

Fricker, M. (2007). Epistemic injustice: Power and ethics of knowing. Hermeneutical injustice. Oxford Scholarship.

Guttmacher Institute. (2020, June,1). An overview of abortion laws. Retrieved from www.guttmacher.org/state-policy/explore/overview-abortion-laws

The Hill. (2019). All the states taking up new abortion laws in 2019. Retrieved September 23, 2019 from https://thehill.com/policy/healthcare/445460-states-passing-and-considering-new-abortion-laws-in-2019

Hogan, S. (1997). *Feminist approaches to art therapy*. New York, NY: Routledge.

Hogan, S. (Ed). (2003). *Gender issues in art therapy*. Philadelphia, PA: Jessica Kingsley Publishers.

hooks, B. (2015). *Feminist theory: From margin to center*. New York, NY: Routledge.

Inhorn, M. C. (2006). Defining women's health: A dozen messages from more than 150 ethnographies. *Medical Anthropology Quarterly, New Series., 20*(3), 245–378.

Lapook, J. (2017). Former team USA gymnasts describe doctor's alleged sexual abuse. Retrieved on Oct 4, 2019 from www.cbsnews.com/news/former-team-usa-gymnasts-describe-doctors-alleged-sexual-abuse-60-minutes-2019-08-09/

Layne. (2003). Unhappy endings: A feminist reappraisal of the women's health movement from the vantage of pregnancy loss. *Social Science and Medicine, 56*(9), 1881–1891.

Madigan, S. P. (1992). The application of Michel Foucault's philosophy of the problem externalizing discourse of Michael White. *Journal of Family Therapy, 14*, 265–279.

Miller, B. (2017). Mothering while poor: Utilizing the reproductive justice framework to build the capacities of young mothers. In L. Ross, L. Roberts, E. Derkas, W. Peoples, & P. Bridgewater Toure (Eds.), *Radical reproductive justice: Foundations, theory, practice, critique* (pp. 355–360). New York, NY: Feminist Press.

O'Connell, K. (2017). We need to talk about disability as a reproductive justice issue. In L. Ross, L. Roberts, E. Derkas, W. Peoples, & P. Bridgewater Toure (Eds.), *Radical reproductive justice: Foundations, theory, practice, critique* (pp. 302–305). New York, NY: Feminist Press.

Reagan, L. (2003). From hazard to blessing to tragedy: Representations of miscarriage in twentieth-century America. *Feminist Studies, 29*(2), 357–477.

Roeder, A. (2019). America is failing its black mothers. *Harvard Public Health Magazine*. Retrieved on October 4, 2019 www.hsph.harvard.edu/magazine/magazine_article/america-is-failing-its-black-mothers/

Romero, D., & Agènor, M. (2017). The welfare family cap: Reproductive rights, control and poverty prevention. In L. Ross, L. Roberts, E. Derkas, W. Peoples, & P. Bridgewater Toure (Eds.), *Radical reproductive justice: Foundations, theory, practice, critique* (pp. 381–396). New York, NY: Feminist Press.

Ross, L., Roberts, L., Derkas, E., Peoples, W., & Bridgewater Toure, P. (Eds). (2017). *Radical reproductive justice: Foundations, theory, practice, critique.* New York, NY: Feminist Press.

Sajnani, N. (2013). The body politic: The relevance of an intersectional framework for therapeutic performance research in drama therapy. *The Arts in Psychotherapy, 40*(382–385). doi:http://dx.doi.org/10.1016/j.aip.2013.05.001

Schneider, A. L., & Ingram, H. M. (Eds.). (2005). *Deserving and entitled: Social construction and public policy.* New York: State of New York Press.

Seftel, L. (2006). *Grief unseen: Healing pregnancy loss through the arts.* Philadelphia, PA: Jessica Kingsley Publishers.

Speert, E. (1992). The use of art therapy following perinatal death. *Art Therapy: Journal of the American Art Therapy Association, 9*(3), 121–128.

Stabile, B. (2016). Reproductive policy and the social construction of motherhood. *Politics and the Life Sciences, 35*(2), 18–29.

Swan-Foster, N. (1989). Images of a pregnant woman: Art therapy as a tool for transformation. *The Arts in Psychotherapy, 16*, 283–292.

Watkins, M., & Shulman, H. (2008). *Towards psychologies of liberation.* New York, NY: Palgrave MacMillan.

White, M., & Epston, D. (1990). *Narrative means to therapeutic ends.* New York, NY: W. W. Norton.

Whitehead, K. (2016). Motherhood as a gendered entitlement: Intentionality, "othering" and homosociality in the online infertile community. *Canadian Sociological Association. CRS/RCS, 53*, 1.

# 16 Addressing Motherhood Issues of Sex Trafficking Survivors Through Art Therapy

*Mary K. Kometiani*

## Introduction to Sex Trafficking

Modern slavery knows no bounds. Slavery prevails in every area of the world (International Labour Office & Walk Free Foundation, 2017), and sex trafficking occurs in each of the states in the United States (National Human Trafficking Hotline, 2019). Although anyone can be targeted, most individuals who are sex trafficked are young females. The International Labour Office and Walk Free Foundation (2017) reported that of the 3.8 million adults and 1 million children who were forced into sexual exploitation, 99% were women and girls. One in four enslaved individuals are children (International Labour Office & Walk Free Foundation, 2017), and 14 to 16 is the average age of entry into sex exploitation (Shared Hope International, 2017). All over the world, female children are vulnerable to the horrendous crimes of sex trafficking.

The United States Victims of Trafficking and Violence Prevention Act of 2000 defines sex trafficking as enlisting, arranging, acquiring, concealing, or moving an individual for the intent of commercial sexual exploitation (2000). When any exploitation of individuals under the age of 18 occurs, with/without power, intimidation or deception, the youth are automatically considered trafficked. Human trafficking is a grave crime that violates human rights of females, males or gender variant people of all ages through the use of force, fraud, and coercion. The malicious techniques used to ensnare vulnerable and at-risk individuals are defined as:

- physical restraint or harm through force as a way to acquire and sustain control
- false promises of love, employment or a better life to vulnerable individuals through fraudulent offers
- coercion through threats or harm to an individual through manipulation, identification confiscation and blackmail to expose an individual to families or others (United States Department of Health and Human Services, 2019).

Globally, sex trafficking occurs in many different forms of exploitation. Gerassi and Nichols (2018) identify the types of sex trafficking as *survival sex* (when individuals sell sex to meet their basic needs), trafficking through family members, partner exploitation after an individual is manipulated into a seeming loving relationship, organized crime or non-intimate exploitation, trafficking through kidnapping or abduction, and false offers of employment and easy money made to unemployed, poor individuals. Sex trafficking occurs in various ways, and numerous, negative consequences quickly ensue that affect survivors' lives and futures.

## Detrimental Outcomes of Sex Trafficking

Although not all individuals who survive exploitation will view their experiences as traumatic (Gerassi & Nichols, 2018), survivors experience a wide range of distressing effects. Individuals who are sex trafficked are maltreated from experiencing lack of complete control over their lives, vast betrayal, uncompromising isolation from continual abuse, and dehumanizing objectification from being sold repeatedly (Hoffman, 2013). The critical consequences of sex trafficking affect an individual's physical, emotional, psychological, mental, and spiritual being. Albeit sex trafficked survivors' situations vary in lengths, exposures, and, from the impact of trauma, devastating long-term outcomes consist of: physical effects from abuse, neglect, and compounded medical issues; psychological trauma, depression, anxiety, and dissociation; social disconnection and emotional consequences that affect an individual's future and relationships; and the weakening of one's spiritual core, which reduces the ability to have a purposeful life (Kometiani, 2020c).

While it is understood that survivors are subject to various physical, mental, emotional, and psychological problems, their reproductive health is often ignored or overlooked in the light of other pressing problems (Freedom Network USA, 2015). Survivors also experience specific problems related to their reproductive systems including not only exposure to STIs (sexually transmitted infections), but the long-term ramifications of these infections that may be left untreated, effects of unsafe procedures from forced abortions, and the aftermath of violent sexual trauma (Campbell, 2002; de Chesnay & Szekes, 2013; Freedom Network USA, 2015; Willis & Levy, 2002). There is a high prevalence of HIV and other STIs in sexually exploited individuals (Freedom Network USA, 2015; United States Department of State Bureau of Public Affairs, 2007), and untreated STIs can lead to chronic pelvic pain, ectopic pregnancy, an increased risk of hysterectomy, and infertility (Willis & Levy, 2002).

These reproductive health problems are due to the high number of forced sexual encounters and the girls' lack of protection, medical advice, and proper hygiene. During exploitation, traffickers may not permit the use of condoms, birth control pills, rings, patches, etc., which require access to medical care; symptoms of STIs are ignored (Freedom Network USA, 2015). As an example of the vast amount of daily abuse, survivors reported being exploited by approximately 13 individuals and with as many as 50 buyers in a day (Lederer & Wetzel, 2014). Another study demonstrated that over 30% of survivors never used a condom because clients pay more money for unprotected sex (Acharya, 2011). Sex trafficking individuals are at particular health risk due to traffickers' greed and their blatant disregard for the exploited survivors' protection or health. Sex trafficked women are dispensable in their controller's mind.

### Effects of Sexual Trauma

There are numerous and devastating end results for survivors of sex trafficking. In addition to using violence and abuse (Acharya, 2011), traffickers may use rape and sexual abuse to terrorize, instill fear, and enforce compliance (Freedom Network USA, 2015). While being held captive, individuals do not have any control over their bodies or sexual lives; they have lost the capacity to make a choice (Freedom Network USA, 2015). After months or years of this repeated abuse and trauma, their damaged mental and physical health consequences are compounded by reproductive system issues.

The most consistent, long-term, and fundamental difference between abused and non-abused women are related to gynecology issues; consequences of forced sex include stress on the immune system, vaginal/anal/urethra trauma, and the effects of unprotected sex (Campbell, 2002). Reproductive system problems stemming from sexual trauma include bleeding, urinary tract infection, pain, discharge, and decreased sexual desire (Acharya, 2011; Lederer & Wetzel, 2014); trafficked individuals are at especially high risk for menstrual cycle issues and permanent injury to their reproductive health, such as loss of fertility (Freedom Network USA, 2015). Sex trafficking and recurrent, unprotected sex result in many painful and disturbing issues that can result in long-term and severe damage in addition to unplanned pregnancies, serious infections and cancer.

### Unplanned Pregnancy and Forced Abortions

Becoming pregnant is the most common health risk experienced by exploited individuals because safe sex is not a choice for the girl or woman (de Chesnay & Szekes, 2013). Many trafficked girls will get pregnant, and forced abortions are a disconcerting reality (Lederer & Wetzel, 2014). In one study, one in four sex trafficked survivors were pregnant (Bick, Howard, Oran, & Zimmerman, 2017). From Lederer and

Wetzel's (2014) study, 47 of 66 women surveyed said that they had at least one pregnancy during trafficking, and 14 women reported five or more pregnancies; about half of these women experienced miscarriages, and more than half said they had aborted or were forced to abort the babies. Unfortunately, multiple pregnancies that end with forced abortions are common for survivors. From Acharya's (2011) survey, 40% of trafficked women experienced unwanted pregnancy with 65% of those having one abortion and 30% having more than one abortion. This report also showed that very few of these abortions were done in a medical clinic and were commonly accomplished by medication administered from the trafficker (Acharya, 2011). Note that the psychological toll of miscarriage or abortion is not considered in these statistics; the findings concentrated solely on the physical injuries to the women.

For exploited individuals, pregnancy and medically authorized/ unauthorized abortions provide further endangerment. Sometimes, individuals are forced to exploit themselves too soon after giving birth, increasing their risk for infection and women who have recently delivered a baby are made to work or make up work missed (de Chesnay & Szekes, 2013). In trafficking, pregnancy does not impart a maternity leave or time to heal from an abortion procedure; exploited women are made to continue selling sex despite pain, swelling, and bleeding (Freedom Network USA, 2015). Traffickers may also attempt to complete abortions without seeking medical care; this is extremely dangerous and can be life-threatening; unsafe abortions can result in further health issues, such as poor wound healing, internal organ damage, infertility, and trauma (de Chesnay & Szekes, 2013).

In addition, there are other potential risks to survivors who become pregnant. Because survivors of sex trafficking are exposed to substandard living conditions and lack adequate nutrition (Farr, 2004), malnutrition and weight loss increases the risk for the baby's lower birth weight or even perinatal mortality (de Chesnay & Szekes, 2013). Lastly, substance use and addiction are common with survivors due to the trafficker's coercion or as a way to endure abuse, trauma, and rape (Office for Victims of Crime, n.d.). Consequently, miscarriage, stillbirth, and birth defects are common for survivors who abuse alcohol and drugs (Groot, 2013). There are multiple, critical consequences for survivors of sex trafficking from the repercussions of STIs, forced abortions from unplanned pregnancies, and sexual trauma in addition to other detrimental complications for the survivor's baby of malnourishment and substance abuse.

Due to the emotional burden and psychological toil of this work, it is necessary for art therapists to practice self-care and resiliency, as well as prioritize their personal well-being. Art therapists who work with survivors of sex trafficking are cautioned regarding the effects of vicarious trauma and the overwhelming nature of this work. Figure 16.1 is an

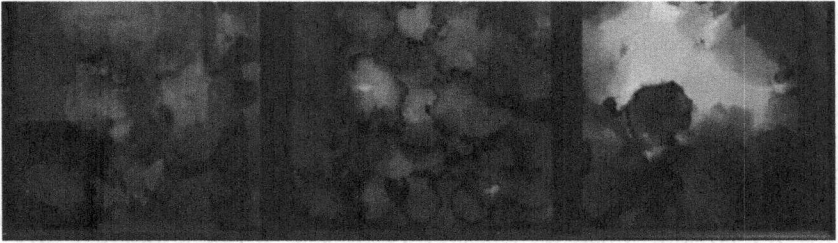

*Figure 16.1* "Illumination to Darkness" alcohol inks.

example of a trio of images that an art therapist created as a reflection of her work with sex trafficked survivors

The art therapist cogitated that as survivors open up about their journeys, their trauma unfolds and the healing begins. For the survivor, light resurfaces and hope replaces the darkness. As art therapists, we create a safe environment for the reduction of suffering for the survivor, and we must remain in the light and not be surrounded by darkness. We need to maintain hope and light not only for the survivor, but for ourselves to continue in this field.

## Sex Trafficking and Motherhood Issues

Sex trafficked survivors face maternity and motherhood issues from a variety of factors. They might be confronted with pregnancy from rape while under control of their exploiters, they may have had children prior to being trafficked, and they may become pregnant after exiting the exploitation. Spouses or family members may have sold the individual into slavery. Once exploited, the woman may feel that she is forced to leave her children, or endure exploitation due to threats of harm that may be done to the children. These complicated dilemmas, interwoven with betrayal, guilt, and shame, beget complicated struggles and distressing emotional situations for survivors.

### Pregnancy and Childbirth

Due the vast and convoluted intricacies of complex trauma and trauma bond, individuals who are trafficked often genuinely believe that they are involved in a loving relationship (Anti Trafficking Monitoring Group, 2016). Traffickers may also deliberately impregnate a woman as means for further domination, threat or to control future generations (de Chesnay & Szekes, 2013). Vulnerable, pregnant women who are sex trafficked have limited options and less control because they are unaware of their rights or denied their rights; they feel powerless as decisions are made by the trafficker leaving the individual without a choice to keep, abort, carry to term or place the child in adoption (de Chesnay & Szekes, 2013). As traffickers often enforce *debt bondage*, coercion into financial burden (National Human Trafficking Hotline, n.d.), the cost of abortion or medication when added to an individual's debt to the trafficker pushes freedom further away (Freedom Network USA, 2015).

Becoming pregnant from rape is complicated and extremely challenging for an individual (de Chesnay & Szekes, 2013). Unwanted pregnancy that is caused during trafficking may be traumatic, hindering to one's recovery and have a lasting negative effect on an individual (Anti Trafficking Monitoring Group, 2016). In the case of rape, mothers may want to terminate the pregnancy, or if they decide to carry the baby full term, they may face difficult births or issues while bonding with the baby (Anti Trafficking Monitoring Group, 2016). While pregnancy can be a stressful time for any female, trafficked survivors are at further risk due to the experience of being exploited and the financial distress that may result with raising a child and care costs (Anti Trafficking Monitoring Group, 2016). Becoming pregnant is a serious health risk for the exploited individual and her baby because prenatal care is not readily available until they have exited their exploited situation (Anti Trafficking Monitoring Group, 2016; de Chesnay & Szekes, 2013). Although pregnancy from rape causes particular challenges, it might also offer potential for an affirming impact, too.

Pregnancy may have a positive effect on survivors who experience new purpose and increased motivation (Anti Trafficking Monitoring Group, 2016). Being pregnant might reduce isolation through prenatal appointments, attention from other women and shopping for baby items; socialization may also have a positive effect on the survivor (Anti Trafficking Monitoring Group, 2016). Becoming a mother is a personal process that provides both opportunities for hope and times of distress depending on the resources and support the pregnant female has and how she views her situation. In addition to further risk for survivors of sex trafficking, pregnancy can increase barriers to recovery.

### Separation from Family

The United Nations Office on Drugs and Crime (2013) recognizes pregnancy as a circumstance that may increase a person's vulnerability to trafficking. In a trafficking situation, a person may be led to believe they will only be working for a short time period, but after they are trapped and exploited, they may be held in bondage until all debts are repaid. The trafficker may prevent the mother's contact with her children after leaving for a promise of a better life, use her children as threats to control and sustain her exploitation or try sell her children into exploitation (Anti Trafficking Monitoring Group, 2016). Some mothers may leave their children and their homes because of this increased risk, or children may also be removed from unfit care by authorities (Anti Trafficking Monitoring Group, 2016). Even in America, it is not unheard for individuals to be trafficked through family members and sold for money, drugs or rent, sold into marriage or forced into exploitation by a spouse (Hoffman, 2013). For survivors of sex trafficking, these varying circumstances contribute to familial separation in both physical and emotional ways; separation and betrayal may severely damage one's view of trust.

While some mothers give up hope and choose not to make any further contact with their children due to the length of time away or reunification challenges, for other survivors, recovery has potential when contact has been made with children and reunion is possible (Anti Trafficking Monitoring Group, 2016). Nonetheless, survivors who are interested in reuniting relationships with their loved ones may be blamed, judged or misunderstood due to unresolved issues from past substance abuse and mental health disorders (Kometiani, 2020b). One hindrance to recovery is the loss of family, which is often accompanied by a deep sense of shame (Tan & Moore, 2020). Ostracism from community, loss of family and estrangement of loved ones can affect one's recovery and reintegration into society.

## Recommended Approaches With Sex Trafficked Survivors

While treating survivors of sex trafficking, a trauma-informed approach is required (United States Department of State, 2018). Trauma-informed care includes cultural competence, focus on safety, understanding the effects of trauma, supporting independence and empowering experiences, and possibility of healing (Gerassi & Nichols, 2018). Gerassi and Nichols (2018) provide the following recommendations for working with sex trafficked survivors:

- strengths-based approach to focus on an individual's positive attributes
- survivor-defined advocacy to allow goal setting that meets an individual's needs
- empowerment through making decisions and experiencing ownership
- rapport building to build trust.

In addition, it is necessary that therapists who work with survivors of exploitation prioritize their health and that they have access to medical care (Campbell, 2002; Hoffman, 2013). The United States Department of State (2012) recommends that survivors of sex trafficking are screened for mental disorders that can be diagnosed as a result of the trauma of trafficking and assessed for suicide. Working towards independence, reintegration with society and the survivor's family, and reestablishing identity reinstates a sense of self-worth for survivors and provides opportunity to experience respect (Campbell, 2002; Hoffman, 2013; United States Department of State, 2012).

Art therapy is an effective way to assist in survivors' recovery (Kometiani & Farmer, 2019; Tan, 2012). Art therapy groups offer a potential for healing relationships, opportunity for empowerment, a way to process familial loss and experience integration of the past, and increase self-identity. Herman (1997) researched how psychological trauma destroys a person's sense of control and connection to others, and recovery happens through empowerment and healing new relationships. During the healing process, survivors trust and connect with supportive individuals, recreate an optimistic view on their life, reconstruct their self, and express reunification or acceptance with their family's level of involvement (Hoffman, 2013). Recovery for survivors of sex trafficking is possible through building a supportive and reintegrated community and constructing a new personal identity with reinstated self-worth.

### Stages of Change

GEMS (Girls Educational and Mentoring Services, 2018), created by survivor Rachel Lloyd, empowers individuals who have survived sexual exploitation. GEMS has applied Prochaska and DiClemente's (1994) stages of change in their treatment model and found it to be extremely effective. A quick and easy change is not realistic with survivors of sex trafficking especially with those who have endured extreme childhood trauma (Lloyd, 2018). The phases of change address current needs and recognize that change is a complex process that occurs at an individual's pace and on a continuum.

Descriptions for Prochaska and DiClemente's (1994) stages are provide in the table below (16.1) with suggestions of application for survivors (Lloyd, 2018), and these have been tailored to art therapists:

## Art Therapy Case Examples

Art therapy rebuilds connection through community, and survivors can experience safety and empowerment through art therapy (Kometiani, 2020a). The following case studies will explore art therapy treatment through vignettes of a pregnant survivor and a survivor who has been separated from her child. These cases examine how art therapy aids in the treatment progress through experiencing a sense of control, emotional processing of trauma and loss, decreasing anxiety and distress, establishing supportive relationships, and increasing hope through developing purpose and vision for the future. In the following vignettes, art

*Table 16.1* Stages of change and recommendations of application for survivors

| | |
|---|---|
| During precontemplation, an individual may act defensive, detached from the problem or uninterested in participating in therapy (Prochaska & DiClemente, 1994). | If an art therapist encounters a survivor during this stage, therapy might be mandated by the court because an individual is not considering change, therefore, instilling trust, active engagement, and a strengths-based approach is suggested (Lloyd, 2018). |
| Action, defined by the change in behaviors and environment, is when progress happens, and this is usually the shortest stage in duration because eagerness regarding change is limited (Prochaska & DiClemente, 1994). | Intensive support is crucial during the action state, and the art therapist needs to address the survivor's feelings of loss because the individual may grieve what was familiar (Lloyd, 2018). |
| A prolonged stage of continuance of change, maintenance, may be marked by an individual's fear of relapse or change and can last months, years, or a lifespan (Prochaska & DiClemente, 1994). | New behavior is sustained during maintenance, and exploration of feelings regarding leaving and a support system is necessary; the art therapist should look out for signs of boredom as this can trigger depression, and the survivor needs to be affirmed for their strength and bravery (Lloyd, 2018). |
| Relapse is evidenced by a return to an original behavior or environment, and subsequently an individual may experience feelings such as weakness, remorse, and failure (Prochaska & DiClemente, 1994). | Both the art therapist and the survivor need to recognize that change is a process and that relapse is normal in recovery; survivors need to be affirmed in their value and previous successes (Lloyd, 2018). |

therapy group services were facilitated by a registered, board certified art therapist. It is imperative to note that the shelter setting also provided extensive weekly trauma counseling, bimonthly dialectical behavior therapy groups, trauma-informed yoga twice a week, addiction support, dental and medical care (including prenatal care when appropriate), and educational and vocational assistance among other supportive services.

## Ali

Ali, in her early twenties, is a Caucasian survivor of sex trafficking. As an adolescent, Ali had been trafficked by her family. Since, she had been diagnosed with comorbid anxiety, mood, and substance use disorders. During art therapy group, Ali presented with a restricted affect, and she seemed detached from her emotions. In one of her first art therapy sessions, she shared that she was pregnant. Even though Ali said she was excited and joyful about her pregnancy, her controlled affect did not match the emotions she was sharing. However, she was adamant to articulate that her baby represented the significant change in her life and was the reason for her to become sober. At this point in her treatment, it appeared that Ali's pregnancy had a positive influence on her.

During the action state of change (Lloyd, 2018) and in the beginning of her art therapy treatment, Ali had her first ultrasound appointment and was grateful to hear her healthy baby's heartbeat. This intrinsic, sensory connection to her baby seemed to help her remain motivated to stay sober despite an escalation of distress. Ali's psychiatrist started to titrate several of her medications, and she began to experience increased anxiety. She was also becoming more concerned for her and her baby's future because of her lack of support, and she was beginning to process the loss of her family as she did not have any contact with them anymore. During an art therapy group session in which the art therapist facilitated an intervention geared to identify and express feelings, Ali painted two separate images. One painting conveyed her anxiety and lack of control with being pregnant and not having any support represented by chaotic, aggressive squiggly lines spiraling out of control. Her second painting was her desired feeling of peace (Figure 16.2).

This round image was a layered pattern of dots in self-soothing colors (aqua, purple, pink, and green). Ali seemed to relax and focus throughout the process of painting the abstract design. Through creating "Peace," Ali was able to experience inner calmness and express peace in her mandala. Ali said she felt peaceful when she was working on her goal of becoming independent to care for her baby and experiencing a sense of control in her life.

During another session, Ali shared that she had found out the sex of the baby. Sharing this news with the other survivors and art therapist brought them together as a community, confirming their supportive relationships with Ali. Finding out that she was going to have a daughter seemed to help her envision her future as a mom. Her strengths-based collage had several main images of how she pictured her future—one large image of a baby playing and one with a mother and baby sitting and playing together. She also used words such as "love," "mother," "togetherness," and "protection." She explained that her main priority as a mother would be to love and protect her daughter in ways that she had not been. Through art therapy group, Ali was able to experience a supportive network that she had not experienced before from her family. She was able to share the joys and concerns of her pregnancy, her motivation and her dreams for the future, and regain a sense of control that had been taken during her exploitation. She was able to replace her anxiety and fear with peace and lack of control with strength. While envisioning her future with her daughter, she moved further from her pain of the past. Art therapy group provided her with an opportunity to get in touch with her emotions and reconnect to

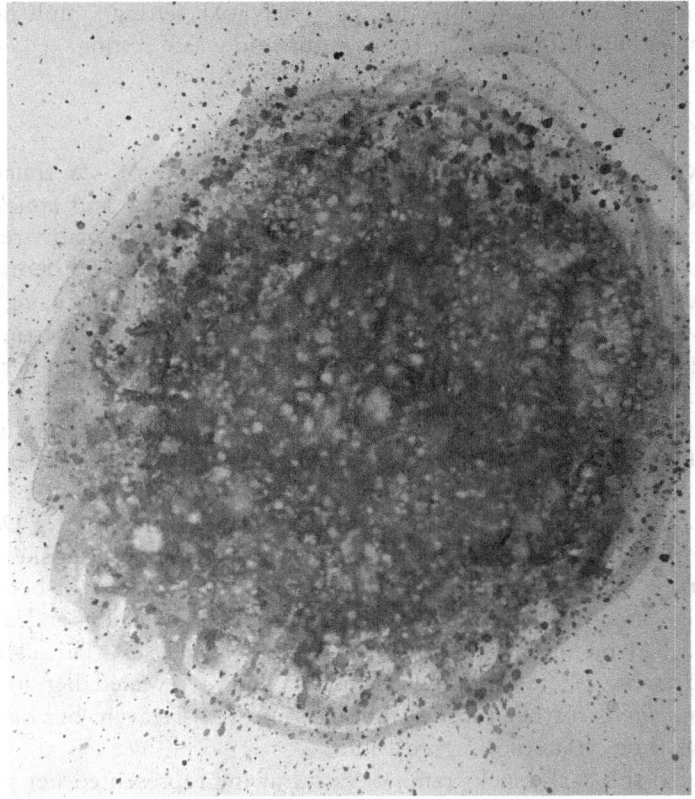

*Figure 16.2* "Peace" watercolor paint.

herself, form connection with others and receive support, which ultimately allowed her to focus on what was most important to her—her
future with her daughter.

Survivor group attendance varies due to multifaceted transition stressors that often result in relapse, running away, and re-trafficking. To
thwart those ends, art therapists are cautioned to provide treatment that
limits further risks, focuses on instilling a safe environment and slowly
builds a trusting relationship for support (Kometiani, 2020b). The nature
of this problem is reflected in sporadic attendance: some survivors may
only attend a few sessions, and others may return to therapy after
a relapse. Therefore, it is imperative that the art therapist not only
model hope, but maintain a positive attitude of hope in the group setting
before survivors who are facing different and difficult stages of change.
There may be times when the art therapist bears this responsibility alone
and represents a single beacon of hope. The intervention of this practice

is not to block survivors from facing a bleak reality, but allowing survivors the chance to practice personal goal setting, implementing dreams, and envisioning their better futures in a safe setting.

## Destiny

Destiny, aged 19, is an African American survivor of sex trafficking. Destiny survived a great deal of violence, sexual abuse, and attachment issues throughout her life; she continued to deal with the many, residual impacts. She was receiving medical treatment for a STI and dental care from repercussion of abuse. Sometimes she had difficulty focusing in art therapy group, or she seemed too exhausted to participate. Destiny also struggled with emotional regulation and with getting along with her peers at times.

In one of her initial sessions, Destiny was very open about sharing her story. During her adolescence, she had moved in with her older sister due to her mother's drug addiction and her father's absence. She began skipping school and hanging out with her sister's friends. After Destiny became pregnant, she moved out on her own in the hopes that she would live her life differently from her own mother and take care of her child. However, after the baby was born, she struggled financially, and, feeling like she had no other options, engaged in survival sex. Through Destiny's drawing, she said that her abstract image revealed her journey, pain, and focus for her future—reunification with Heaven, her daughter who was three years old (Figure 16.3).

She said the dark black frame of her drawing represented her painful past; the red was her pain represented by the color of "blood," and the radiating yellow and white in the center was representative of her daughter. She engaged easily with the provided materials and verbalized the cathartic release that highlighted the center of the image.

During another session, Destiny and the other group members were provided with jewelry making supplies and were encouraged to make themselves a symbolic gift of a necessity. Destiny made a necklace to represent the grief she was dealing with over the loss of her mother's presence in her life. Her mother had struggled with a drug addiction and had been unable to care for Destiny. Using letter beads, she spelled out "HOPE," and she explained that although she never felt love from her mom, she was trying to forgive her and have hope that she could be present for her own daughter. After finishing, Destiny seemed attached to her necklace and the meaning it held; she fastened the chain and didn't take it off after group ended. She also made a keychain for the "house mom" of the safe house and wrote out "MOM" in letter beads. Although Destiny felt unsupported by her biological mother, she had supportive figures like the "house mom" who helped her feel nurtured and loved, and exemplified aspects of motherhood. This empowering

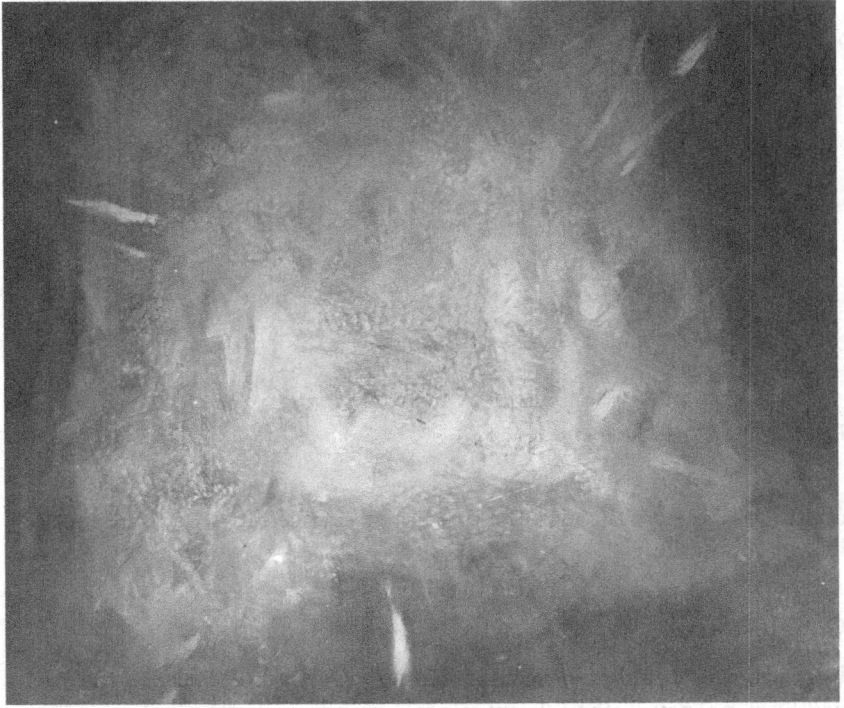

*Figure 16.3* "Light from the Darkness" oil pastel.

intervention was a tangible representation of Destiny's connection to others—a healing new relationship that was aiding in forgiveness for a past, estranged relationship and the hope she had for renewing her relationship with her daughter.

Despite her progress in art therapy, Destiny was struggling in her recovery, and she relapsed from treatment. Upon her return in a following session, the art therapist provided supplies to make mantras, hopeful sayings or special words of meaning to affirm one's self-worth. Destiny chose "Love" to express her commitment to recreating her family. Through this word, Destiny expressed her goal and focus in her recovery to reunite with her child and regain custody in the future (Figure 16.4).

Through participating in art therapy and in her process towards change, Destiny processed her personal journey through symbolic colors, initiated forgiveness and acceptance of her past, increased self-reflection, and expressed hope in creating a brighter future for her own family. Despite her relapse, Destiny's art confirmed she was able to

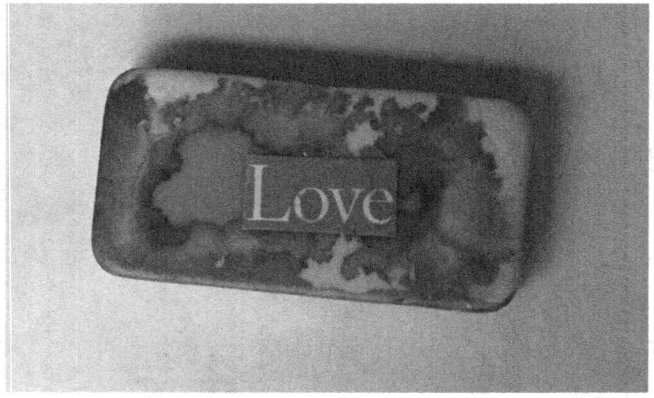

*Figure 16.4* "Love" altered domino.

continue to evolve through the process of change rather than be motionless or immobile.

## Conclusion

Reproductive healthcare needs are often overlooked because the focus has been on psychological, emotional, or physical effects of trafficking; however, giving survivors access to reproductive healthcare and prioritizing their health can improve their self-image and support their therapy (Freedom Network USA, 2015). Survivors who are facing motherhood issues require holistic and trauma-informed care to treat the multifaceted consequences of sexual trauma. When survivors' needs are met, they can begin their journey to recovery and make progress towards change, and art therapy is a vital way to help meet a survivor's emotional, psychological, and social needs.

Ali and Destiny's case studies demonstrate that art therapy can assist survivors in recognizing their pasts, processing their emotions, and creating visions for the future. When provided with a safe setting where recovery and change are possible, survivors can move towards brighter futures and venture beyond their dark pasts. Art therapy offers potential for mending relationships through experiencing acceptance, building new connections, empowering opportunities to reclaim control and developing self-identity. Although motherhood is different for each survivor (Anti Trafficking Monitoring Group, 2016), becoming a mother is an opportunity to make the world better and brighter by choosing joy over pain, light over darkness, love over abuse, and life over death.

# Terms

**Debt bondage**  Coercive technique to enforce financial burden.
**Sex trafficking**  forced sexual exploitation of an individual
**Survival sex**  When individuals sell sex to meet their basic needs.
**Victims of trafficking and Violence Protection Act of 2000 (TVPA)**  The first federal law in the United Sates to address human trafficking regarding deterrence, safety, and prosecution.

## Recommendations for Art Therapists

- When art therapists have information regarding a trafficking situation, they can contact the National Human Trafficking Resource Center at 1 (888) 373–7888.
- Art therapists are ethically responsibility to be aware of how their own beliefs may affect a therapeutic relationship (American Art Therapy Association, 2013), and sensitive care is required for this complex population when dealing with issues such as sexual exploitation, rape, pregnancy, abortion, etc.
- Motherhood is a complicated transformation for survivors of sex trafficking, and an art therapist's role is to provide opportunities for empowerment, emotional processing, and hope for the future.
- Art therapists are encouraged to seek supervision, support, and apply strategies for self-care such as making personal art while working within the many intricate needs of this population.
- For a more in-depth exploration of this topic, art therapists are encouraged to reference *Art Therapy Treatment for Sex Trafficked Survivors: Facilitating Empowerment, Recovery and Hope.*

## References

Acharya, A. K. (2011). Trafficking of women in Mexico: Sexual exploitation and reproductive health status. In R. L. Dalla, L. M. Baker, J. DeFrain, & C. Williamson (Eds.), *Global perspectives on prostitution and sex trafficking: Europe, Latin America, North America, and Global* (pp. 109–122). Lanham, MD: Lexington Books.

American Art Therapy Association. (2013, December 4). Ethical principles for art therapists. Retrieved from https://arttherapy.org/wp-content/uploads/2017/06/Ethical-Principles-for-Art-Therapists.pdf

Anti Trafficking Monitoring Group. (2016, February). Time to deliver: Considering pregnancy and parenthood in the UK's response to human trafficking. Retrieved from www.antislaverycommissioner.co.uk/media/1254/time-to-deliver.pdf

Bick, D., Howard, L. M., Oran, S., & Zimmerman, C. (2017, November 22). Maternity care for trafficked women: Survivor experiences and clinicians' perspectives in the United Kingdom's National Health Service. *PLoS One, 12* (11), e0187856. doi:10.1371/journal.pone.0187856.

Campbell, J. C. (2002, April). Health consequences of intimate partner violence. *The Lancet, 359,* 1331–1336.

de Chesnay, M., & Szekes, L. (2013). Pregnancy and termination of pregnancy. In M. de Chesnay (Ed.), *Sex trafficking: A clinical guide for nurses* (pp. 191–202). New York, NY: Springer Publishing Company.

Farr, K. (2004). *Sex trafficking: The global market in women and children.* New York, NY: Worth Publishers.

Freedom Network USA. (2015, April). Human trafficking and reproductive rights. Retrieved from https://freedomnetworkusa.org/app/uploads/2018/07/HT-and-Reproductive-Rights.pdf

Gerassi, L. B., & Nichols, A. J. (2018). *Sex trafficking and commercial sexual exploitation: Prevention, advocacy, and trauma-informed practice.* New York, NY: Springer Publishing Company.

Girls Educational and Mentoring Services. (2018). Our story. Retrieved from www.gems-girls.org/our-story

Groot, K. (2013). Drug-abused women and children. In M. de Chesnay (Ed.), *Sex trafficking: A clinical guide for nurses* (pp. 203–238). New York, NY: Springer Publishing Company.

Herman, J. L. (1997). *Trauma and recovery: The aftermath of violence- from domestic abuse to political terror* (2nd ed. ed.). New York, NY: Basic Books.

Hoffman, K. (2013). Surviving sex trafficking: Recovery and healing. In J. Pritchard (Ed.), *Good practice in promoting recovery and healing for abused adults* (pp. 117–136). London: Jessica Kingsley Publishers.

International Labour Office & Walk Free Foundation. (2017). Global estimates of modern slavery: Forced labour and forced marriage. Retrieved from www.ilo.org/wcmsp5/groups/public/@dgreports/@dcomm/documents/publication/wcms_575479.pdf

Kometiani, M., & Farmer, K. (2019). Exploring resilience through case studies of art therapy with sex trafficked survivors and their advocates. *The Arts in Psychotherapy.* Advance online publication. doi: 10.1016/j.aip.2019.101582.

Kometiani, M. K. (2020a). Beauty in the disorder: Art therapy with sex trafficking survivors in Ohio, United States. In M. K. Kometiani (Ed.), *Art therapy treatment for sex trafficked survivors: Facilitating empowerment, recovery and hope* (pp. 97–112). New York, NY: Routledge.

Kometiani, M. K. (2020b). Challenges and future considerations of treatment for sex trafficked survivors. In M. K. Kometiani (Ed.), *Art therapy treatment for sex trafficked survivors: Facilitating empowerment, recovery and hope* (pp. 211–228). New York, NY: Routledge.

Kometiani, M. K. (2020c). Deceptive tactics and adverse consequences of sex trafficking. In M. K. Kometiani (Ed.), *Art therapy treatment for sex trafficked survivors: Facilitating empowerment, recovery and hope* (pp. 17–32). New York, NY: Routledge.

Lederer, L. J., & Wetzel, C. A. (2014). The health consequences of sex trafficking and their implications for identifying victims in healthcare facilities. *Annals of Health Law, 23*(1), 61–91.

Lloyd, R. (2018). Change is a process: Using the transtheoretical model with commercially sexually exploited and trafficked youth and adults. In

A. J. Nichols, T. Edmond, & E. C. Heil (Eds.), *Social work practice with survivors of sex trafficking and commercial sexual exploitation* (pp. 51–69). New York, NY: Columbia University Press.

National Human Trafficking Hotline. (2019). The facts. Retrieved from https:// polarisproject.org/human-trafficking/facts

National Human Trafficking Hotline. (n.d.). *Federal Law*. Retrieved from https:// humantraffickinghotline.org/what-human-trafficking/federal-law

Office for Victims of Crime. (n.d.). *Substance abuse needs*. Retrieved from www. ovcttac.gov/taskforceguide/eguide/4-supporting-victims/44-comprehensive-victim-services/mental-health-needs/substance-abuse-needs/

Prochaska, J. O., & DiClemente, C. C. (1994). *The transtheoretical approach: Crossing traditional boundaries of therapy*. Malabar, FL: Krieger Publishing Company.

Shared Hope International. (2017). What is sex trafficking? Retrieved from http:// sharedhope.org/wp-content/uploads/2017/07/What-is-Sex-Trafficking-Printable-Handout.pdf

Tan, L. A. (2012). Art therapy with trafficked women. *Therapy Today, 23*(5), 26–31.

Tan, L. A., & Moore, T. M. (2020). The women's transformational program: An art therapy, life skills, and reproductive health program in Nepal. In M. K. Kometiani (Ed.), *Art therapy treatment for sex trafficked survivors: Facilitating empowerment, recovery, and hope* (pp. 163–186). New York, NY: Routledge.

United Nations Office on Drugs and Crime. (2013, April). Position paper: Abuse of a position of vulnerability and other "means" within the definition of trafficking in persons. New York, NY. Retrieved from www.unodc.org/docu ments/human-trafficking/2012/UNODC_2012_Issue_Paper_-_Abuse_of_a_Posi tion_of_Vulnerability.pdf

United States Department of Health and Human Services. (2019). What is human trafficking? Retrieved from www.acf.hhs.gov/otip/about/what-is-human-trafficking

United States Department of State. (2018, June 18). Implementing a trauma-informed approach. Retrieved from www.state.gov/documents/organiza tion/283795.pdf

United States Department of State Bureau of Public Affairs. (2007, August 8). Health consequences of trafficking in person. Retrieved from https://2001-2009. state.gov/documents/organization/91537.pdf

United States Department of State Office to Monitor and Combat Trafficking in persons. (2012, June). Addressing the internal wounds: The psychological aftermath of human trafficking. Retrieved from www.state.gov/j/tip/rls/fs/2012/ 194719.htm

Victims of Trafficking and Violence Protection Act of 2000. (2000). Pub. L. No. 106-386, 114 Stat. 1464. Retrieved from www.govinfo.gov/content/pkg/PLAW-106publ386/pdf/PLAW-106publ386.pdf

Willis, B. M., & Levy, B. S. (2002, April 2). Child prostitution: Global health burden, research needs, and interventions. *The Lancet, 359*(9315). doi:10.1016/ S0140-6736(02)08355-1

# Appendix 1
## Art Therapy and Antenatal Period

1. Assessment of antenatal emotional states through art therapy requires psychological knowledge, training with art materials and processes and clinical art therapy experience with continued education in trauma and childbearing issues (Appendix 3).
2. There is no need to force any model, including the archetype of initiation, *onto* the pregnant woman, which only objectifies her and disguises her true inner experiences. Instead, the art therapist observes and tracks archetypal patterns/images emerging spontaneously through her art and dreams that support her changing maternal identity. Trust that the images and her psyche have innate healing capacities.[1]
3. Within a liminal space, the art therapist may notice shifting relationship with time, space, and focus of the work—softening boundaries echo somatic softening—use supportive, respectful, collaborative communication.
4. The therapist may be induced to reveal traumatic childbearing stories or use a sharp tongue (anger, envy, or jealousy) in reaction to the uncertainty and the differences that exist within the dyadic intersubjective field. This echoes archaic initiation rites of inflicting pain on an initiand[2] and exercising power. Instead, tolerate and seek support for her own feelings and judgments that are associated with medical history, antenatal experiences, trauma, death, loss, ambivalence, and uncertainty.
5. Serious mental health issues and socioeconomic challenges are susceptible to overwhelm or over-identification with archetypal energies that may be expressed through suicidal thoughts, substance use, dissociation, neglect, dominance, self-harm, or violence towards others. Physical changes or incidences within the antenatal journey can mirror and trigger early childhood trauma and PTSD flashbacks. A trauma-informed protocol supports her immediate stability and her long-term well-being.[3]
6. Track ego strength. A softening ego consciousness is different from an ego with poor ties to reality. If a woman loses touch with reality

and daily events, depth work is contraindicated during pregnancy. Instead, use ego-strengthening interventions, specific materials and tasks, and refer or seek additional psychosocial resources so that she and her baby are safe; put plans in place for postpartum.

7. Offer clear options regarding scheduling that suit her situation: specifically focused sessions prior to childbirth, postpartum check in, additional appointments. Always encourage an expanded support system.

8. Trust and listen to the pregnant woman: she often knows what is best for her (support mother's intuition).

9. Empowerment and trauma: Although her body changes without her, she can exercise decision-making with materials, how and what she will create, whether or not she will make art at all and how long she will continue prenatal and postnatal sessions. Discern whether or not her closure of therapy is a defensive reaction to avoid feelings of shame, failure or traumatic memories (Simpkin & Klaus, 2004/2018).

10. The art therapist's job is to encourage conscious decisions and choices and to minimize shame and failure while encouraging areas of strength, success, confidence, and self-respect and dignity. Shame and failure are often explored if the woman is interested, and if she has adequate ego strength.

## Notes

1 Swan-Foster, N. (2018). *Jungian art therapy: A guide to dreams, images, and analytical psychology.* New York, NY: Routledge.
2 A person who is about to or is in the process of an initiation.
3 Simkin, P., & Klaus, P. (2004/2018). *When survivors give birth: Understanding and healing the effects of early sexual abuse on childbearing women.* Seattle, WA: Classic Day Publishing.

# Appendix 2
## Art Therapy with High-Risk Pregnancy and Antenatal Depression and Anxiety

Psychological or physical issues can define a pregnant woman as "high risk" and are diagnosed when a woman has one or more factors that raise her or her baby's chances for health problems such as, but not limited to, mood disorders (prenatal anxiety/depression), toxic stress, multiples, maternal age, preterm labor, high blood pressure, toxemia, genetic defects, or physical abnormalities with the baby or previous issues with a pregnancy. Stress is highly modifiable and can impact medical conditions; art therapy is a viable modality that normalizes an environment, provides visual stimulation and anchors and clarifies cognitive behaviors. If severe, the mother and/or baby are put on bed rest and/or hospitalized and monitored on a regular basis, sometimes for months. High-risk pregnancies can result in bed rest at home or in the hospital. When hospitals with a wellness and/or art therapy department offer integrative and collaborative care, the medical environment can serve as a maternal holding environment for the pregnant woman. Women at home may at times be more isolated and at greater risk for mood disorders.

While most women are happily anticipating motherhood, many pregnant women are living with tremendous stress, feelings of loneliness, resentment, guilt, and uncertainty. Consequently, prenatal mood must always be considered.

### Prenatal Depression and Anxiety

The Mayo Clinic reports that about 7% of women experience depression while pregnant.[1] It is sometimes difficult to get an honest read from women because shame, social and cultural expectations, and fear prevent them from revealing what is behind their protective persona. A trained art therapist and counselor interview is required.

### Important High-Risk Factors

- increased anxiety and/or depression
- life stress (typically three or more events in the year prior to and during pregnancy)

- history of abuse: trans-generational, medical, physical or sexual abuse
- unintended pregnancy
- intimate partner violence
- chronic mental or physical illness
- race, immigration or exile status, and language barriers.

## Additional Factors

- excessive anxiety about the baby
- low self-esteem
- lack of joy in usual activities
- poor response to reassurance
- poor adherence to prenatal care
- smoking, alcohol use or illicit drugs
- poor weight gain due to inadequate diet
- suicidal thoughts.

Prenatal depression and anxiety are now known to be possible predictors for postpartum depression and in rare cases postpartum psychosis (immediate hospitalization). Early concerns are assessed and appropriately treated with increased regular self-care (massage, acupuncture, exercise, prenatal yoga groups, extra childcare support, and creative arts therapy—including individual or group counseling). Such services, unless covered by Medicaid, are not economically possible for all women. In some cases, additional pharmacology from a psychiatrist is needed. Medical reasons for bed rest are comorbid and have complicating factors. Typically, women have renewed energy during the second trimester, while the first, third, and fourth trimesters seem to be the most frequently assessed for mental health concerns. While some anxiety, depression, and grief are normal aspects of maternal adjustment that benefit from mental health support, prolonged toxic stress and the inability to shift her mood are significant indicators that may also reveal themselves in art therapy.

Prenatal art therapy for women on bed rest can indirectly address stress, anxiety, guilt, resentment, sadness, and fears by offering a nonverbal outlet. Hospitalization for weeks or months can lead to feelings of isolation and missing her family life and regular routine. She can feel like a failure, have anger about her body and medical treatments and turn it towards herself or the baby. Art therapy interventions that give her encouragement and hope are essential.

## Art Therapy and Medical Staff

Developing collaborative professional relationships with the medical staff is essential.

Addressing a woman's emotions is important, but may concern the doctors and nurses who are working towards medical goals and are protective of their patients. Art therapy treatment should not focus on emotional discovery or trauma work. Should a woman discuss difficult emotions, the art therapist can offer visual resourcing and strength-building. For instance, decorating a box to put difficult feelings in may help someone become regulated. Art therapists need a trauma-informed approach so as to minimize dysregulation, dissociation and activating stress levels.

## What Art Therapy Offers

To build bridges with medical staff, art therapists can explain that the clinically supported art therapy:

- helps to build confidence and patience as well as normalize the sterile medical environment with interesting tasks and materials
- offers potential assessment information that supports her care and bridges with medical team
- gives creative expression that enlivens a woman's depressed mood or calms an anxious one
- documents her hospital stay while giving recognition and encouragement through productive projects that take her mind off medical worries and fears
- connects her with other high-risk women, which is occasionally arranged through art therapy groups or shared art via phone apps
- focuses on relationships and the well-being of her baby or babies through handwork, such as beading or cross-stitching
- collaborates with her on creating projects of interest and supporting her autonomy
- creates projects that are focused on decreasing anxiety and help her feel hopeful, productive and connected to loved ones.

## Additional Suggestions

- Nontoxic materials and adjustments made for medical and bed rest requirements.
- Project ideas: beading, knitting, pre-cut collage, boxes, notecards, trading cards, daily mandala journal.

## Note

1 Mayo Clinic Staff. (2019, Oct 15). *Life style week by week.* Retrieved from: www.mayoclinic.org/healthy-lifestyle/pregnancy-week-by-week/in-depth/depres sion-during-pregnancy/art-20237875

# Appendix 3
## Postpartum Depression Checklist

Although recognized by women, midwives, and doctors, postpartum depression (PPD) was first introduced in 1994 in the American Psychological Association's (APA) Diagnostic and Statistical Manual (*DSM IV*) under Major Depressive Disorder with "postpartum onset." A more sophisticated version occurred in 2013 with the *DSM-V* under Unspecified Depressive Disorder with "peripartum onset and mood symptoms during pregnancy."

### Perinatal Mood and Anxiety Disorder, Baby Blues and Variations on Postpartum Depression

**Perinatal mood and anxiety disorder (PMAD)** is used to describe disturbing feelings from conception through the first year of the baby's life. This term is often used to replace postpartum depression because depression and anxiety, once thought to be only occurring during postpartum, is found prior to and during pregnancy. PMAD also acknowledges that women may present with mixed anxiety and depression, and/or obsessive compulsive symptoms within six months onset in postpartum.

**"Baby blues"** is a term for normal mood fluctuations after the birth of the baby. Some 50 to 70% of women to experience this for a few days to a few weeks after the birth while her hormones adjust, and she and her baby settle into a rhythm. Midwives often recommend that women stay home for several weeks with limited activity so that their bodies can heal; they prioritize the bonding process between the mother and baby and maternal self-care often called *Matrescene*[1] because initially, the physical, emotional and psychological process of becoming a mother benefits from low-stress and supportive environments.

**Post-traumatic stress (PTSD)** occurs following a traumatic pregnancy or childbirth; a woman will experience flashbacks and specific physical and emotional symptoms associated with these flashbacks. In addition, a woman will avoid situations that remind her of the event, which can cause disruptions in maternal focus and regulation of moods.

Depression following the birth of a baby is referred to as **postpartum depression (PPD)** and this affects one in seven women in the United States and does not go away on its own. The stigma of PPD can interfere with treatment, and because of its very complicated nature, women may never recognize it or may be slow to seek medical and mental health support. **Postpartum psychosis** is far less common, but is an extreme version of PPD with psychotic thoughts, paranoia, dissociation, mania, and delusions, all of which put the baby at extreme risk. Immediate care and hospitalization is necessary.

## Postpartum Depression Checklist:[2]

Kleiman and Raskin (2013) offer the following questions in their book for preliminary assessment. "If a woman agrees with four or more of these symptoms and they last for two or more weeks she would be a candidate for postpartum depression" (pp. 5–6). (This is only a guideline.)

1. I can't shake feeling depressed no matter what I do.
2. I cry at least once a day.
3. I feel sad most or all of the time.
4. I can't concentrate.
5. I don't enjoy the things that I used to enjoy.
6. I have no interest in making love at all, even though my doctor says I'm physically able to resume sexual relations.
7. I can't sleep, even when my baby sleeps.
8. I feel like a failure all of the time.
9. I have no energy; I am tired all the time.
10. I have no appetite and no enjoyment of food (or, I am having sugar and carbohydrate cravings and compulsively eating all the time).
11. I can't remember the last time I laughed.
12. Every little thing gets on my nerves lately. Sometimes, I am even furious at my baby. Often, I am angry with my [partner].
13. I feel that the future is hopeless.
14. It seems like I will feel this way forever.
15. There are times when I feel that it would be better to be dead than to feel this way for one more minute.

## Note:

• If a woman is at risk, the abrupt ending of medical appointments with doctors and nurses and classes can cause greater risk of the onset of lack of sleep, loneliness, isolation, and disorientation. The greater use of midwives and doulas in the US could result in expanded continuity of care and home visits and a lowering of mood disorders.

- If a woman has risk factors such as intimate partner abuse, early sexual abuse, and/or depression, anxiety and PTSD symptoms, the sudden loss of medical attention, structure and emotional support may be even more problematic (Appendix 1).

## Notes

1 Dr. Dana Raphael, an anthropologist, coined the terms *matrescene* and *doula* to frame a holistic model of care that valued the antenatal woman.
2 Kleiman, K., & Raskin, V. (2013). *This isn't what I expected: Overcoming postpartum depression.* Boston, MA: DaCapo Life Long Books.

# Appendix 4
## Resources and Training Opportunities[1]

National Advocates or Pregnant Women
http://advocatesforpregnantwomen.org/main/about_us/about_us.php

Pregnant Association
https://americanpregnancy.org/

The Association for Pre and Perinatal Psychology
https://birthpsychology.com/

Postpartum Support International
www.postpartum.net/professionals/certification/

Seleni: Perinatal Mental Health Training
www.seleni.org/advice-support/2018/3/16/the-need-for-perinatal-mental-
    health-training

The Reproductive and Maternal Wellbeing Track of the SWG Certificate
http://swgproject.org/blog/2016/1/7/reproductive-maternal-wellbeing-curri
    culum-is-launched

International Perinatal Association
www.nationalperinatal.org/

When Survivors Give Birth
www.whensurvivorsgivebirth.net

Doula International
www.dona.org/

National Black Doulas Association
https://blackdoulas.org/

Childbirth and Postpartum Professional Association
https://cappa.net/

Maternal Health Task Force at Harvard Chan School
www.mhtf.org/topics/perinatal-mental-health/

Midwives Alliance of North America
https://mana.org/

American College of Nurse-Midwives
www.midwife.org/

Every Mother Counts
https://everymothercounts.org/

National Human Trafficking Hotline
https://humantraffickinghotline.org/

## Note

1 This limited selection was created with the intent to inspire readers to investigate and support local resources and trainings as well as consider the range of relevant options that are applicable to the childbearing period.

# Index

Printed in the United States
by Bookmasters

Printed in the United States
By Bookmasters